Akiyashi Funato • Tomohiro Ishikawa

4D Implant Therapy: Esthetic Considerations for Soft Tissue Management

4D Implant Therapy:

Esthetic Considerations for Soft Tissue Management

Akiyashi Funato, DDS
Private practice
Kanazawa, Kanazawa
Japan

Tomohiro Ishikawa, DDS
Private practice
Hamamatsu, Shizuoka
Japan

Quintessence Publishing Co, Ltd
London, Berlin, Chicago, Tokyo, Barcelona, Beijing, Istanbul, Milan,
Moscow, New Delhi, Paris, Prague, São Paulo, Seoul and Warsaw

Title of the original edition:
"4-D Concept"

Quintessence
British Library Cataloguing in Publication Data

Funato, Akiyashi.
4D implant therapy : esthetic considerations for soft tissue management.
1. Dental implants. 2. Dentistry--Aesthetic aspects.
I. Title II. Four-dimensional implant therapy
III. Ishikawa, Tomohiro.
617.6'93-dc22

First published in Japanese in 2008 by Quintessence Publishing Co, Ltd, Tokyo.

ISBN 978-1-85097-201-3

QUINTESSENCE PUBLISHING

Quintessence Publishing Co. Ltd,
Grafton Road, New Malden, Surrey KT3 3AB,
Great Britain
www.quintpub.co.uk

Editorial coordination: Bryn Grisham, Quintessence Publishing Comp. Inc., Chicago, USA
Figure reproduction: Quintessenz Verlags-GmbH, Berlin, Germany
Production: Jens Girke, Quintessenz Verlags-GmbH, Berlin, Germany
Printing: Bosch-Druck GmbH, Landshut

Printed in Germany

Contents

Preface

The field of implant dentistry has experienced dramatic changes in the past decade. New implant designs and surface technologies allow for much faster osseointegration and modulation of bone reaction specific to the dental implant. Immediate implant placement and immediate implant loading potentially reduce the overall treatment period. Alveolar ridge preservation and augmentation are now more predictable as a result of new innovations in techniques and materials. Advances in computer technology have enabled better examination, diagnosis, and treatment planning with three-dimensional (3D) imaging and simulation software and the fabrication of custom abutments with computer-aided design/computer-assisted manufacture (CAD/CAM) technology. As this evolution of implant therapy has occurred, there has been widespread recognition of the need for a restoration-driven approach that considers the placement of implants in bone and soft tissue from a 3D perspective. Through our own clinical experience, we have found that for optimal esthetics and patient satisfaction, a fourth dimension—timing—must be given equal weight in implant treatment planning. Hence we developed the four-dimensional (4D) approach to implant therapy described in this book.

Our collaboration began when we met in dental school almost 30 years ago. After several years in private practice, we both attended the Japan Institute for Advanced Dental Studies to pursue our growing interest in periodontal treatment. There we had the privilege of studying periodontal prostheses under Drs Yoshihiro Ono, Kimio Nakamura, and Yasukazu Miyamoto. Since then we have been pursuing excellence in patient care, especially in esthetic implant therapy. Although our treatment methods have evolved, all aspects of our patient care and implant therapy are based on the fundamental concepts and principles of the periodontal prosthesis that we learned from our mentors. As a result, clinical periodontology is the core principle that guides our dental practice, which is aimed at preserving the patients' alveolar bone, dentition, function, and esthetics over the long term. We believe that we, as dentists, must be able to respond to patients' natural desire to maintain their own teeth whenever possible. Our primary mission must be to save the remaining dentition through the proper execution of periodontal treatment. We emphasize that both esthetic implant treatment and proper periodontal treatment must be provided to each patient.

We have learned much about implant dentistry in the past decade from leaders in the field such as Drs Ueli Grunder, Maurice Salama, Massimo Simion, Sascha Jovanovic, Joseph Kan, Carlo Tinti, and many others. It was during the course of this experience that we developed the 4D approach to implant therapy. We first published this method in 2007 and presented it at the Academy of Osseointegration annual meeting in 2008. We hope that by further explaining the details of the approach in this book, we will aid readers in treating challenging esthetic implant cases predictably and effectively and in providing better service to their patients. We also hope to continue to share our experiences and knowledge and to improve patient care for years to come.

Acknowledgments

We express our deep appreciation to Drs Yahihiro Ono, Kimio Nakamura, Yasukazu Miyamoto, and Myron Nevins for their mentoring over the years. We offer our sincere gratitude to Dr Maurice Salama for his friendship and for introducing us to esthetic implant treatment. We also express appreciation to Drs Hajime Kitajima, Masahiro Minami, Kazuhiro Fukunishi, Satoru Urano, and Kahei Hasegawa for their friendship. We thank the following dental technicians for their excellent work: Takeshi Kamibayashi, Yoshimi Nishimura, Kiyoshi Nakajima, Hiroshi Shigemura, Shougo Yamamoto, Tomio Kawata, Toshiya Kishimoto, Ryuji Tsuji, Shigeki Shinya, and Sumie Takabayashi. We express our thanks to Dr Kousuke Nonoyama for his advice in creating the illustrations found in this book. We thank Mr Kazutaka Sasaki, Ms Megumi Hata, Mr Yasumichi Kitamine, and Mr Hiroki Tada of Quintessence Japan and Ms Tomoko Tsuchiya of Quintessence USA. In addition, we thank Dr Hidetada Moroi for his effort in the English translation of this book and for his continuing friendship, and we thank the staffs of the Nagisa Dental Clinic and the Ishikawa Dental Clinic for their daily support. Finally, we express our deep gratitude to our families for their understanding and support.

Chapter 1

4D Concept and Strategy

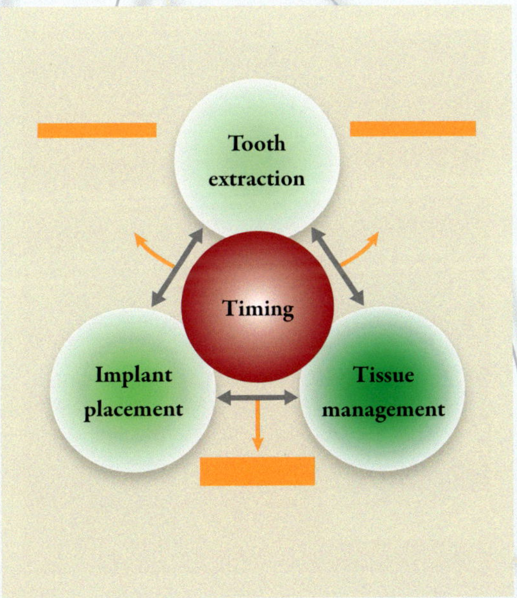

In this chapter the timing of the treatment sequence, which is the key element in the four-dimensional (4D) concept of esthetic implant treatment, is introduced.

Traditional Restoration-Driven Implant Treatment

Goals of implant treatment

There are four major goals in implant therapy:

- Esthetic results
- Short treatment period
- Minimally invasive treatment
- Affordability

Each of these goals is consistent with the typical demands of implant treatment patients; however, we are rarely able to satisfy all of these demands at the same time. For example, one measure of the success of implant treatment is whether both the clinician and the patient view the implant restorations as esthetically pleasing. However, when a patient has several missing teeth, esthetic implant treatment will often require the clinician to reconstruct missing bone and soft tissue to provide support for the definitive restoration. This process requires an appropriate healing period and prolongs the overall treatment time.

A patient-centered approach

The key to successful restoration-driven implant therapy is appropriate examination, diagnosis, and treatment planning to achieve optimal functional and esthetic results. Most importantly, patients must be at the heart of this process (Box 1-1). Clinicians must present patients with all possible treatment methods, outlining the advantages and disadvantages of each (eg, treatment period, morbidity, outcome predictions) so that patients understand their options and can make well-informed decisions. Dentists should work with patients to develop a realistic treatment plan. They should not force a particular treatment plan upon a patient. Nor should they allow patients to have unattainable or unrealistic expectations. Instead, they should be able to offer a wide variety of treatment options to meet a patient's specific wants and needs.

Rationale for Development of the 4D Concept

Esthetic challenges

Most patients undergoing implant treatment imagine that their definitive restorations will look just like natural teeth. However, there are many challenges that must be overcome to meet these expectations and many ways in which the restorations may fail to meet the patient's and the clinician's esthetic standards. Grunder[1] has identified five categories of possible failures in esthetic implant treatment (Box 1-2).

The authors have tried many techniques to overcome these hurdles to esthetic outcomes. Over the course of their experience, they came to realize that in order to provide minimally invasive treatment and achieve more successful and predictable esthetic outcomes, the timing of the treatment sequence (Box 1-3) was just as important as the considerations taken into account in the traditional three-dimensional (3D) approach, ie, management of implant position and bone and soft tissue requirements. The authors therefore add time to the traditional 3D axes and describe their approach herein as the *4D concept for esthetic implant therapy* (Fig 1-1).

Box 1-1 Restoration-driven implant therapy as a patient-centered approach

Clinicians and patients share responsibility for the treatment:

- Clinicians must present patients with all possible treatment options.
- Patients must understand their treatment options so that they can make well-informed decisions.

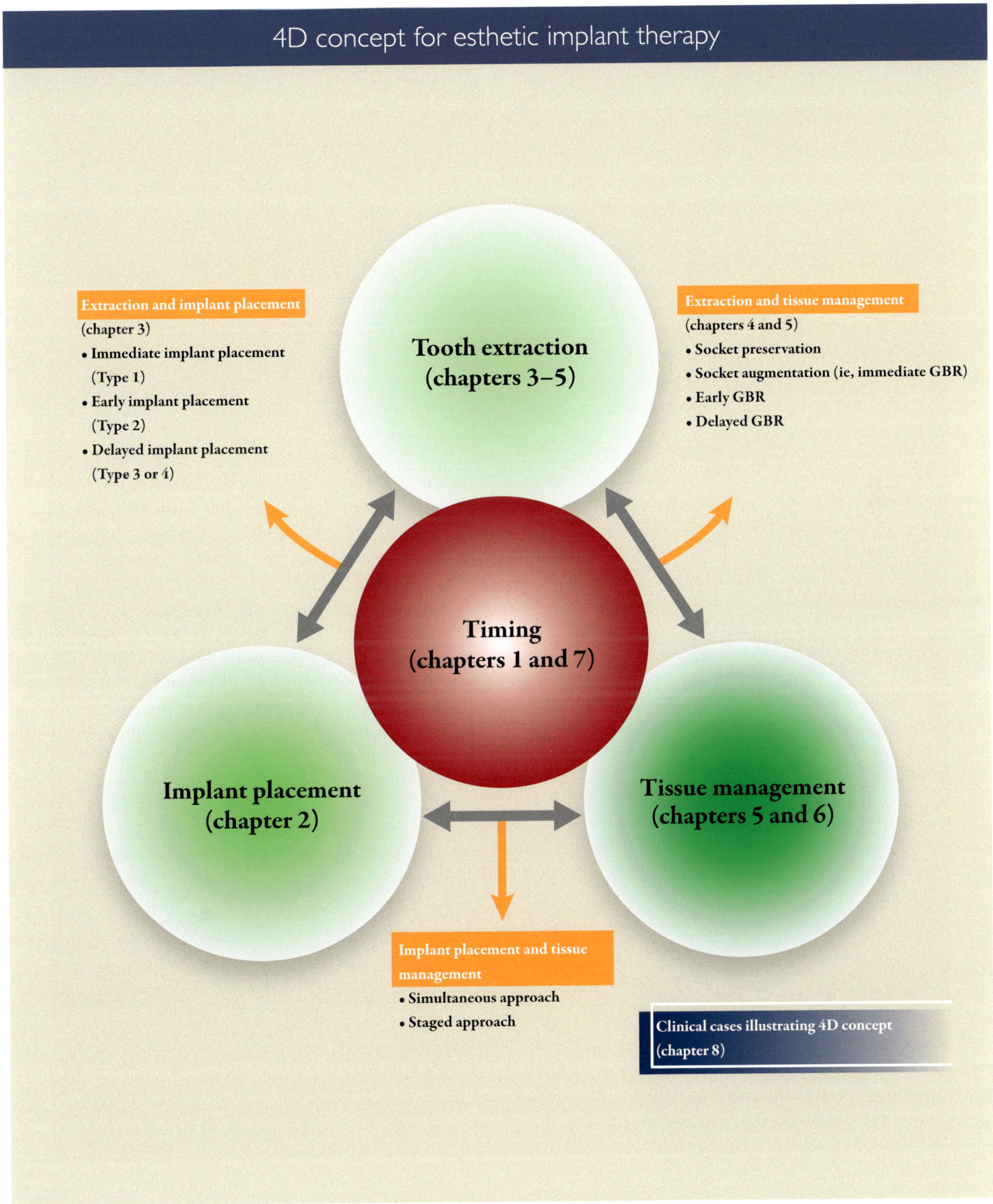

Fig 1-1 The 4D concept for esthetic implant therapy, as presented and organized in this book. In addition to the traditional 3D management of bone, soft tissue, and implant positioning, the fourth dimension of timing is critical. GBR—guided bone regeneration.

Box 1-2 Possible failures in esthetic implant treatment*

- Irregular soft tissue contour
- Scar tissue
- Missing papillae
- Missing buccal volume
- Soft tissue discoloration

*Based on Grunder.[1]

Box 1-3 Critical timing issues in the 4D concept

- Tooth extraction
- Hard and soft tissue management: Preservation or augmentation
- Implant placement: Immediate, early, or delayed
- Stage-two surgery and abutment connection
- Tissue sculpting
- Definitive restoration

Importance of timing

The new, expanded concept of 4D implant treatment planning, ie, giving due consideration to the timing of implant treatment sequences, is necessary for predictable and esthetically pleasing treatment outcomes. For example, when dealing with a hopeless tooth that needs to be extracted and replaced with a dental implant, the timing of the tooth extraction and implant placement must be carefully assessed. Immediately placing an implant into a fresh extraction socket may produce a result that is not esthetically pleasing. To avoid an undesirable outcome, practitioners may *(1)* preserve the extraction site, *(2)* engage in early or delayed site development with or without orthodontic tooth extrusion prior to extraction, or *(3)* perform a root submergence technique.

To achieve optimal esthetic results, the timing of site development, soft tissue management, tissue sculpting, and definitive restoration must be considered as part of a comprehensive treatment plan (Box 1-4).

Multiple-tooth implant treatment

Esthetic implant treatment requires detailed examination and proper diagnosis, which together form the basis of a restoration-oriented treatment plan. To restore multiple-tooth defects, the process is even more complex. First, the practitioner must conduct facial, smile, and functional analyses to determine the 3D position of the incisal edge of the maxillary central incisors. The proper shape, form, and dimension of the teeth as well as the arch form should thereafter be determined. At that stage, it is possible to evaluate the bone and soft tissue requirements necessary to support an ideal esthetic definitive restoration. Those requirements must be met either surgically or through the use of tissue-colored dental materials. If the requirements are to be met surgically, patient and clinician must understand the necessary surgical procedures, treatment period, costs, and possible risks and complications. Clinicians must go beyond selecting the most appropriate clinical techniques and armamentarium. In addition to the traditional 3D management of implant position and bone and soft tissue requirements, they must consider a fourth dimension: the timing of the treatment sequence. That consideration is necessary to minimize surgical morbidity and the length of the treatment period and to maximize treatment predictability and positive outcomes.

Summary

Today, implant therapy is in a state of critical review. The notion that anterior esthetic implant treatment should be fast, easy, and universally applied must be revisited. The authors' goal is not to facilitate the speed or the ease of implant treatment, nor is it to present implant therapy as a panacea. Rather, the aim of this book is to introduce the new 4D concept for esthetic implant therapy and to reexamine the traditional implant treatment sequence so that practitioners and patients can achieve an optimal esthetic result (Box 1-5).

Box 1-4 4D treatment planning sequence

Step 1: Assessing existing bone and dentition

A. Edentulous alveolar ridge assessment: Determination of vertical and horizontal alveolar ridge resorption through diagnostic wax-up

B. Evaluation of remaining dentition and determination of whether to extract

C. Determination of bone level for augmentation

- Extraction: The amount of bone loss, the degree of decay, previous or required endodontic treatment, and the tooth position will determine the prognosis of the tooth.
- Periodontal treatment (regenerative or resective), caries control, endodontic treatment, and orthodontic treatment might be necessary for preserving the remaining dentition.

Step 2: Determining implant position and number

- Definitive implant restoration design (functional and esthetic considerations): For better esthetics in multiple tooth implant cases, insert pontics when possible to avoid placing adjacent implants.
- Provisional restoration design: When periodontal and periapical infection of the abutment teeth can be controlled, a fixed provisional restoration provides better esthetics and function during the treatment period.

Step 3: Evaluating abutment teeth that may be extracted after provisional restoration

- Determine the timing of extraction and treatment protocol.
- Decide whether the extraction site should be an implant or pontic site.

Timing options

Implant:
- Immediate implant placement
- Early implant placement with GBR (6 to 8 weeks after extraction)
- Delayed implant placement with GBR (3 to 4 months after extraction)
- Two-stage implant placement with GBR (stage one with GBR 8 weeks after extraction, stage two at least 4 months after extraction)

Pontic:
- Socket preservation
- Immediate GBR
- Root submergence technique
- GBR 8 weeks after extraction

Additional considerations

1. Determine the classification for immediate implant placement (see Fig 3-10):
   - Class 1 or 2: Perform immediate implant placement.
   - Class 3: Perform immediate implant placement with socket preservation.
2. For pontic sites, consider using the root submergence technique.
3. If immediate implant placement is contraindicated:
   - Perform socket preservation.
   - Use the two-stage approach to reduce potential complications.
4. With either immediate implant placement or staged implant placement, GBR usually will be performed 8 weeks after extraction. In the authors' practices, the majority of cases are treated with GBR rather than immediate implant placement.

Step 4: Comprehensive treatment planning based on steps 1 to 3 with the goals of efficient treatment and an esthetic final result

Decision-making factors:

Local factors:

- Control of existing chronic infection
- Evaluation of residual bone anatomy
- Evaluation of the condition of the soft tissue

(Note: Immediate implant placement is a viable option, but considering the factors listed above, most teeth are not indicated for this option in the authors' practices.)

Global factors:

- Provisional restoration design (see chapter 7).
- Definitive restoration design: Staged immediate implant placement allows for the preservation of interproximal tissue.
- Incision and flap design: Early or delayed GBR allows larger and simpler incision and flap design for better predictability.
- Implant placement: Multiple implants should be placed at the same time for greater precision in overall implant positioning.

Box 1-5 Summary of the 4D concept for esthetic implant therapy

3D Consideration of Bone and Soft Tissue + 3D Implant Positioning + Timing Efficiency

=

Optimal Diagnosis, Strategy, and Sequence

Application of 4D Concept

The 4D concept for esthetic implant therapy is demonstrated in the two clinical cases shown in Figs 1-2 and 1-3.

Reference

1. Grunder U. Strategies for achieving predictable esthetic results in challenging implant cases. Presented at the 9th International Symposium on Periodontics and Restorative Dentistry, Boston, 8 June 2007.

Application of 4D concept: Case 1

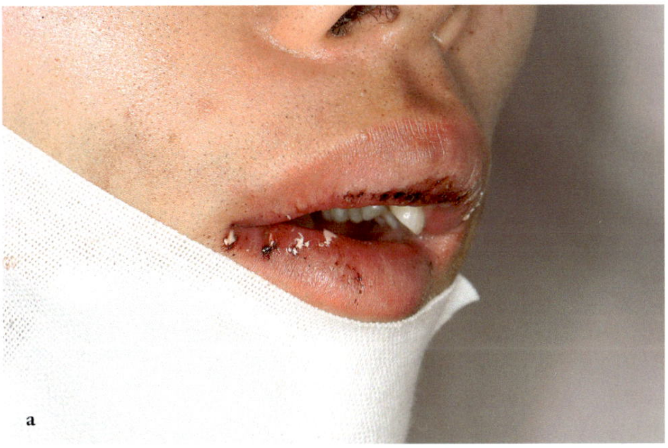

Figs 1-2a to 1-2d A 20-year-old man wanted to replace his maxillary teeth that were damaged in an accident. The right lateral incisor and its entire surrounding buccal bone had been lost. The right central incisor had a subgingival fracture and was thought to be restorable with orthodontic extrusion and crown lengthening; however, the definitive crown would not match the left incisor. The treatment plan included implant treatment in the right central and lateral incisor sites and a crown restoration on the left central incisor.

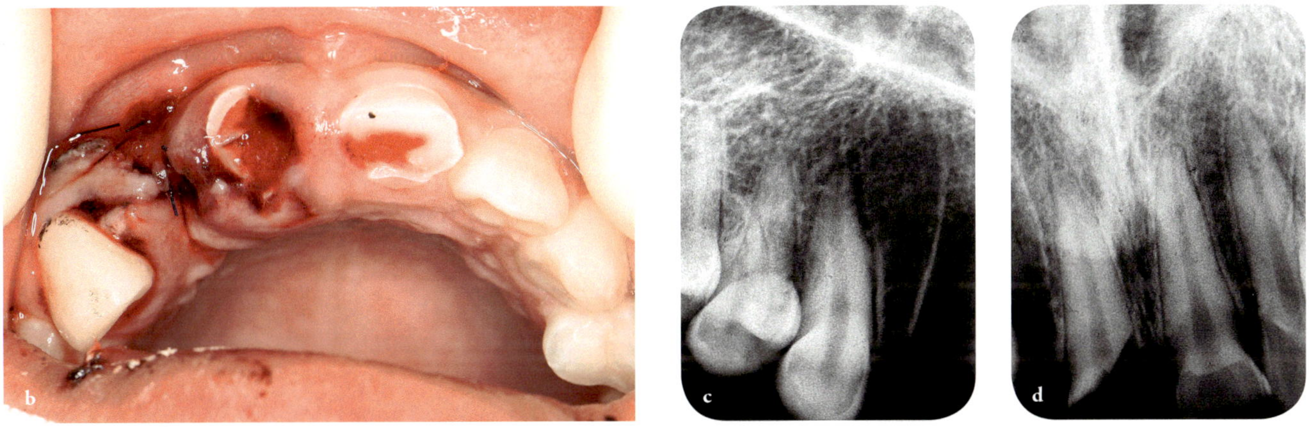

↓ Application of 4D concept ↓

A staged approach was planned for placement of two adjoining implants to create a papilla between them with effective augmentation and preservation of surrounding bone and soft tissue.

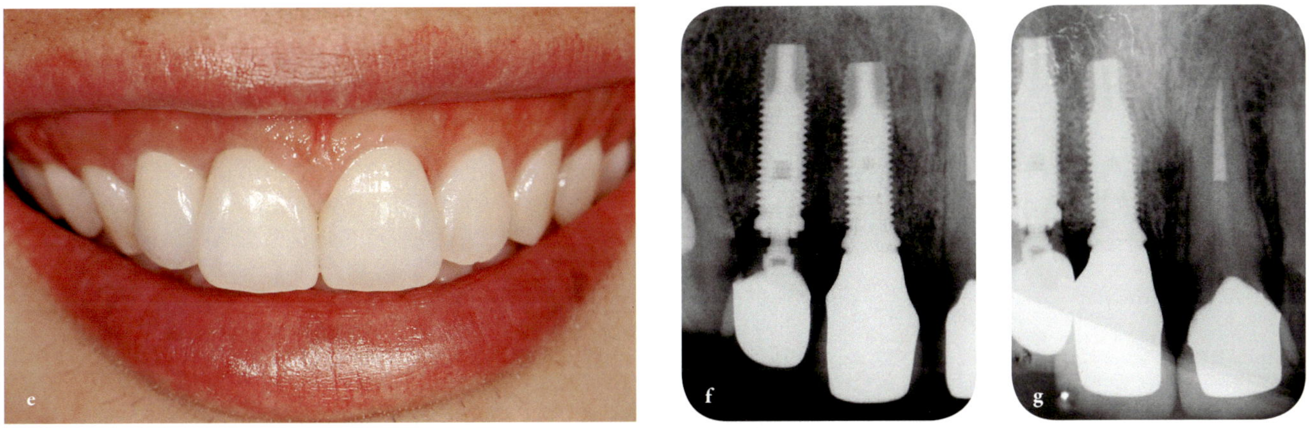

Figs 1-2e to 1-2g Definitive restorations. With careful consideration of the timing of implant placement and of bone and soft tissue augmentation and preservation, an acceptable result was obtained in a patient with a challenging high smile line.

Application of 4D concept: Case 2

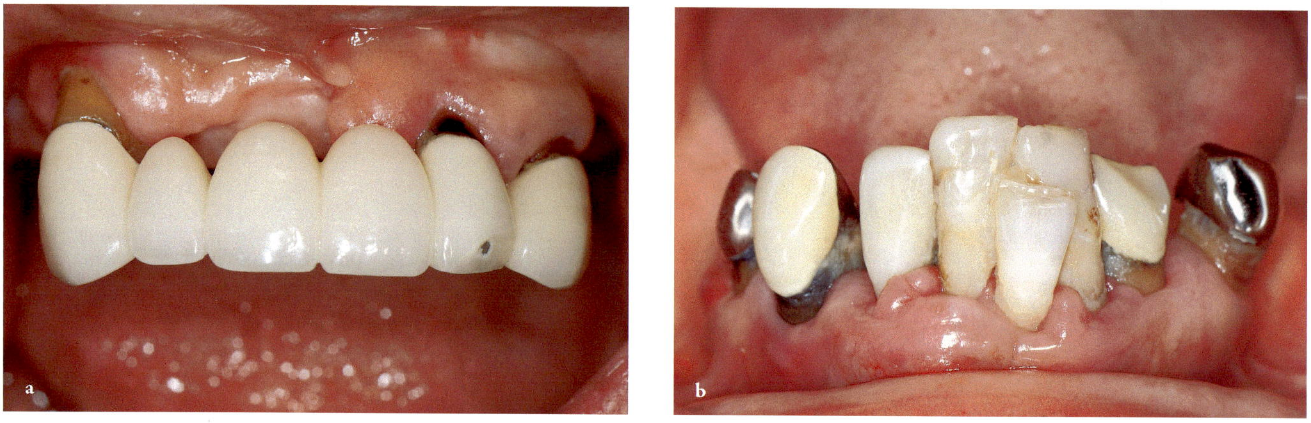

Figs 1-3a and 1-3b At the initial visit, the patient's chief complaint was mobility of the anterior teeth. The patient requested esthetic implant treatment.

Application of 4D concept

The timing of the extraction of anterior teeth and of bone and soft tissue augmentation and preservation was critical for an esthetic definitive restoration.

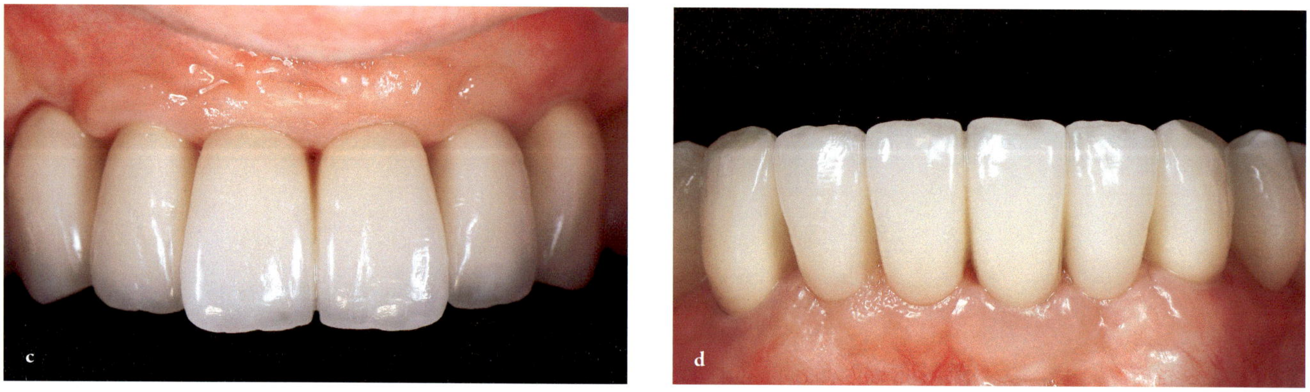

Figs 1-3c and 1-3d Clinical appearance at the 2-year follow-up of the definitive restoration. An esthetic result was obtained through the application of the 4D concept.

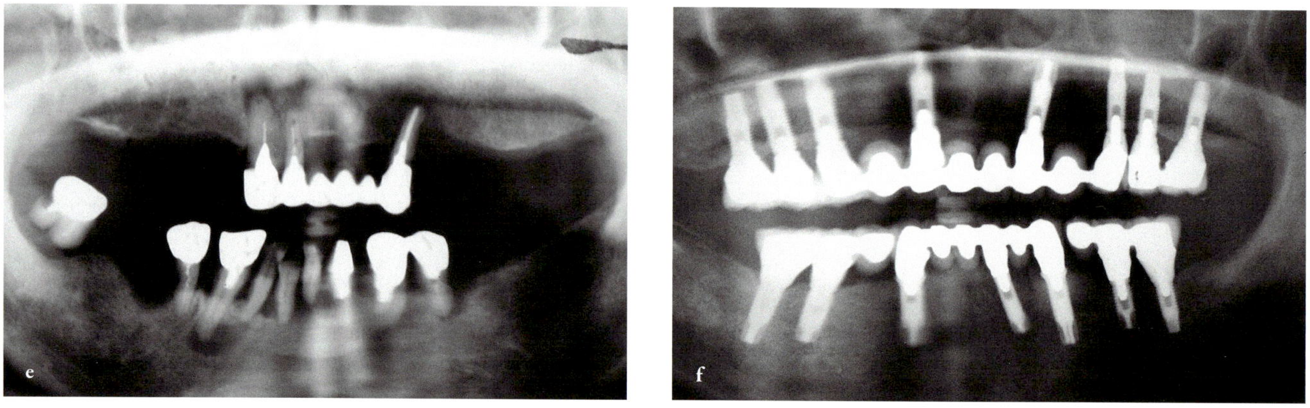

Figs 1-3e and 1-3f Comparison of panoramic radiograph obtained *(e)* at the initial visit with that obtained *(f)* at the 2-year 6-month follow-up.

Chapter 2

3D Implant Placement

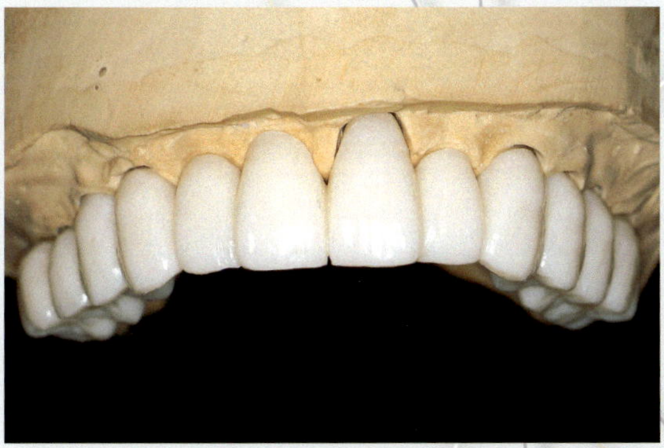

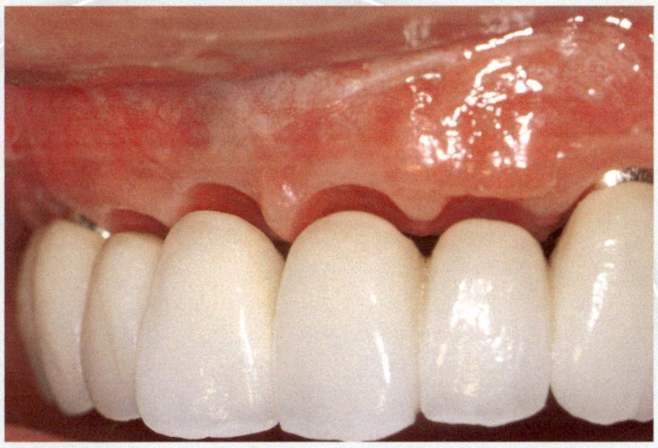

In this chapter, traditional three-dimensional (3D) management of implant positioning for optimal esthetic and functional implant treatment is discussed.[1–3] It is critical to understand these concepts prior to adding the fourth dimension of timing to the treatment sequence.

Mesiodistal Position

The implant should be placed in the mesiodistal center of the definitive restoration, which can be located with the aid of a surgical guide.

Effect on papilla height

According to Tarnow et al,[4] bone remodeling and resorption occur at the implant-abutment junction with a horizontal range of 1.3 to 1.4 mm. Therefore, if the implant is placed less than 1.5 mm from the natural tooth, it could potentially compromise the supporting bone of the adjacent tooth[5,6] (Fig 2-1). In addition, if the distance between adjoining implants is less than 3 mm, the height of the alveolar bone between them could decrease[7,8] (Figs 2-2 and 2-3). It is therefore critical to maintain appropriate distance between a natural tooth and an implant or between adjoining implants.

Blood supply in peri-implant soft tissue is compromised compared to the supply in the gingiva around a natural tooth, which has additional blood supply from the periodontal ligament space. Papilla height between adjoining implants is supported only by alveolar bone. The morphology of this bone is important to achieving an esthetic soft tissue frame. Funato et al[9] have developed a classification system for the predicted height of papillae in six different restorative environments (Table 2-1). This classification system allows the clinician to develop a plan for an esthetic soft tissue frame by selecting appropriate restorative options. Note that the data indicated that the vertical height of papillae between two implants (3.5 mm) was significantly less than in other environments.

Salama et al[10] evaluated and classified the area of bone between the implant and a natural tooth, called the *interproximal height of bone* (IHB) (Fig 2-4). The papilla height between the implant and the natural tooth is determined by the height of the periodontal attachment apparatus of the natural teeth.[11,12] In the clinical case shown in Fig 2-5, papilla height was maintained despite attachment loss. In the case presented in Fig 2-6, appropriate examination, diagnosis, and treatment planning was performed to prevent papilla loss as a result of implant placement.

Buccolingual Position

As mentioned earlier, bone remodeling and resorption occur at the implant-abutment junction within a 1.3- to 1.4-mm horizontal range.[1] Spray et al[13] reported that facial marginal bone will resorb and reduce in height with flap elevation and implant placement if its thickness is less than 1.8 to 2.0 mm. Grunder et al[14] stated that there must be at least 2 mm, or ideally 4 mm, of labial alveolar bone beyond the body of the implant to achieve an esthetic treatment result.

Positioning the implant lingually facilitates maintenance of adequate labial bone thickness; if the practitioner considers the buccolingual width of the teeth and the necessary prosthetic space, the implant platform should be placed 2 mm lingual to the free gingival margin (Fig 2-7).

Distance between implant and adjacent tooth

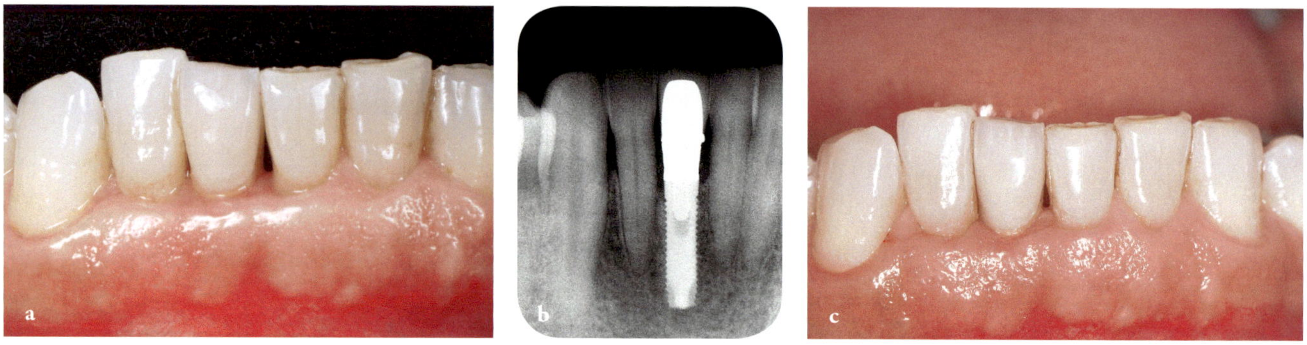

Fig 2-1 *(a and b)* Single-tooth implant placed in anterior mandible less than 1.5 mm from the adjacent tooth. *(c)* Papilla is still missing at the 3-year follow-up.

Distance between adjoining implants

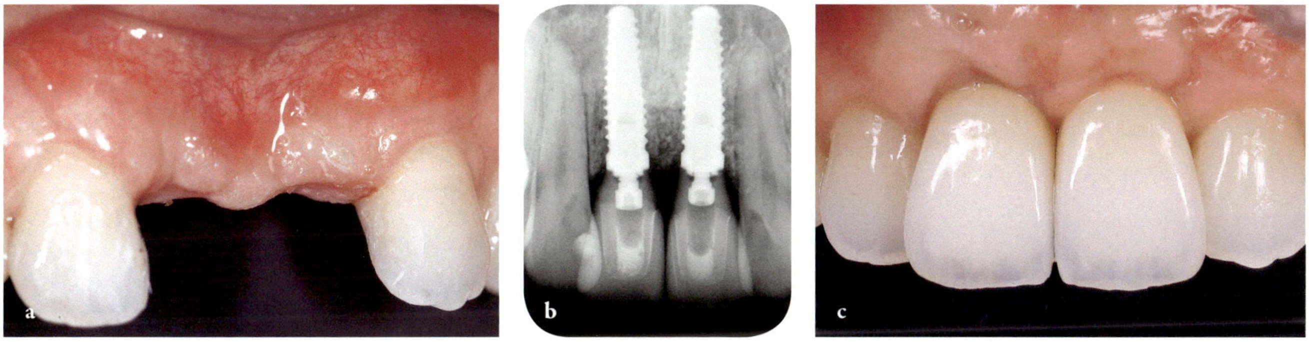

Fig 2-2 *(a)* A 37-year-old woman lost her central incisors as well as some buccal bone. One month later, implant placement with bone and soft tissue augmentation was done. The distance between the implants was only 3 mm because of space limitations. *(b and c)* At the 1-year follow-up, there was enough buccal tissue, but the bone height between the implants was only at the platform level, and the papilla height was more apical than that of the papillae between natural teeth.

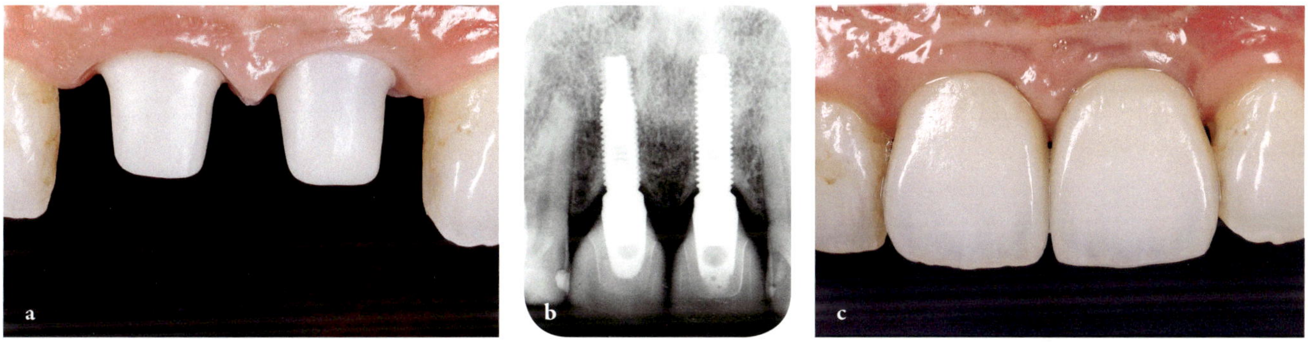

Fig 2-3 *(a)* The central incisors of a 55-year-old woman were replaced with implants. The distance between the adjoining implants was about 4 mm. *(b and c)* At the 6-year follow-up, the bone height between the implants was coronal to the platform level, and the papilla height matched that of adjacent teeth.

Table 2-1 Classification of predicted interdental papilla height*

Class	Restorative environment	Proximity limitation (mm)	Vertical soft tissue limitation (mm)
1	Tooth-Tooth	1.0	5.0
2	Tooth-Pontic	NA	6.5
3	Pontic-Pontic	NA	6.0
4	Tooth-Implant	1.5	4.5
5	Implant-Pontic	NA	5.5
6	Implant-Implant	3.0	3.5

NA—not applicable.
*Reprinted from Funato et al[9] with permission.

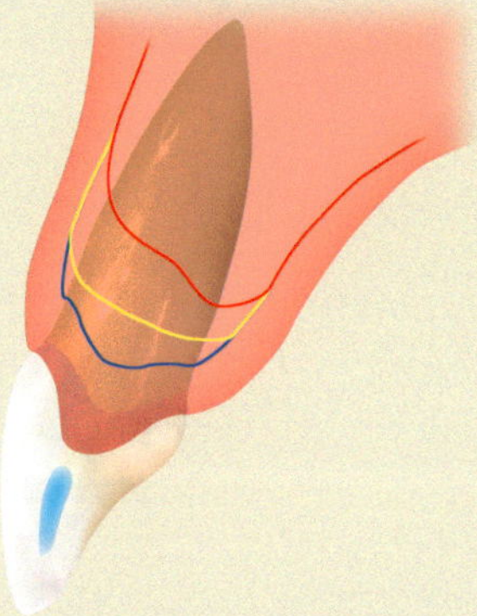

- Class 1 (optimal prognosis):
  2 mm from CEJ and 4–5 mm from the contact point
- Class 2 (uncertain prognosis):
  4 mm from CEJ and 6–7 mm from contact point
- Class 3 (poor prognosis):
  > 5 mm from CEJ and > 7 mm from contact point

Fig 2-4 Classification of IHB, based on its distance from the cementoenamel junction (CEJ) of the natural tooth and from the contact point between the implant and the natural tooth.

IHB Class 1

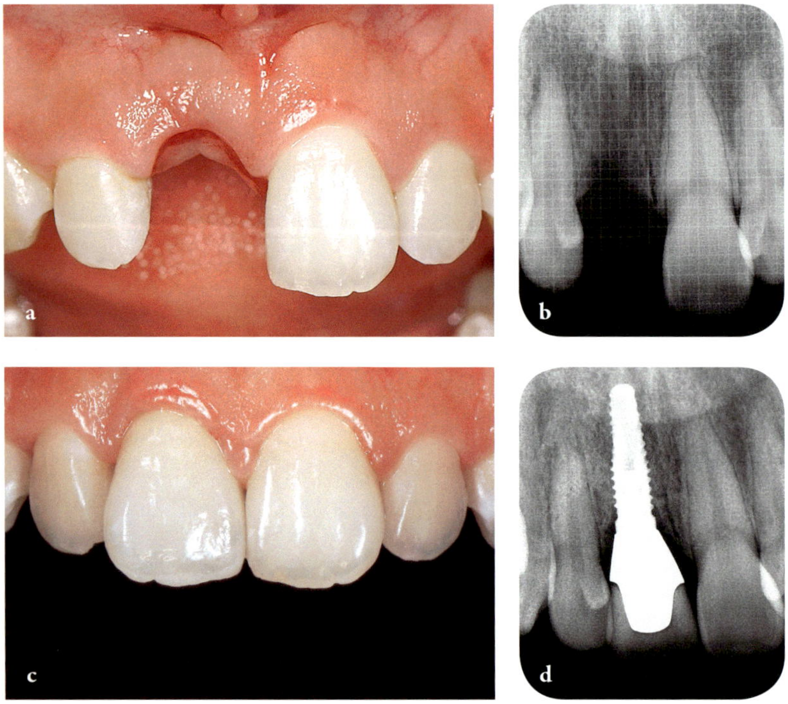

Fig 2-5a Two months after extraction, soft tissue healing was completed. There was buccal alveolar ridge resorption.

Fig 2-5b IHB is Class 1 for both adjacent teeth.

Fig 2-5c One-year follow-up with definitive restoration.

Fig 2-5d Papilla height was very well maintained.

IHB Class 3 with orthodontic extrusion to create IHB Class 2

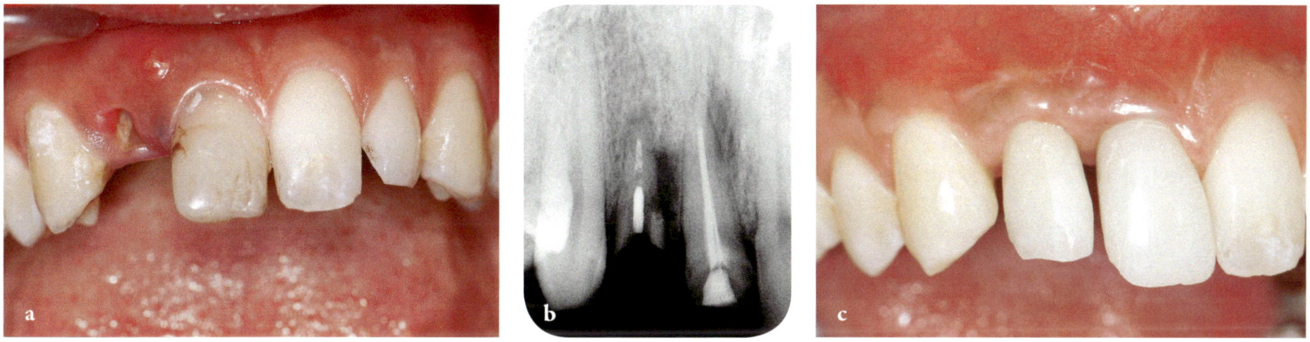

Figs 2-6a to 2-6c Fracture of the maxillary right lateral incisor. The IHB on the distal of the maxillary right central incisor was Class 3. An implant was placed following guided bone regeneration. Papillae were flat.

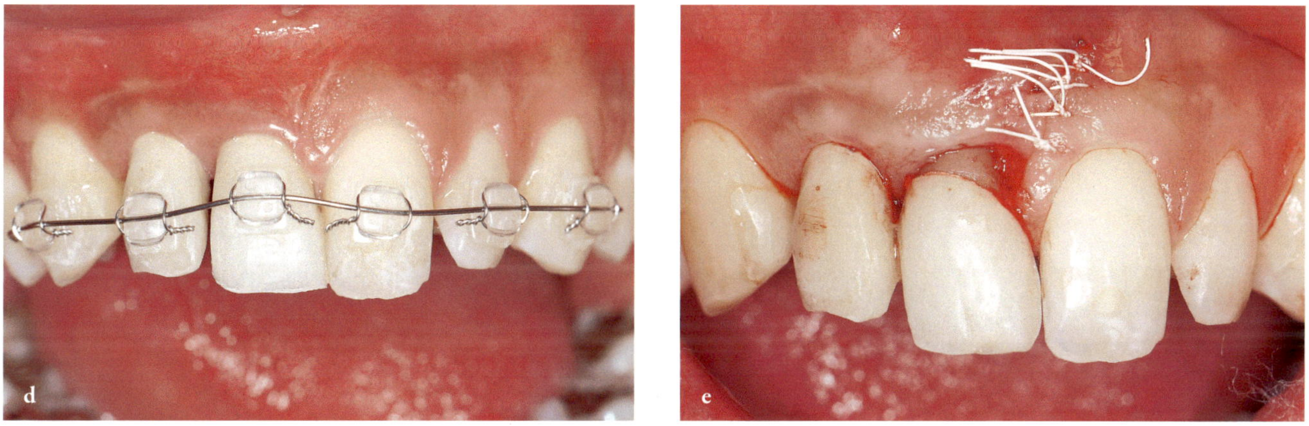

Figs 2-6d and 2-6e The distal bone crest was moved coronally with orthodontic extrusion of the maxillary right central incisor to achieve change in IHB from Class 3 to Class 2.

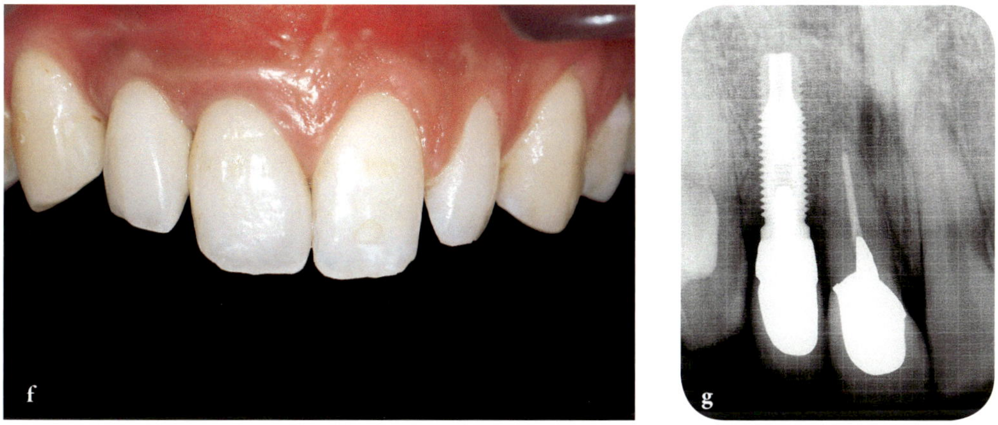

Figs 2-6f and 2-6g At the 2-year follow-up, adequate papilla height was maintained.

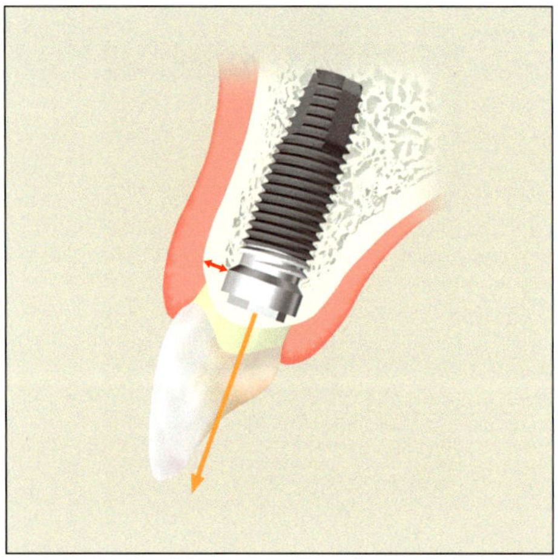

Fig 2-7 The implant platform should be located 2 mm lingual to the free gingival margin, with at least 2 mm of alveolar bone labial to the implant body.

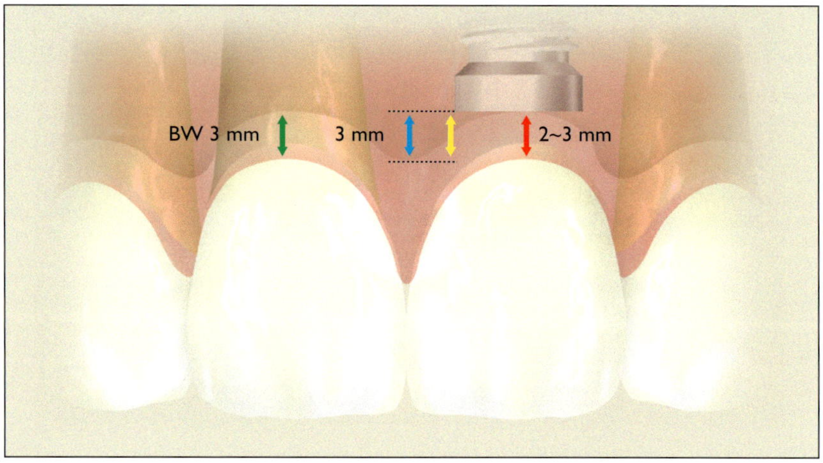

Fig 2-8 The biologic width (BW), measured from the free gingival margin to the bone crest, should be about 3 mm *(green arrow)*. The measurement from the bone crest to the IHB should also be about 3 mm *(blue arrow)*. The implant platform should be 2 to 3 mm apical to the IHB *(yellow arrow)* and the free gingival margin *(red arrow)*.

Vertical Depth of Implant Platform and Direction of Long Axis

The platform of the implant should be located 2 to 3 mm apical to the midfacial aspect of the free gingival margin, with the extended long axis directed lingual to the incisal edge of the definitive restoration.

Vertical depth of implant platform

The vertical prosthetic space must be 2 to 3 mm to create a smooth transition from the round implant platform to the natural root and scalloped cervical anatomy. In natural teeth, the crestal bone level typically follows the cementoenamel junction (CEJ). This creates a scallop-shaped bone anatomy. The bone crest is located approximately 3 mm apical to the IHB.

Ideally, the implant platform adjacent to a natural tooth should be positioned at the bone crest level, 2 to 3 mm apical to the free gingival margin at the facial aspect, to maintain both biologic width and an adequate prosthetic space (Fig 2-8). It should also be positioned 2 to 3 mm apical to the IHB.

Bone remodeling at an implant platform and discrepancies between the flat nature of the implant platform and the naturally scalloped alveolar crest anatomy could result in interdental papilla loss and a much deeper soft tissue profile in proximal surfaces.[15,16] The following concepts were proposed to help maintain crestal bone height in proximal surfaces:

- Platform switching (ie, using different implant and abutment diameters)[17–20]
- Scallop-shaped implant platform[21]
- Conical and internalized seal design[22,23]
- One-piece implant

Direction of long axis

When the long axis of the implant is inclined too labially, the subgingival contours of the abutment or restoration will tend to deflect the gingival margin apically.[24] To correct this problem, a custom abutment with a straight or convex contour, extending from implant platform to free gingival margin, is necessary.

The extended long axis of an ideally placed implant will pass through the cingulum and be slightly lingual to the incisal edge of the definitive restoration. Figure 2-9 illustrates the classification of implant positioning based on the extended long axis of the implant. Figure 2-10 presents a case in which the left central incisor implant was in a Class 3, Division 1 position.

Class 1: Ideal implant platform position with presence of more than 2 mm of buccal bone

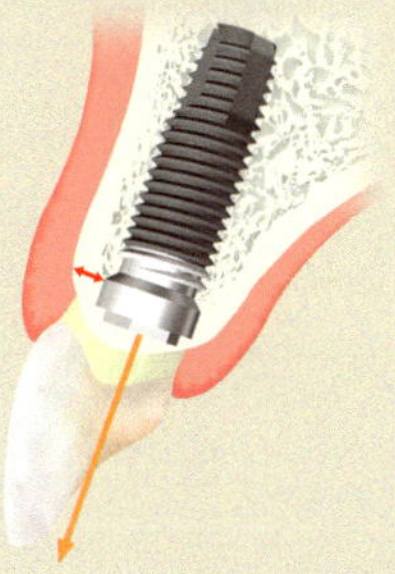

Division 1

Extended long axis of the implant is between the incisal edge and the cingulum. Allows for ideal implant placement, high degree of freedom in selection of abutment design, and thicker buccal tissue.

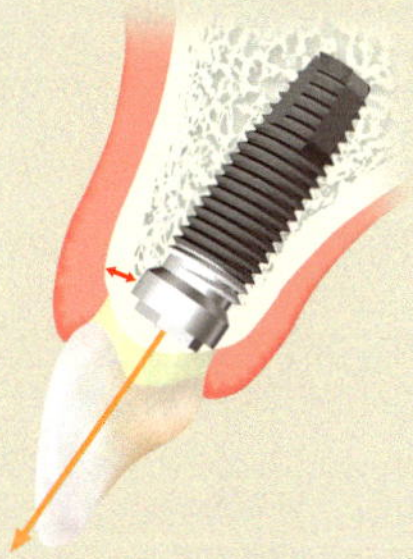

Division 2

Extended long axis of the implant is facial to the incisal edge. Requires selection of a custom abutment with a flat to convex subgingival contour. Because it engages more palatal bone, it potentially prevents a facial fenestration-type defect.

Class 2: Ideal implant platform position with presence of less than 2 mm of buccal bone

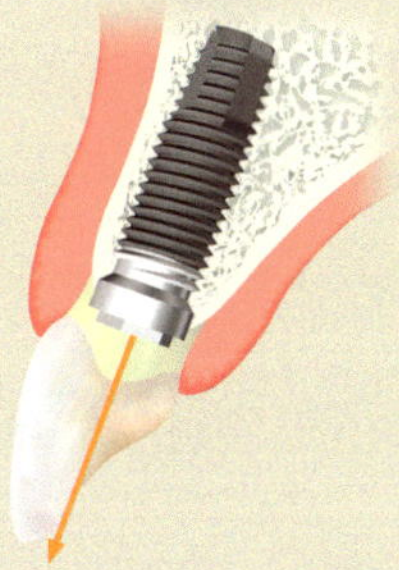

Division 1

Implant positioned the same as Class 1, Division 1. Potential risk for more gingival recession. Requires more facial soft tissue thickness.

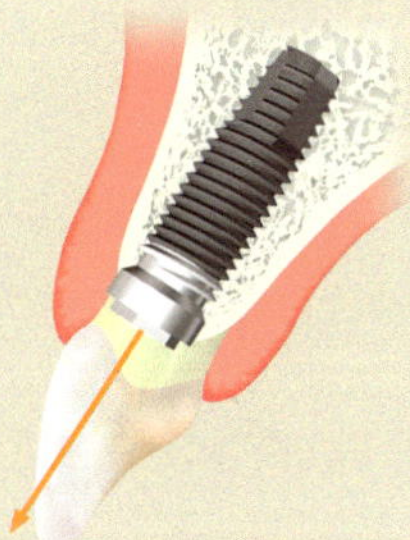

Division 2

Implant positioned the same as Class 1, Division 2. Facial tissue tends to become even thinner.

Class 3: Inadequate implant position

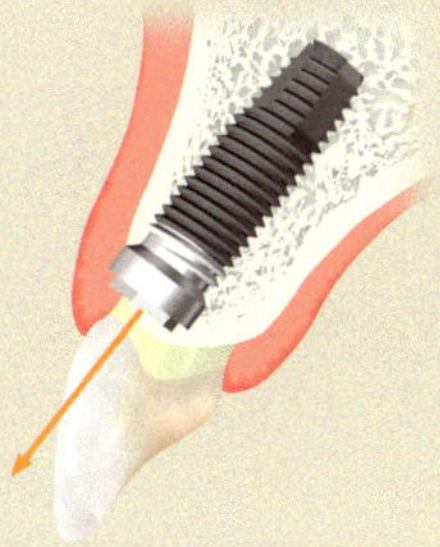

Division 1

Extended long axis of the implant is too facially inclined. Definitive restoration will have to be very long, or implant must be submerged or removed.

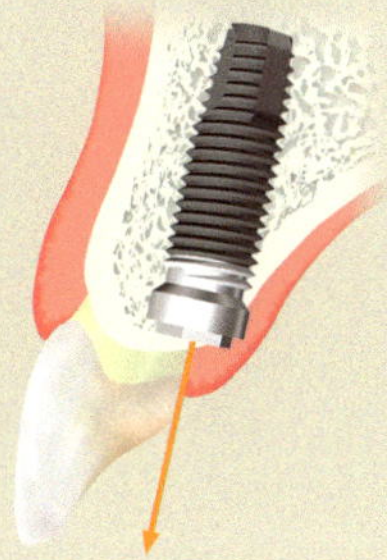

Division 2

Extended long axis of the implant is too palatally inclined. Definitive restoration will have to be short. Phonetics and anterior guidance might be compromised.

Fig 2-9 Classification of implant placement based on the extended long axis of the implant.

Learning from failure: Esthetic and functional problems

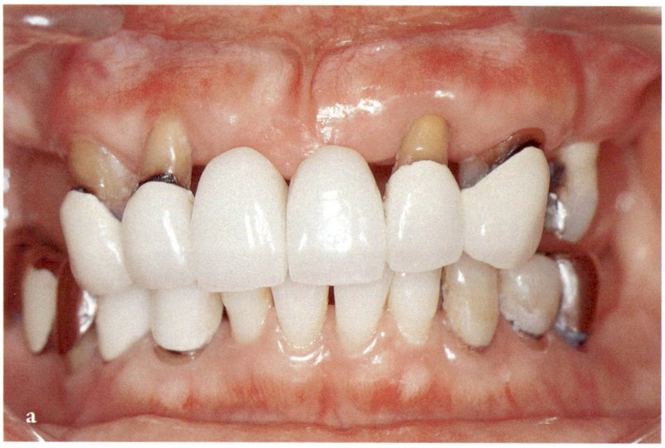
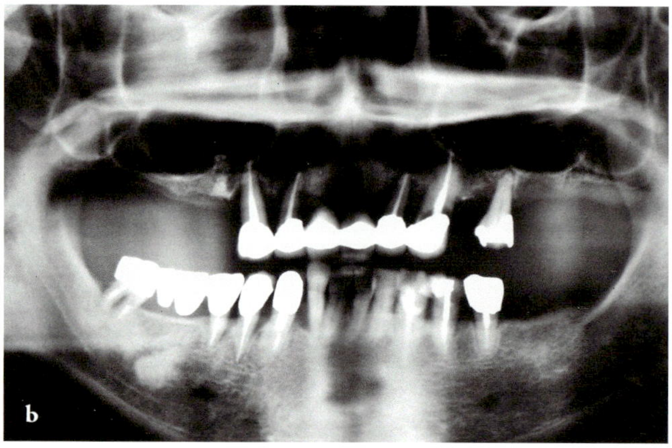

Figs 2-10a and 2-10b Patient requested implant treatment. All maxillary dentition was hopeless.

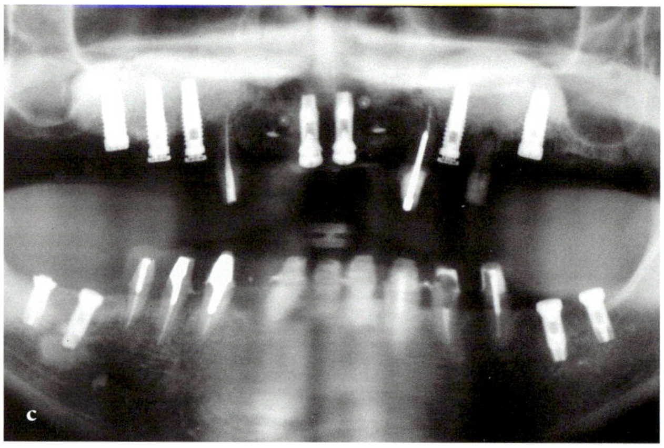

Fig 2-10c Seven implants were placed in the maxilla.

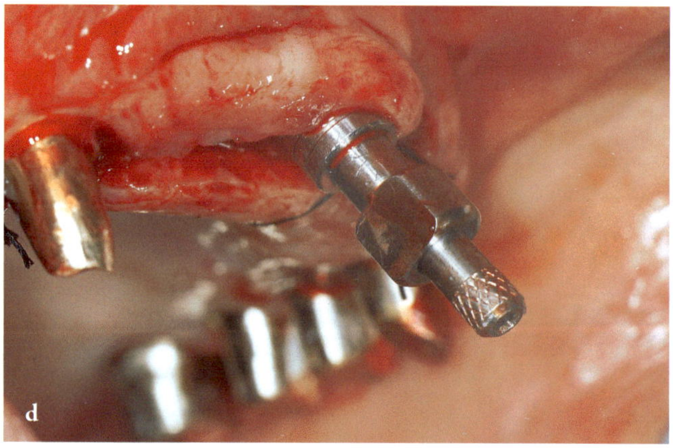

Fig 2-10d Immediate implant placement was performed in the canine and left second premolar sites. Due to the close proximity of the implants, only one implant was selected for abutment connection.

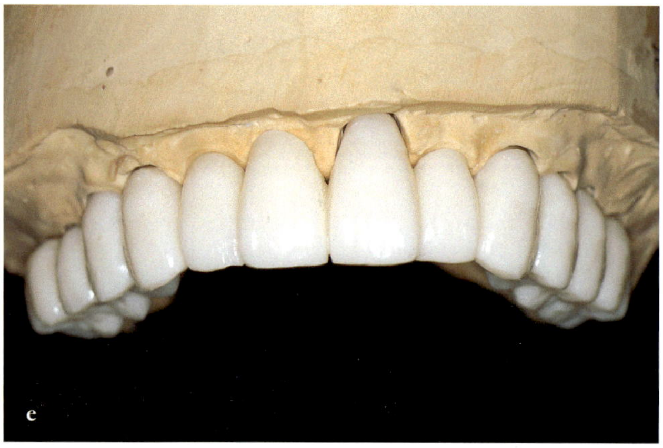

Fig 2-10e The implant at the site of the left central incisor was in a Class 3, Division 1 position. The provisional restoration requires a very long crown.

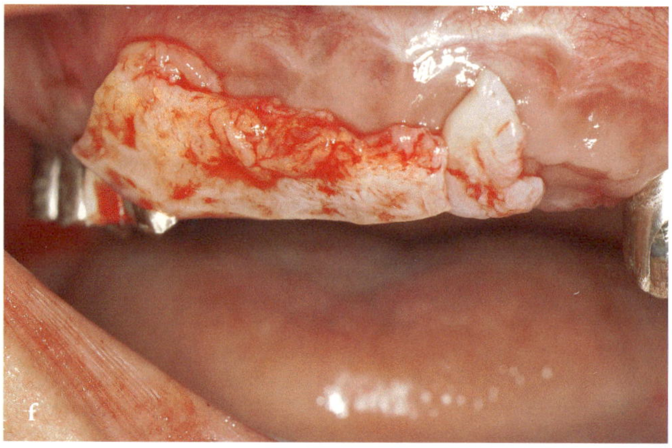

Fig 2-10f The implant at the site of the left central incisor was submerged with a connective tissue graft.

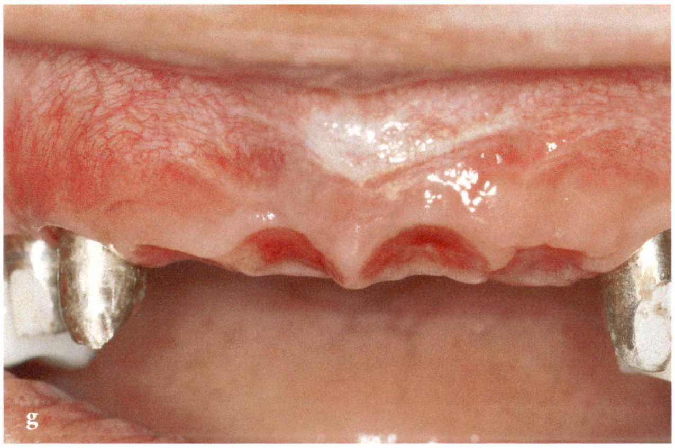

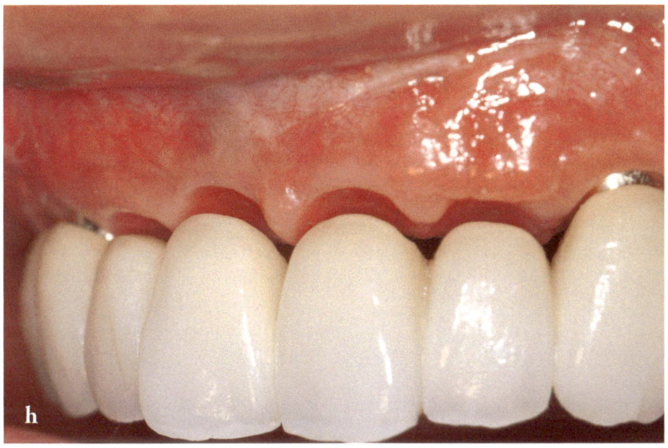

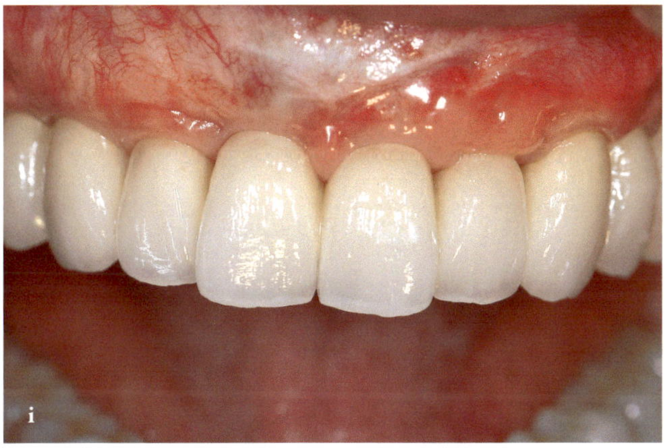

Figs 2-10g to 2-10j Two months after connective tissue grafting. The implant was completely covered with soft tissue. The soft tissue was sculpted using ovate pontics. An acceptable final result was obtained.

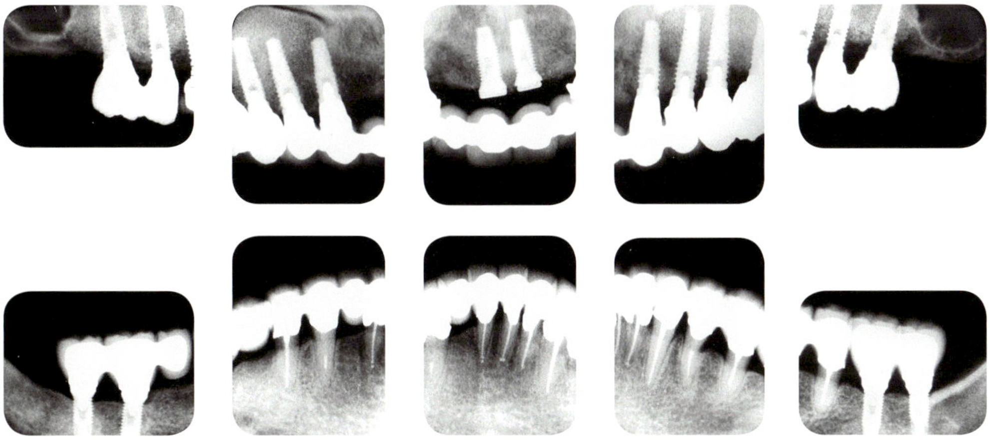

j

☞ Clinical tips

- Implant position may become too facial during immediate implant placement.
- Implant placement should be planned as a staged approach.
- Avoid adjoining central incisor implants for a better soft tissue profile.

References

1. Garber DA. The esthetic dental implant: Letting restoration be the guide. J Am Dent Assoc 1995;126:319–325.
2. Garber DA, Belser UC. Restoration-driven implant placement with restoration-generated site development. Compend Contin Educ Dent 1995;16:796,798–802,804.
3. Buser D, Martin W, Belser UC. Optimizing esthetics for implant restorations in the anterior maxilla: Anatomic and surgical considerations. Int J Oral Maxillofac Implants 2004;19(suppl):43–61.
4. Tarnow DP, Cho SC, Wallace SS. The effect of inter-implant distance on the height of inter-implant bone crest. J Periodontol 2000;71:546–549.
5. Esposito M, Ekestubbe A, Gröndahl K. Radiological evaluation of marginal bone loss at tooth surfaces facing single Brånemark implants. Clin Oral Implants Res 1993;4(3):151–157.
6. Adell R, Lekholm U, Brånemark PI, et al. Marginal tissue reactions at osseointegrated titanium fixtures. Swed Dent J Suppl 1985;28:175–181.
7. Tarnow D, Elian N, Fletcher P, et al. Vertical distance from the crest of bone to the height of the interproximal papilla between adjacent implants. J Periodontol 2003;74:1785–1788.
8. Scarano A, Assenza B, Piattelli M, et al. Interimplant distance and crestal bone resorption: A histologic study in the canine mandible. Clin Implant Dent Relat Res 2004;6(3):150–156.
9. Funato A, Salama MA, Ishikawa T, Garber DA, Salama H. Timing, positioning, and sequential staging in esthetic implant therapy: A four-dimensional perspective. Int J Periodontics Restorative Dent 2007;27:313–323.
10. Salama H, Salama MA, Garber D, Adar P. The interproximal height of bone: A guidepost to predictable aesthetic strategies and soft tissue contours in anterior tooth replacement. Pract Periodontics Aesthet Dent 1998;10:1131–1141.
11. Grunder U. Stability of the mucosal topography around single-tooth implants and adjacent teeth: 1-year results. Int J Periodontics Restorative Dent 2000;20:11–17.
12. Kan JY, Rungcharassaeng K, Umezu K, Kois JC. Dimensions of peri-implant mucosa: An evaluation of maxillary anterior single implants in humans. J Periodontol 2003;74:557–562.
13. Spray JR, Black CG, Morris HF, Ochi S. The influence of bone thickness on facial marginal bone response: Stage 1 placement through stage 2 uncovering. Ann Periodontol 2000;5:119–128.
14. Grunder U, Gracis S, Capelli M. Influence of the 3-D bone-to-implant relationship on esthetics. Int J Periodontics Restorative Dent 2005;25:113–119.
15. Berglundh T, Lindhe J. Dimension of the periimplant mucosa. Biological width revisited. J Clin Periodontol 1996;23:971–973.
16. Cochran DL, Hermann JS, Schenk RK, Higginbottom FL, Buser D. Biologic width around titanium implants. A histometric analysis of the implanto-gingival junction around unloaded and loaded nonsubmerged implants in the canine mandible. J Periodontol 1997;68:186–198.
17. Baumgarten H, Cocchetto R, Testori T, Meltzer A, Porter S. A new implant design for crestal bone preservation: Initial observations and case report. Pract Proced Aesthet Dent 2005;17:735–740.
18. Lazzara RJ, Porter SS. Platform switching: A new concept in implant dentistry for controlling postrestorative crestal bone levels. Int J Periodontics Restorative Dent 2006;26:9–17.
19. Cappiello M, Luongo R, Di Iorio D, Bugea C, Cocchetto R, Celletti R. Evaluation of peri-implant bone loss around platform-switched implants. Int J Periodontics Restorative Dent 2008;28:347–355.
20. Jung RE, Jones AA, Higginbottom FL, et al. The influence of non-matching implant and abutment diameters on radiographic crestal bone levels in dogs. J Periodontol 2008;79:260–270.
21. Wohrle PS. Nobel Perfect esthetic scalloped implant: Rationale for a new design. Clin Implant Dent Relat Res 2003;5(suppl 1):64–73.
22. Novaes AB Jr, de Oliveira RR, Muglia VA, Papalexiou V, Taba M. The effects of interimplant distances on papilla formation and crestal resorption in implants with a morse cone connection and a platform switch: A histomorphometric study in dogs. J Periodontol 2006;77:1839–1849.
23. Wennström JL, Ekestubbe A, Gröndahl K, Karlsson S, Lindhe J. Implant-supported single-tooth restorations: A 5-year prospective study. J Clin Periodontol 2005;32:567–574.
24. Saadoun AP, Le Gall M. Selection and ideal three-dimensional implant positioning in the anterior aesthetic zone. Int Mag Oral Implantol 2003;4(4):8–18.

Chapter 3

Immediate Implant Placement

in Extraction Sockets in the Esthetic Region

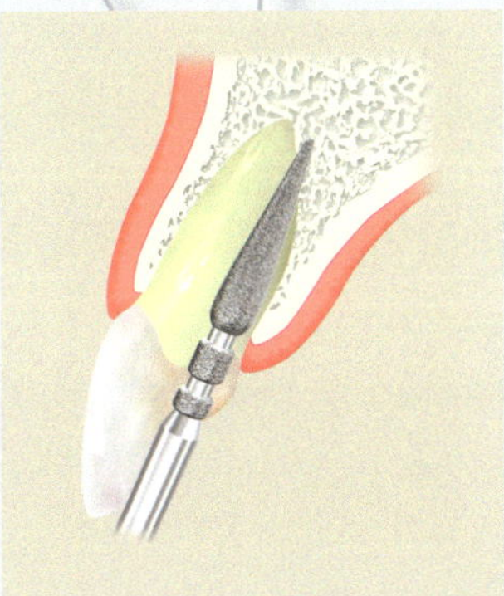

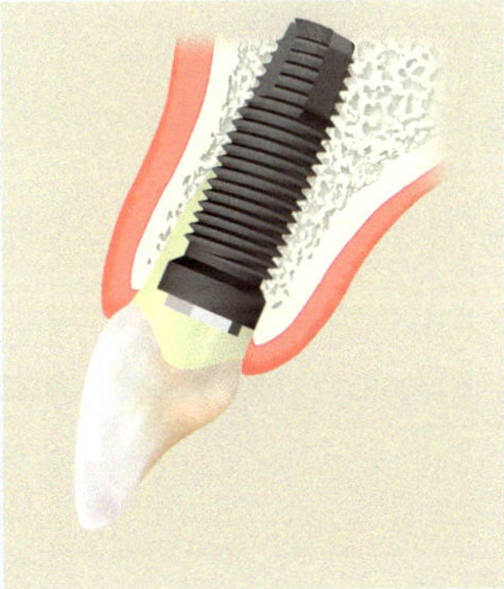

Immediate implant placement into the extraction socket could reduce the number of surgical visits and the treatment period. It could also potentially reduce the extraction socket's labial bone resorption. Many studies demonstrate that immediate implant placement is comparable to the staged approach in terms of its efficacy and high predictability. Ongoing advances in resorbable membranes have helped to expand the potential indications of immediate implant placement with decreased complications. However, the staged approach is still indicated for many cases. In this chapter, the timing of extraction is discussed in addition to the traditional three-dimensional (3D) management of implant positioning and surrounding bone and soft tissue.

Indications for Immediate Implant Placement

Classification of the timing of tooth extraction and implant placement

Table 3-1 presents the classification of the timing of tooth extraction and implant placement according to Hämmerle et al.[1]

Target tooth for immediate implant placement

A tooth targeted for immediate implant placement should first be diagnosed as unsalvageable for at least one of the following reasons: endodontic failure, internal and/or external resorption, subcrestal extensive caries, or root fracture. The targeted tooth should demonstrate no osseous compromise. The bone on the immediately adjacent teeth should be evaluated to determine the relative height of the interproximal height of bone (IHB).

Full understanding of the indications for immediate implant placement will aid the clinician in determining an appropriate treatment plan, including the timing of individual tooth extractions and implant placement.

Predictability of immediate implant placement

When immediate implant placement was introduced, it was embraced by patients and clinicians because it requires fewer surgical and restorative interventions and a shorter treatment period. However, with immediate implant placement, just as with the staged approach, incorrect implant selection, inaccurate 3D implant positioning, and unexpected bone and soft tissue remodeling and resorption may result in esthetic problems.[2–6] Fewer surgical and restorative interventions and a shorter treatment period should not be the only reasons to opt for immediate implant placement. Immediate implant placement is effective and predictable only when clinicians understand its indications and limitations.[7–9] Long-term follow-up and evaluation of immediate implant placement cases are presented in Figs 3-1 and 3-2.

Table 3-1 Classification of timing of extraction and implant placement*

Classification	Timing	Description
Type 1	Occurs at time of extraction using flapless technique or flap elevation with simultaneous CTG and/or GBR	Immediate implant placement
Type 2	Occurs 6 to 8 weeks after extraction to allow soft tissue healing over the extraction socket; may be performed with simultaneous GBR	Early implant placement
Type 3	Occurs 3 to 4 months after extraction, ie, following socket preservation	Delayed implant placement
Type 4	Occurs more than 4 months after extraction, ie, following immediate or early GBR	

CTG—connective tissue graft, GBR—guided bone regeneration.
*According to Hämmerle et al.[1]

Extraction and immediate implant placement with 10-year follow-up

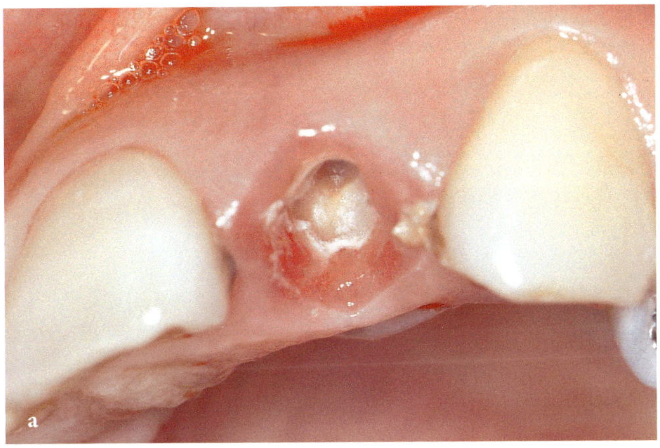

Fig 3-1a The left lateral incisor was diagnosed as unrestorable.

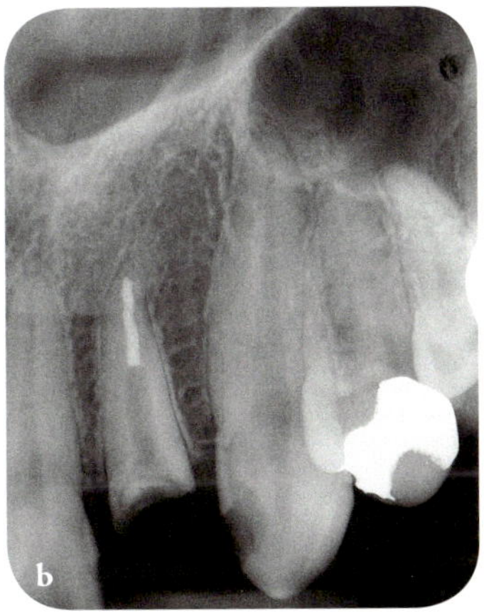

Fig 3-1b Radiograph at initial examination.

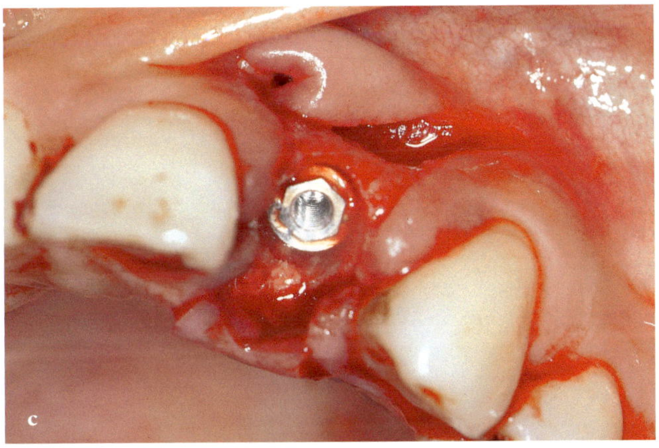

Fig 3-1c A machined-surface 3.75- × 13-mm implant was immediately placed into the extraction socket. A nonresorbable membrane was used.

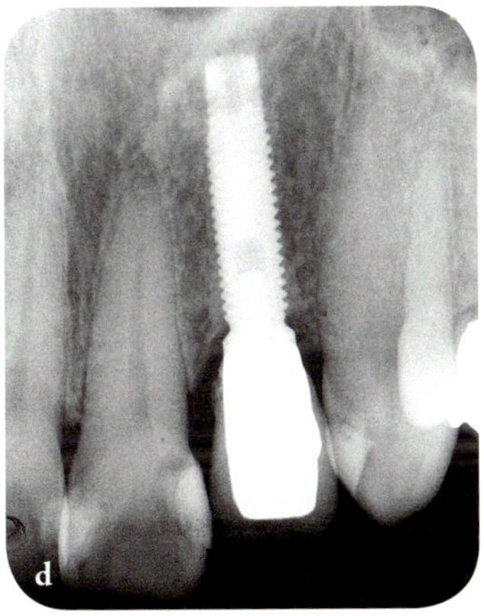

Fig 3-1d Radiograph at 7-year follow-up.

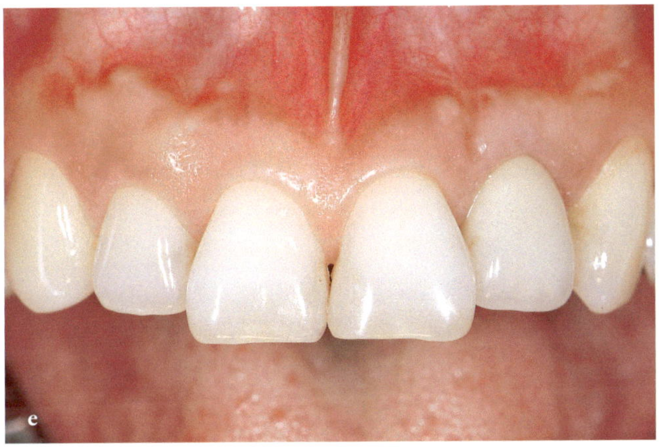

Fig 3-1e Clinical appearance at the 7-year follow-up, before connective tissue grafting (CTG).

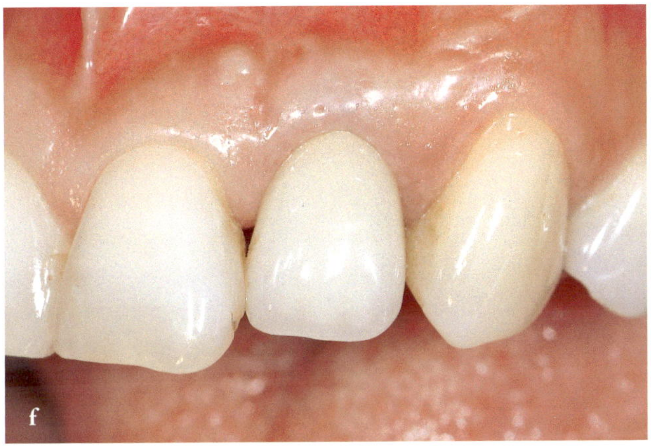

Fig 3-1f Clinical appearance 3 years after CTG, 10 years after implant placement.

Immediate implant placement with buccal bone resorption

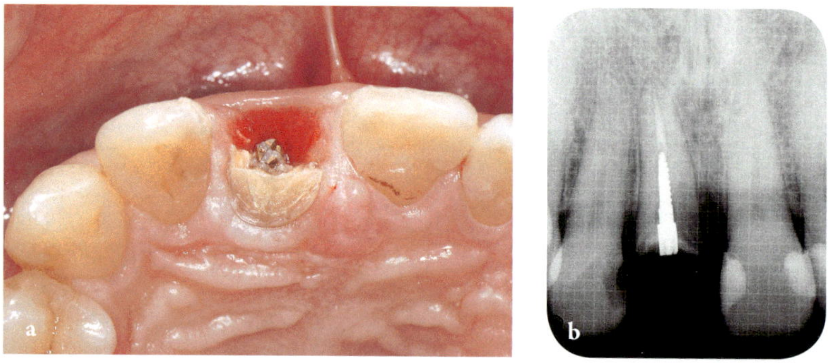

Figs 3-2a and 3-2b The patient presented with a broken restoration and a fractured tooth.

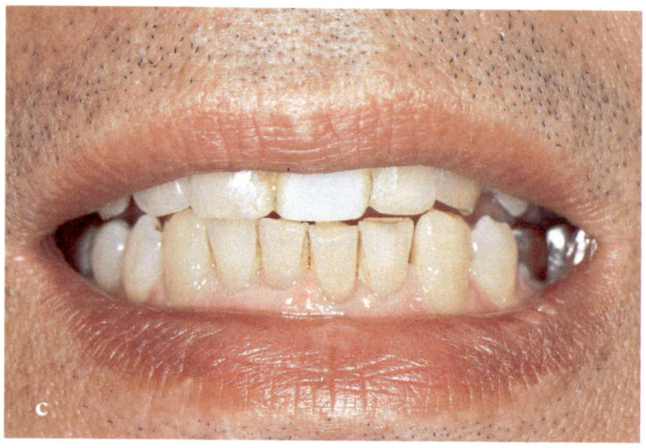

Fig 3-2c The patient had a low smile line.

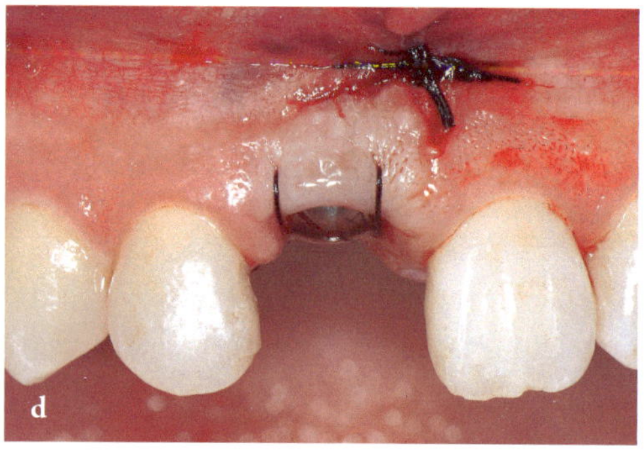

Fig 3-2d The patient did not want to undergo orthodontic extrusion and chose the quickest option—immediate implant placement—with the understanding that the definitive restoration would be longer than the adjacent teeth because of the presence of buccal bone loss.

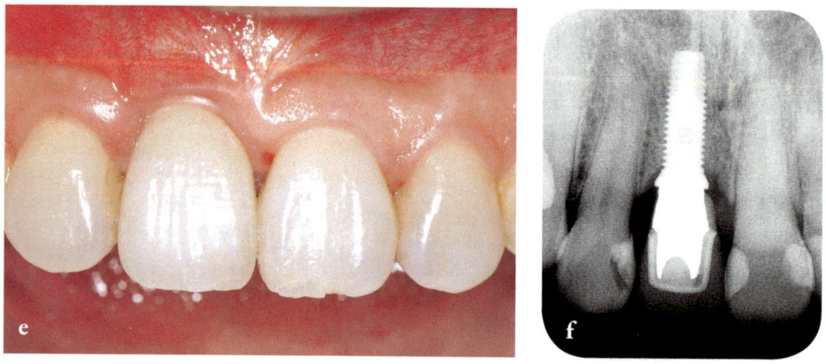

Figs 3-2e and 3-2f *(e)* Clinical and *(f)* radiographic views of the definitive restoration, which was longer than the adjacent teeth as predicted.

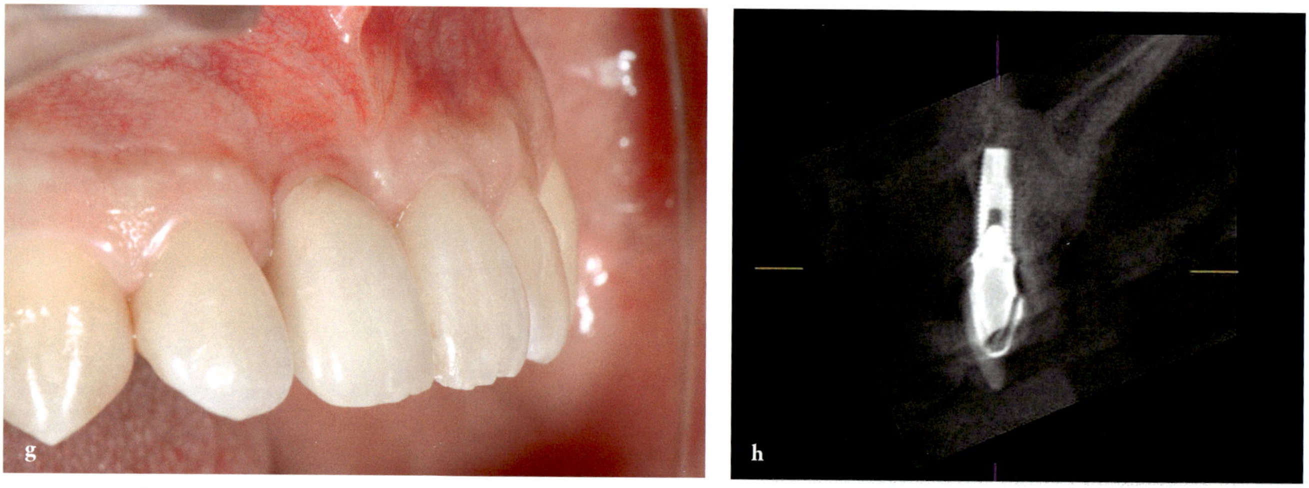

Figs 3-2g and 3-2h At the 4-year follow-up, the soft tissue seems stable, but the computed tomographic evaluation shows buccal bone resorption and four to five exposed threads.

Alveolar Ridge Alteration Following Extraction and Immediate Implant Placement

Araújo and Lindhe[10] reported that in the early stages following extraction of the mandibular premolar in dogs, the bundle bone in the alveolar ridge, which had lost its function, was resorbed and replaced with woven bone (Fig 3-3). Since the crest of the buccal bone wall was comprised solely of bundle bone, this remodeling resulted in substantial vertical reduction of the buccal crest height. Then, subsequent resorption from the outer surfaces of both buccal and lingual bone walls resulted in horizontal resorption and possibly contributed to the vertical reduction. Botticelli et al[11] studied the healing of marginal bone defects that occurred around implants placed in fresh extraction sockets as compared with surgically created defects. They concluded that immediate implant placement was unable to prevent alteration to the alveolar ridge following tooth extraction (Fig 3-4).

It is critically important to understand the nature of the crestal bone remodeling process that follows tooth extraction. The authors strongly believe that orthodontic extrusion should precede immediate implant placement in the esthetic region to compensate for the bone loss that is inevitable with extraction (see Fig 3-2). This is particularly necessary in Asian patients, who often have extremely thin labial bone plates in the maxillary anterior region. In these thin, scalloped periodontal biotypes, alveolar ridge height and width reduction occurs even if particulate bone graft materials are placed in the extraction socket. Following implant placement, 1 to 3 mm of gingival recession invariably occurs over time following the connection of the abutment because of hard and soft tissue remodeling around the implant platform.

Therefore, immediate implant placement is possible in the esthetic region only if the following criteria are met:

- Intact extraction socket wall (except buccal wall)
- Sufficient bone volume around the extraction socket for implant primary stability
- Preemptive orthodontic extrusion to assure the two criteria above.

Overall advantages and disadvantages of immediate implant placement are listed in Box 3-1.

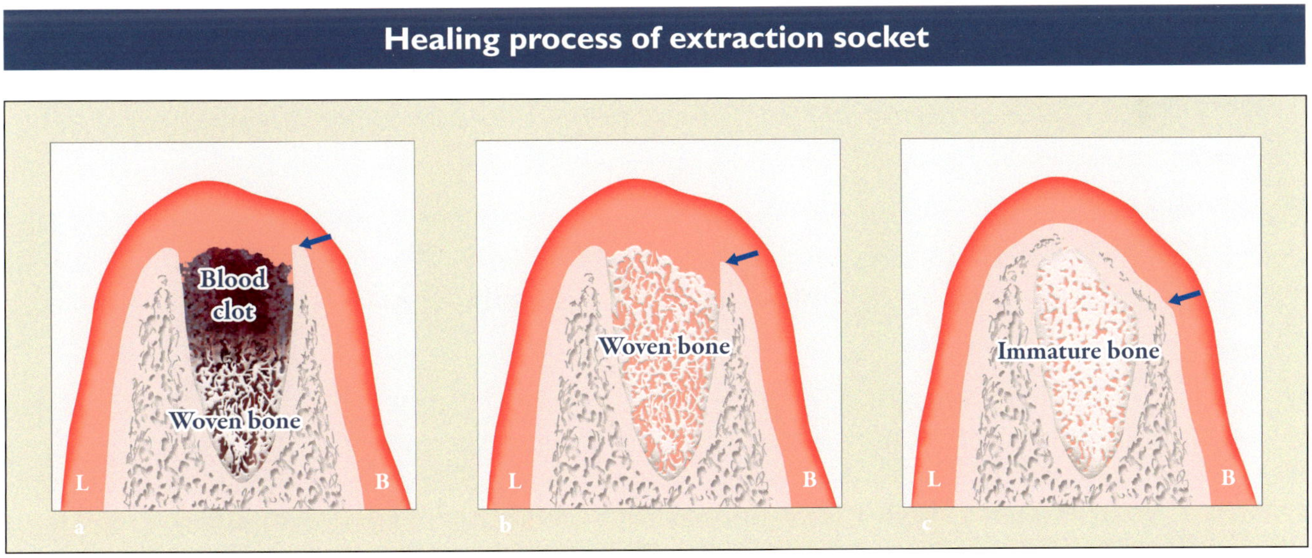

Fig 3-3 Healing process of dog extraction socket at 2- *(a)*, 4- *(b)*, and 8-week *(c)* observation. Most of the crestal portion of the buccal bone *(arrow)* is comprised of bundle bone, which will be resorbed after tooth extraction as it loses its function. L—labial, B—buccal.

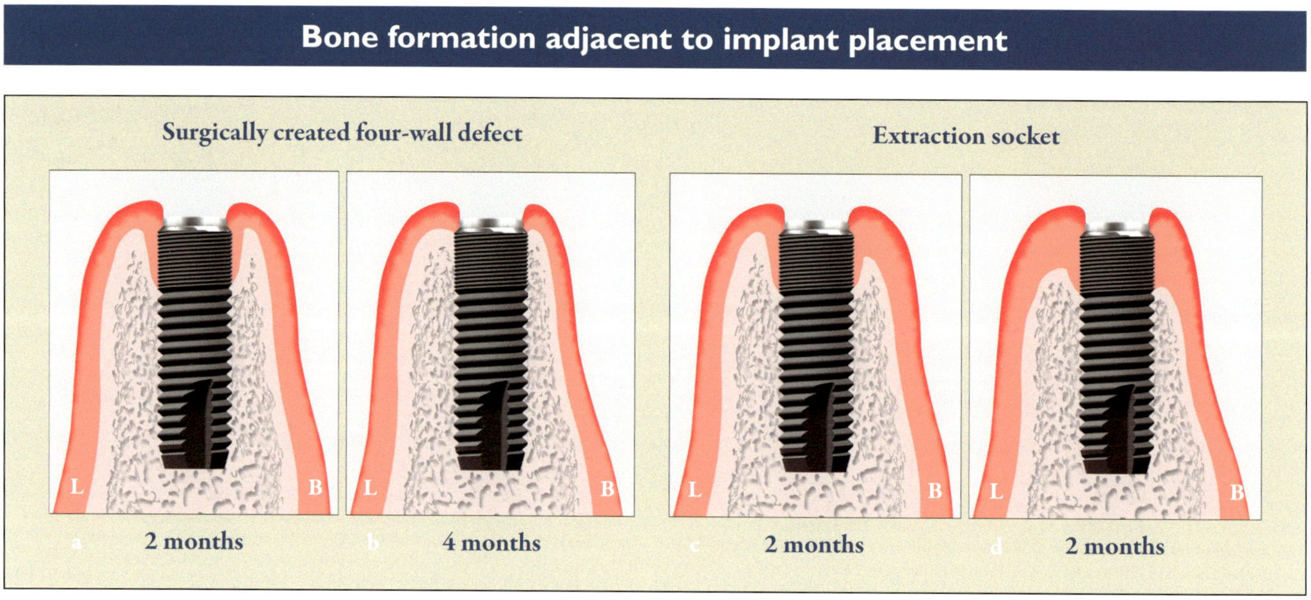

Fig 3-4 *(a and b)* Implant placement in surgically created four-wall defect. Complete bone fill is observed in the gap between implant and defect, and there are no crestal bone level changes. *(c and d)* Implant placement in an extraction socket. Significant lingual (L) and buccal (B) crestal bone resorption is observed.

Box 3-1 Advantages and disadvantages of immediate implant placement

Advantages
- Shorter treatment period
- Less surgical intervention
- Preservation of papilla form with an immediate provisional restoration
- Immediate replacement of abutment teeth

Disadvantages
- Difficulty of achieving ideal 3D implant positioning
- Impossibility of maintaining alveolar bone anatomy using a bone graft inside the extraction socket only
- Possibility that immediate implant placement will have to be canceled depending upon the condition of extraction socket
- Frequent results of compromised esthetics

Immediate implant placement sequence and positioning

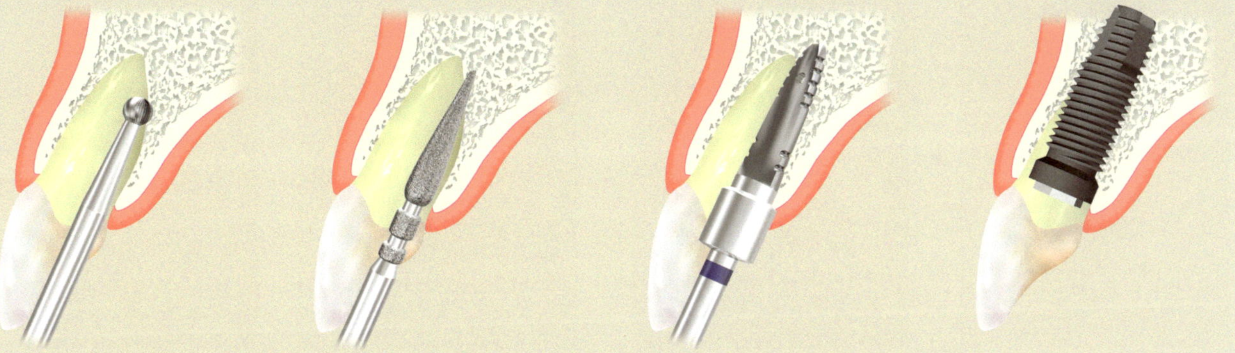

1. After orthodontic extrusion, atraumatic extraction is performed with a periotome and forceps.
2. The extraction socket is thoroughly debrided.
3. Initial drilling is performed with a long shank diamond bur (2710-0).
4. Drilling is continued with a 2710-1 or 2710-2 bur with careful attention to the long axis.
5. Final drilling is accomplished with a twist drill or shaping drill.
6. The implant is placed, maintaining a gap between the implant and buccal bone to avoid buccal inclination.
7. The gap is filled with bone graft. A provisional restoration can be placed if primary stability is adequate.

Fig 3-5 The extended long axis of the implant is placed in a Class 2, Division 1 position (see Fig 2-9) to create a harmonious gingival margin.

Immediate Implant Positioning

An ideally placed immediate implant should engage the palatal wall of the extraction socket and leave a gap between the buccal bone wall and the implant body (Fig 3-5).

Evans and Chen[12] retrospectively analyzed the esthetic outcomes of 42 nonadjacent, single-unit restorations on immediately placed implants. The mean time in function was 18.9 months. Those with a thin periodontal biotype showed slightly greater recession than those with a thick periodontal biotype, but the difference was not statistically significant. Implants with a buccal shoulder position showed three times more recession than implants with a lingual shoulder position. That difference was highly statistically significant.

Chen et al[13] evaluated the healing of marginal defects with immediate implant placement. Thirty immediate implants in the maxillary anterior extraction site randomly received a bone graft only, a bone graft and a resorbable membrane, or no graft. Bone grafting significantly reduced horizontal resorption of buccal bone. This study also found that mucosal recession was more significantly associated with buccally positioned implants than with lingually positioned implants.

During immediate implant placement, 3D implant positioning—especially control of the angulation of the long axis of the implant—becomes very difficult. As described in many publications, the extended long axis of the implant should be slightly lingual to the incisal edge of the definitive restoration. An immediately placed implant with a labially inclined long axis, as illustrated in Fig 3-6, could be acceptable; however, a custom abutment with a straight or convex contour is necessary to prevent buccal mucosal recession. The direction of the long axis of the implant can be determined by the position of the screw access hole on the abutment, which should not be visible from the buccal aspect. In addition, the implant platform should not be positioned too lingually.

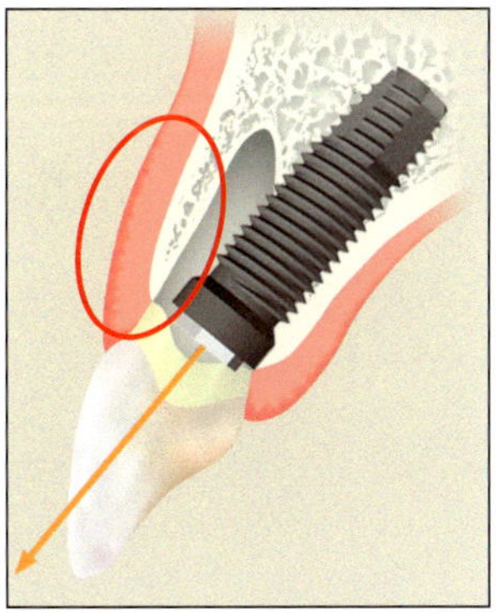

Fig 3-6 Immediate implant with a labially inclined long axis.

Advantages of orthodontic extrusion

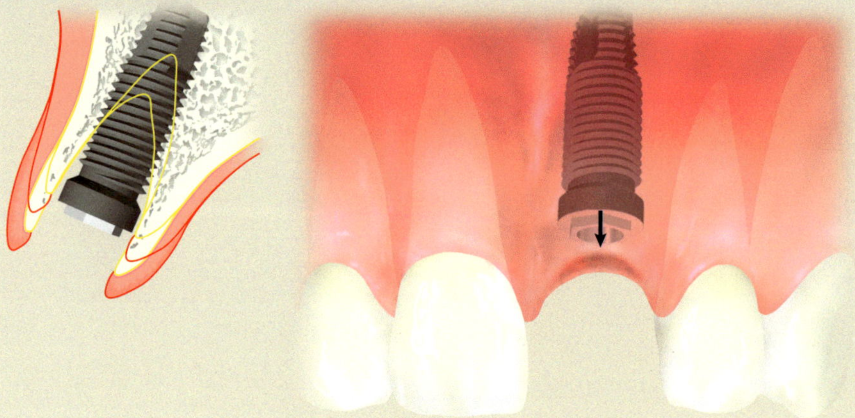

1. Compensation for buccal bone resorption, which occurs after extraction (with intact buccal bone)
2. Fewer complications with immediate GBR
3. Minimization of the gap between the implant and the extraction socket
4. Better primary implant stability
5. Facilitation of extraction through loosening of the tooth

Fig 3-7 Coronal augmentation of the alveolar bone and gingiva created by orthodontic extrusion. GBR—guided bone regeneration.

Orthodontic Extrusion and Immediate Implant Placement

Future extraction sites are routinely augmented vertically by orthodontic extrusion as a preliminary step to immediate implant placement.[14] The advantages of orthodontic extrusion include the following (Fig 3-7):

- It augments the crestal alveolar bone height and width as well as the overlying gingival tissue, decreasing the negative impact of postoperative alveolar resorption and gingival recession.
- It decreases or minimizes the "gap" between the implant body and the extraction socket.[15]
- It helps to enhance primary stability in the alveolus by developing the alveolar bone beyond the root apex.[16,17]
- It helps facilitate extraction by loosening the tooth.

Orthodontic extrusion should be used to generate at least 2 mm of additional vertical gingival tissue beyond the gingival margin of the future definitive restoration. To accomplish this, appropriate retention (approximately 12 weeks) is necessary prior to extraction and immediate implant placement (Figs 3-8 and 3-9).

Preservation of buccal tissue volume with orthodontic tooth extrusion

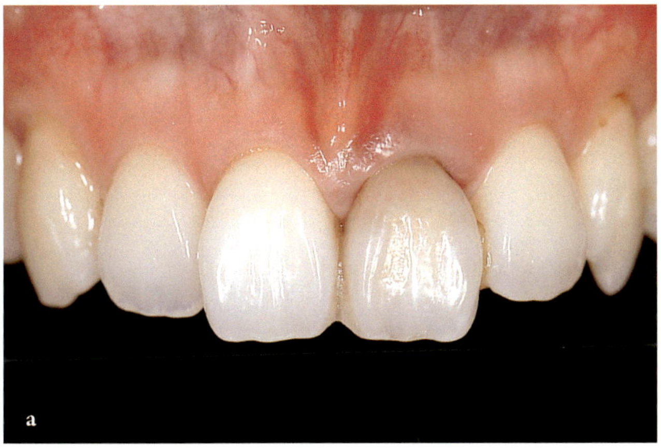

Fig 3-8a Initial examination.

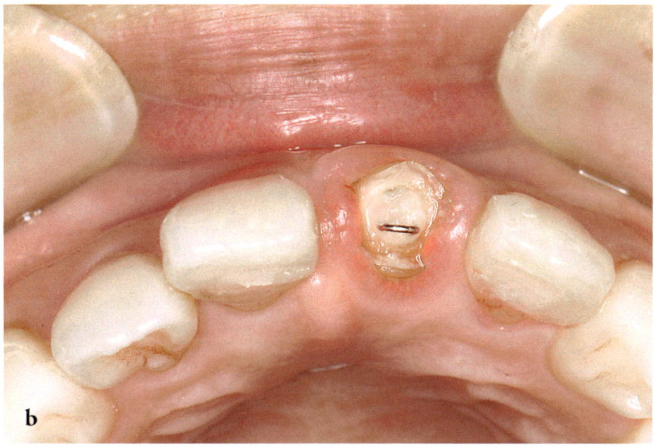

Fig 3-8b Occlusal view following 12-month retention after orthodontic extrusion.

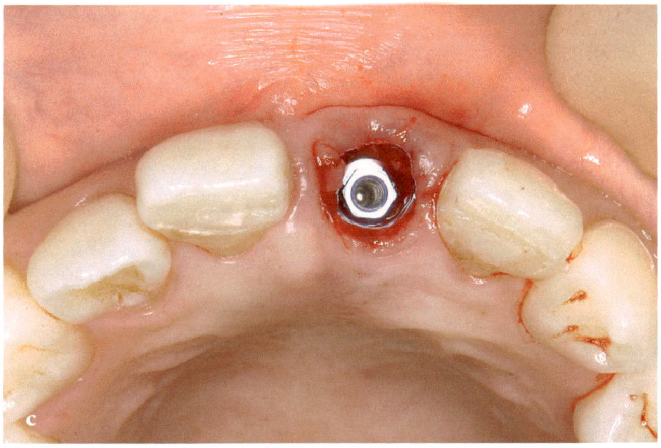

Fig 3-8c Overcorrection of buccal tissue with immediate implant placement.

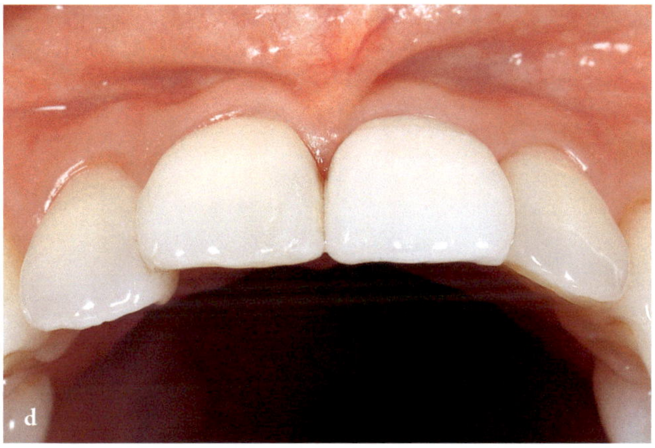

Fig 3-8d Occlusal view at 2-year follow-up of definitive restoration. There is slight buccal tissue volume reduction, but it is at an acceptable level.

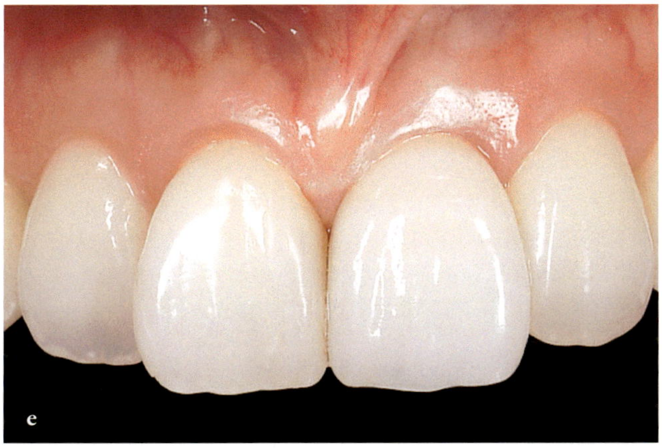

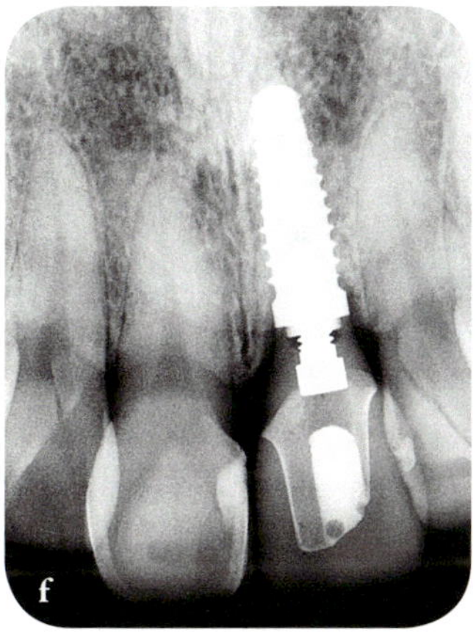

Figs 3-8e and 3-8f Frontal *(e)* and radiographic *(f)* views at the 2-year follow-up visit.

Orthodontic extrusion with guided bone regeneration (GBR)

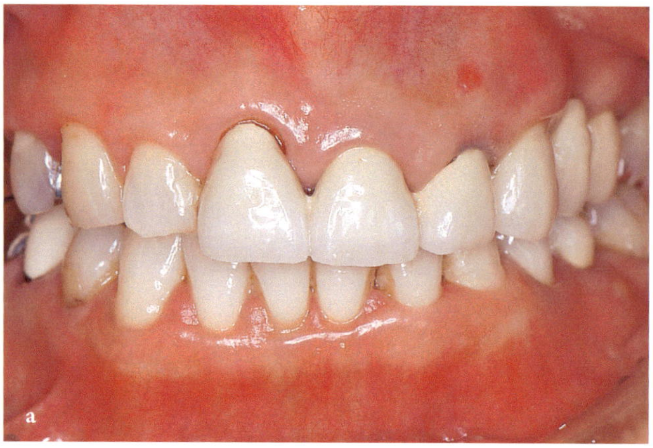

Fig 3-9a Initial examination.

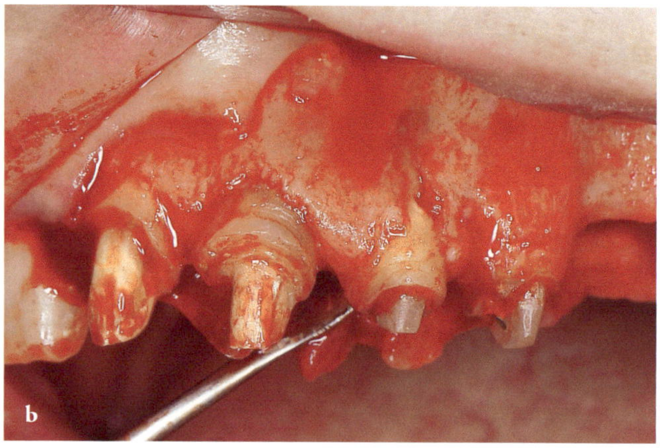

Fig 3-9b After extrusion, a coronal shift of the alveolar bone can be observed at the left lateral incisor and first premolar sites.

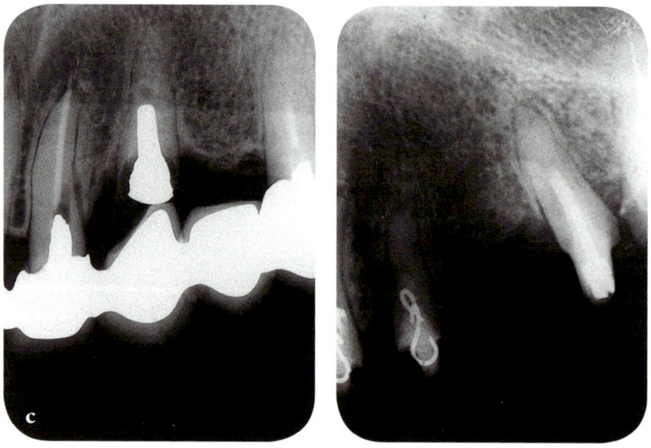

Fig 3-9c Radiographs taken before extrusion *(left)* and after 13 weeks of retention following extrusion *(right)*.

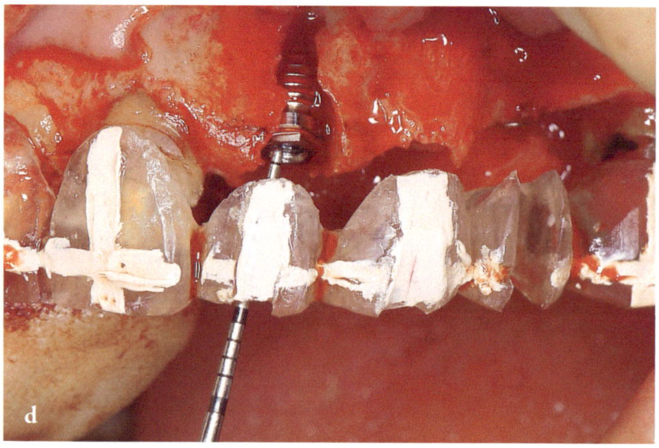

Fig 3-9d Precise implant positioning with a surgical guide. A coronal shift of the alveolar bone is evident.

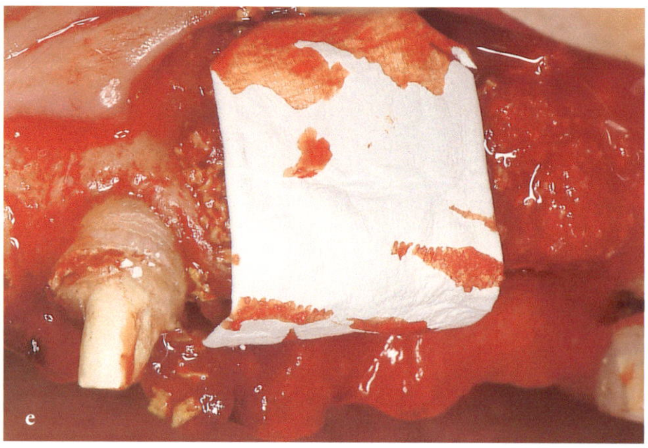

Fig 3-9e GBR with a xenograft and resorbable membrane.

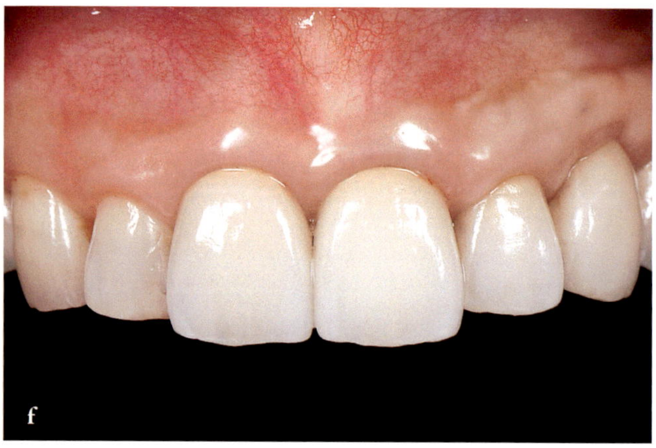

Fig 3-9f Buccal tissue volume was maintained at the left lateral incisor and premolar sites 4 years after treatment completion.

Classification of Immediate Implant Placement Sites

The classification of immediate implant placement sites according to Funato et al[18] is detailed in Fig 3-10. Clinical case examples are shown in Fig 3-11 (Class 1), Figs 3-12 and 3-13 (Class 2), Fig 3-14 (Class 3), and Fig 3-15 (Class 4).

The importance of a thorough evaluation of the periodontal biotype prior to immediate implant placement is supported in the literature. Maynard and Wilson[19] related the risk of potential gingival recession to the periodontal biotype and underlying alveolar bone. They indicated that a periodontal biotype with thin gingival tissue and thin alveolar bone has the highest risk of gingival recession. Kan et al[20] reported that the thick periodontal biotype has a more coronal level of gingival margin, with greater predictability than the thin periodontal biotype. Kois[21] reported the advantages of the thick, flat periodontal biotype for better esthetic definitive restoration.

With the thin periodontal biotype, connective tissue grafting may be necessary to compensate for compromised soft and hard tissue. Care must be taken to ensure that the clinician's attempts to expedite implant placement within the extraction socket do not result in an implant that tends to extrude labially. The extended long axis of the implant should be placed lingual to the incisal edge whenever possible.

Classification of immediate implant placement sites

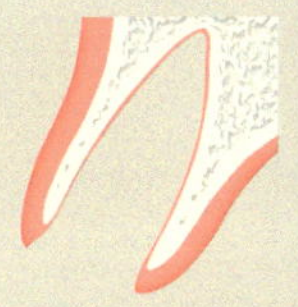	**Class 1: Optimal results**	• Intact buccal bone • Thick periodontal biotype • Immediate implant placement without flap reflection
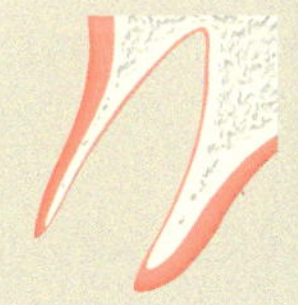	**Class 2: Good results**	• Intact buccal bone • Thin periodontal biotype • Immediate implant placement with CTG or staged CTG
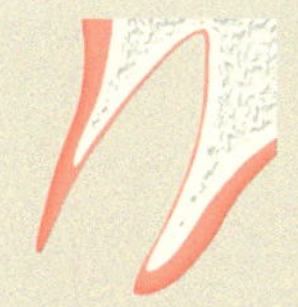	**Class 3: Acceptable results**	• Deficient buccal bone • Implant placement possible in remaining alveolar housing of extraction socket with simultaneous GBR and CTG or followed by staged CTG • Staged early implant placement should be considered for better esthetic results
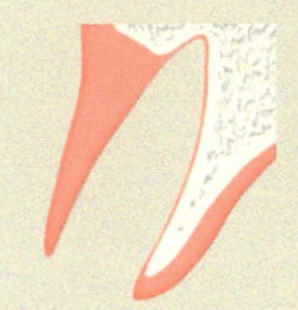	**Class 4: Poor or unacceptable results**	• Deficient buccal bone • Implant placement may deviate from alveolar housing • Delayed implant placement

Fig 3-10 Classification of immediate implant placement sites based on bone sounding or computed tomographic evaluation after orthodontic extrusion, according to Funato et al.[18] CTG—connective tissue grafting, GBR—guided bone regeneration.

Class 1: Optimal results

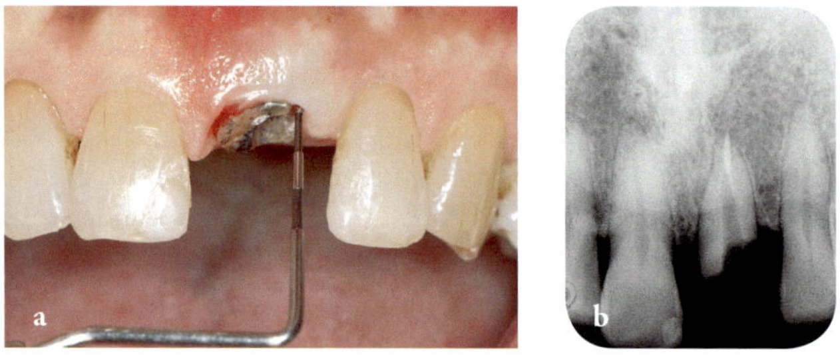

Figs 3-11a and 3-11b The patient presented with a fractured tooth. The buccal bone was evaluated using bone sounding, and the site was determined to be Class 1.

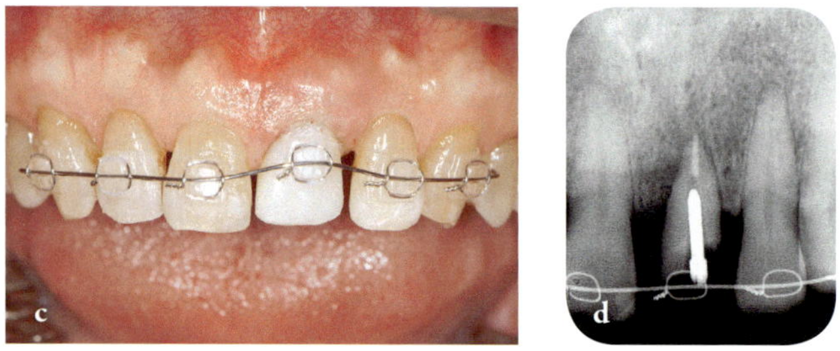

Figs 3-11c and 3-11d Orthodontic extrusion was performed prior to extraction.

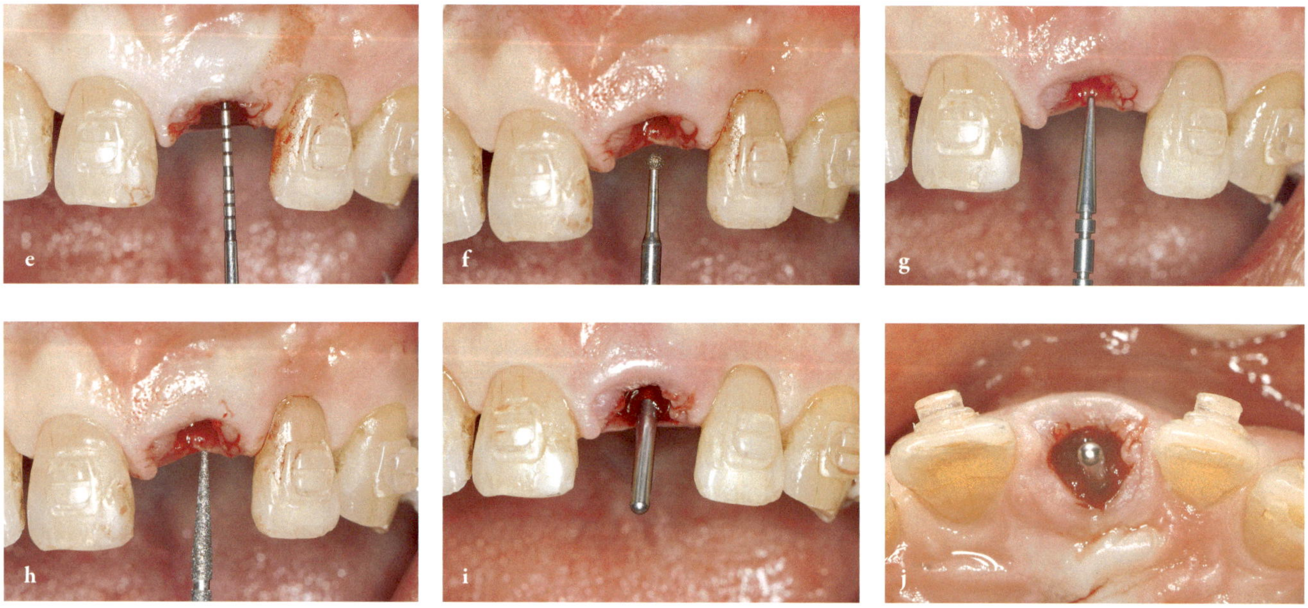

Figs 3-11e to 3-11j Implant site osteotomy was initiated in the palatal wall of the extraction socket with a long shank diamond bur. An implant was placed using an incisionless procedure, ie, without flap reflection.

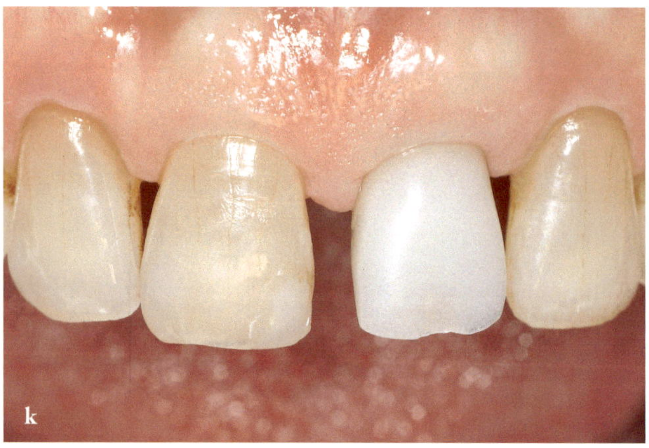

Fig 3-11k A provisional restoration was placed immediately after implant surgery.

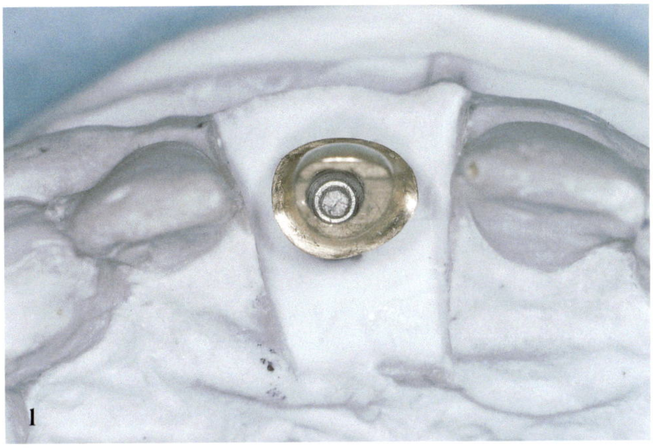

Fig 3-11l The location of the abutment access hole indicates that the extended long axis of the implant is lingual to the incisal edge of the definitive restoration.

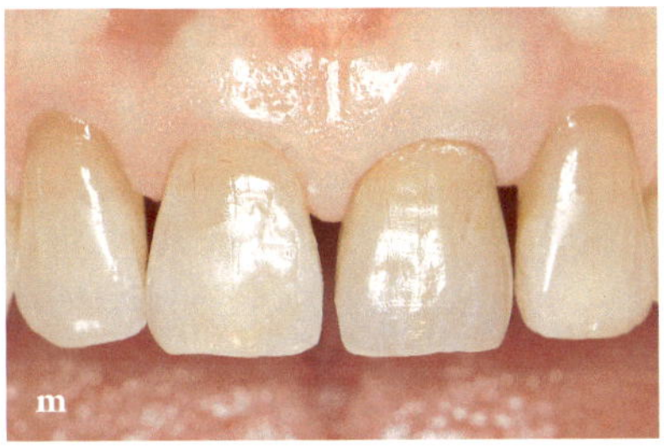

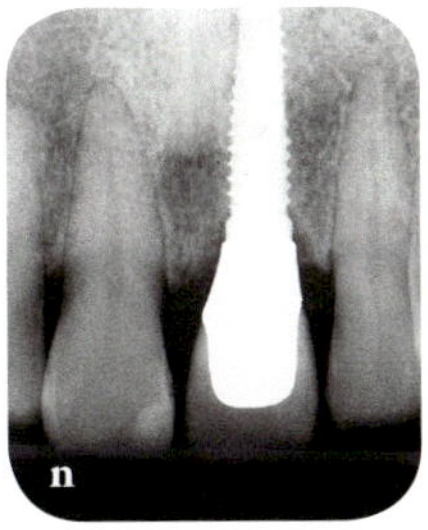

Figs 3-11m and 3-11n Facial view of the definitive restoration.

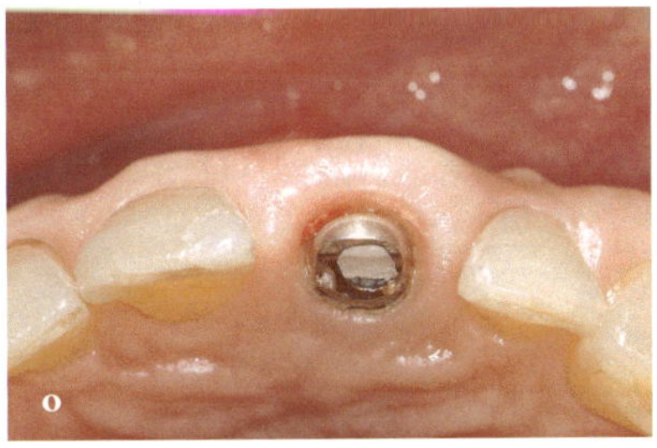

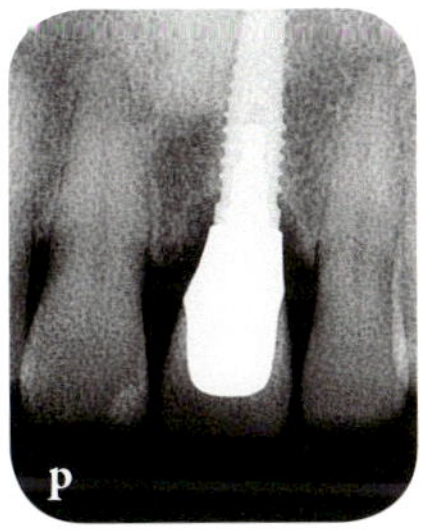

Figs 3-11o and 3-11p At the 2-year follow-up, buccal tissue volume was maintained.

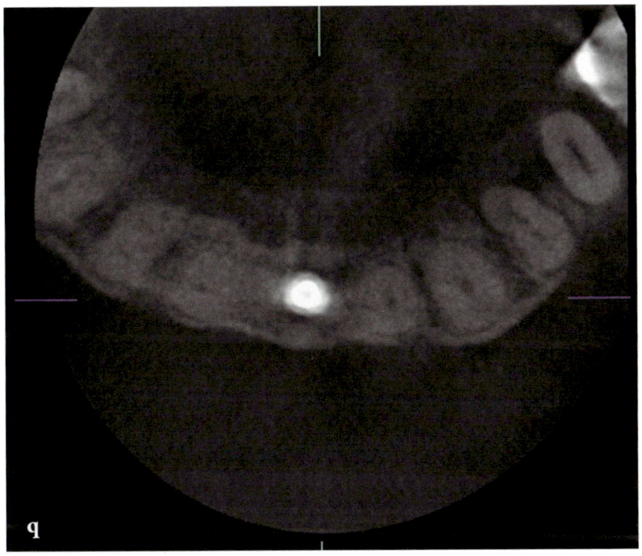

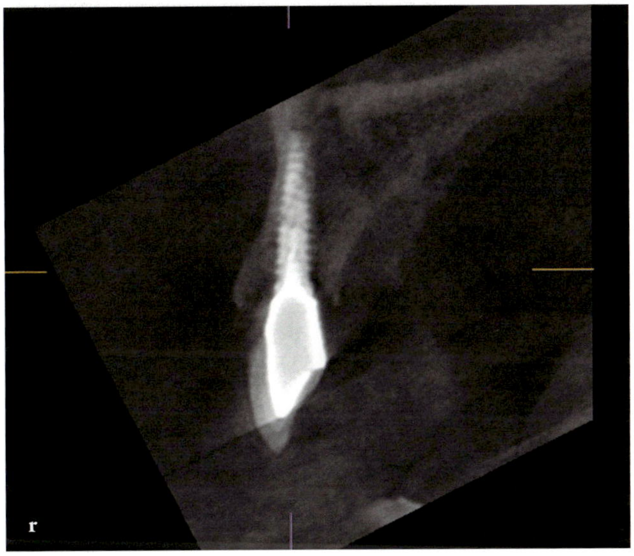

Figs 3-11q and 3-11r Computed tomographic evaluation 2.5 years after implant placement confirmed adequate buccal bone thickness.

Class 2: Good results (Case 1)

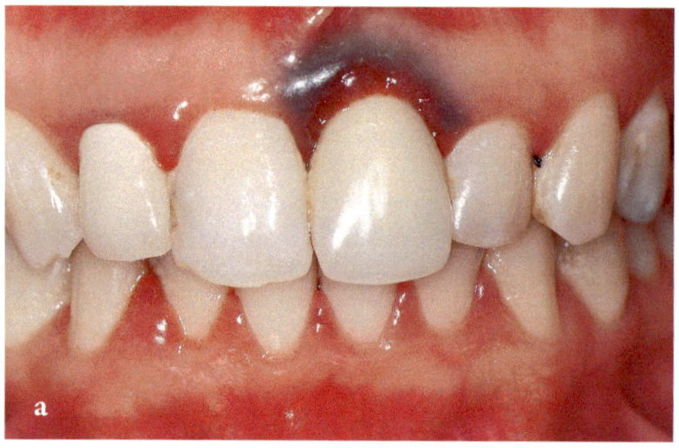

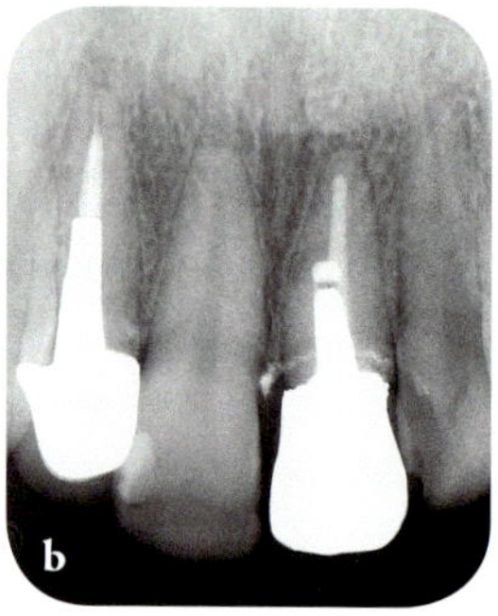

Figs 3-12a and 3-12b Facial view at initial examination. Gingival discoloration and perforation of root canal were observed.

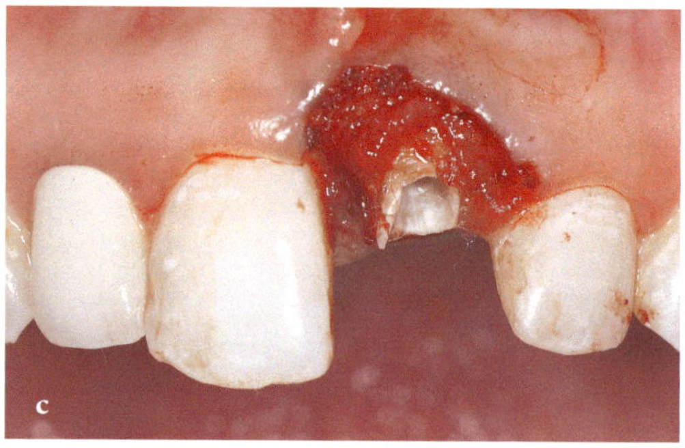

Fig 3-12c Gingival discoloration was excised.

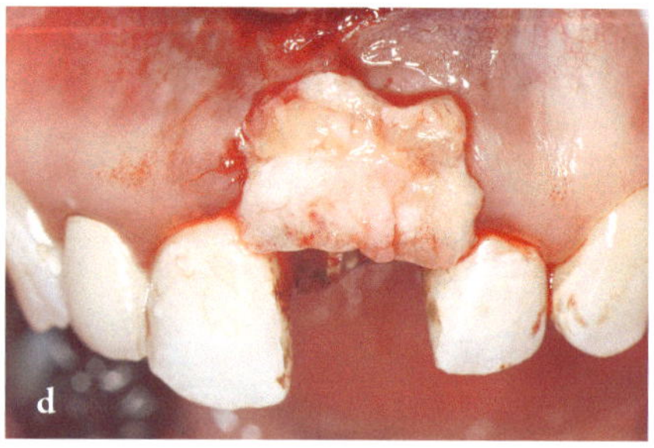

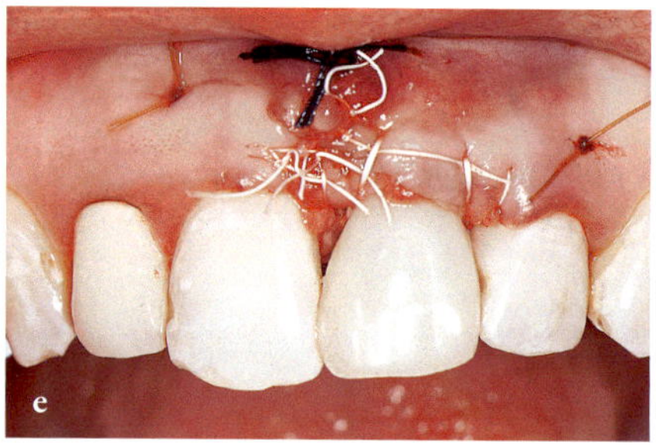

Figs 3-12d and 3-12e Following 1 month of healing, connective tissue grafting (CTG) was performed.

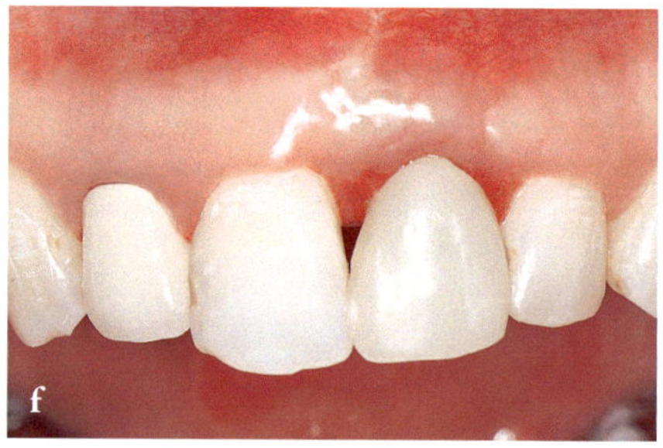

Fig 3-12f Three months after CTG.

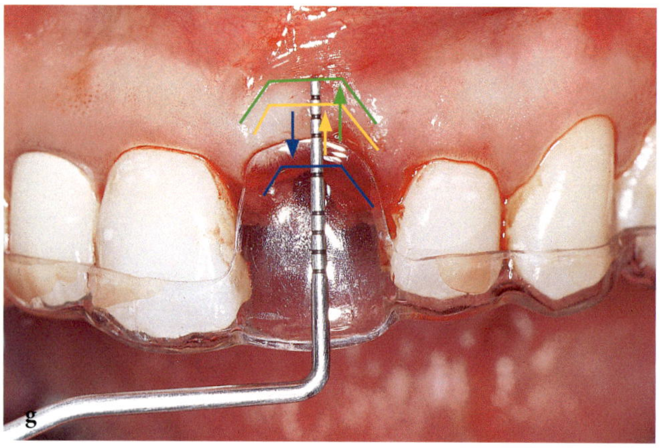

Fig 3-12g Orthodontic extrusion was started 3 months after CTG. The three goals of orthodontic extrusion to allow immediate implant placement without flap reflection are illustrated. *(blue line and arrow)* Gingival margin must be augmented 2 mm coronal to the margin of the definitive restoration. *(yellow line and arrow)* Ideally, the bone crest must be located 3 mm apical of the augmented gingival margin. *(green line and arrow)* Implant platform must be positioned 3 mm apical of the margin of the definitive restoration.

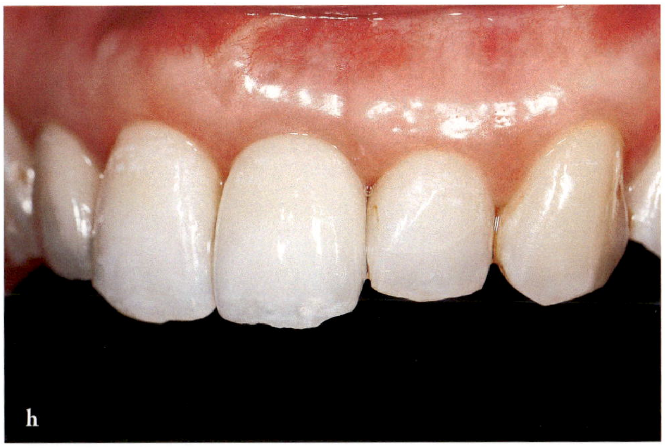
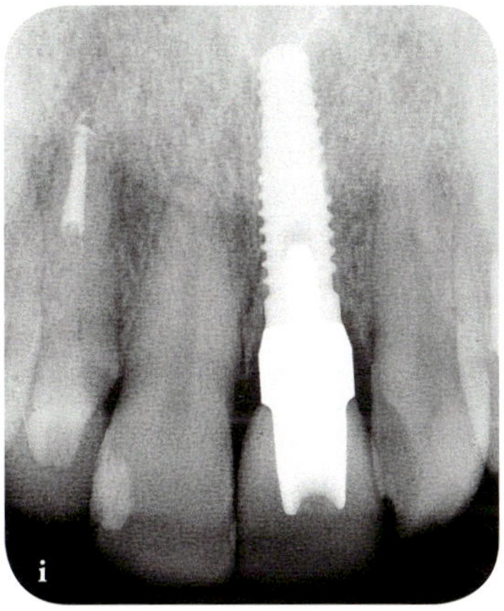

Figs 3-12h and 3-12i Lateral view *(h)* and periapical radiograph *(i)* of the definitive restoration.

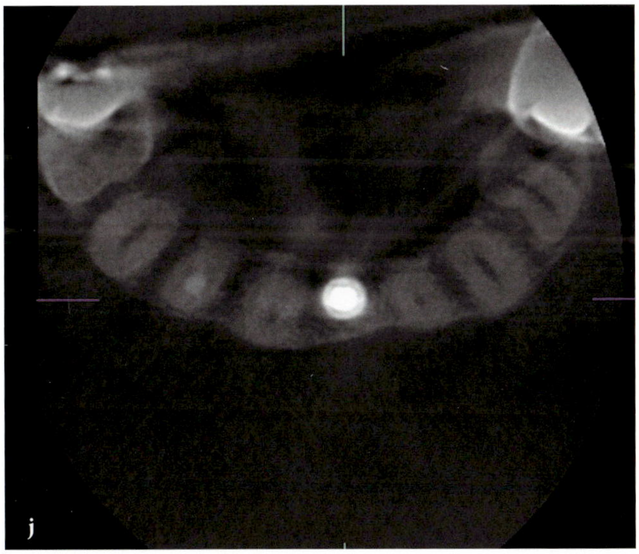
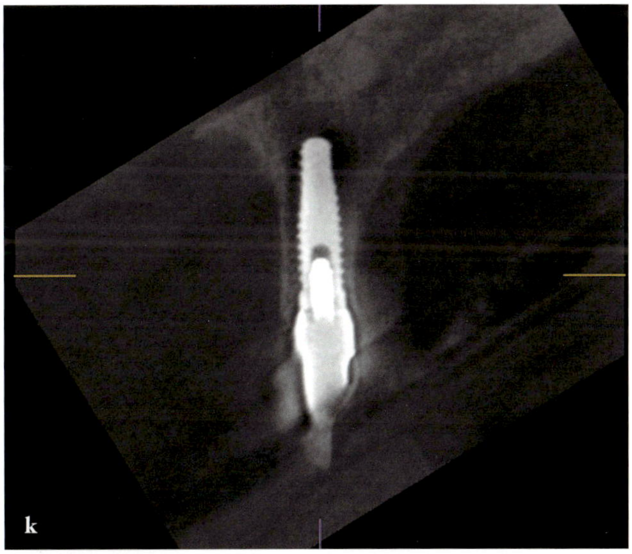

Figs 3-12j and 3-12k Computed tomographic evaluation 4 years after implant placement shows slight buccal bone resorption but maintenance of adequate thickness.

Class 2: Good results (Case 2)

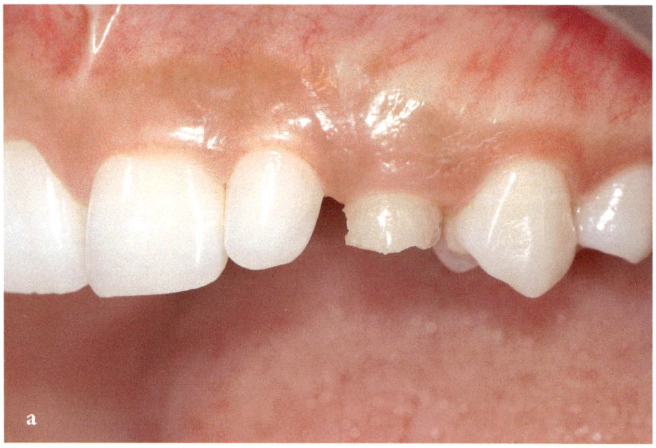

Fig 3-13a The patient presented with an unesthetic retained primary canine and a high gingival margin.

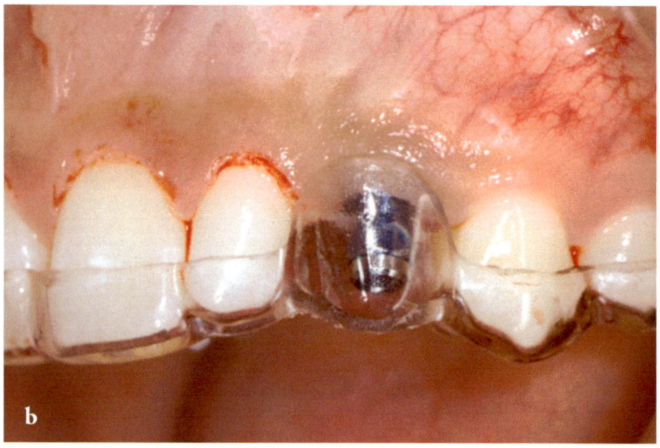

Fig 3-13b Immediate implant placement was performed without flap elevation.

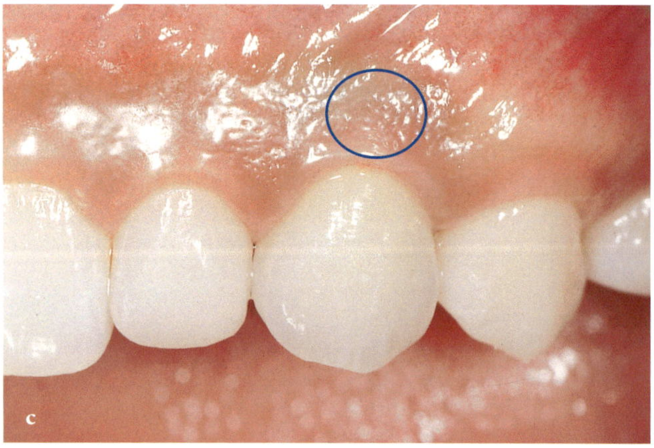

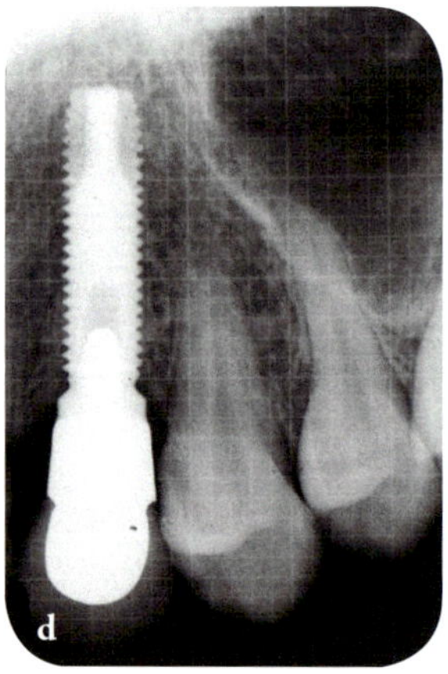

Figs 3-13c and 3-13d At the 3-year follow-up, a perforation *(blue circle)* was observed in the thin buccal soft tissue at the implant-abutment connection.

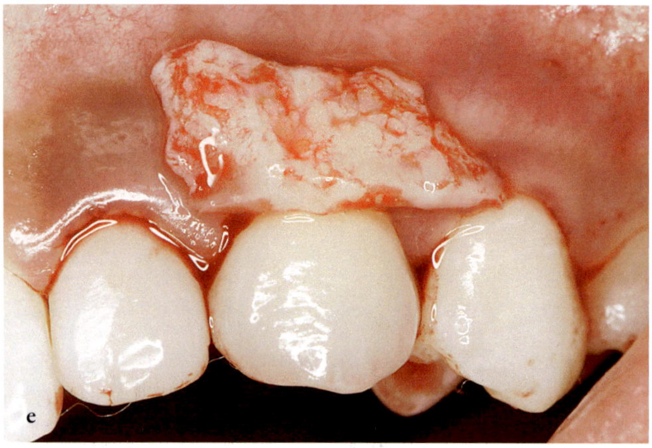

Fig 3-13e CTG was performed to augment the soft tissue thickness. This should have been done prior to the definitive restoration placement.

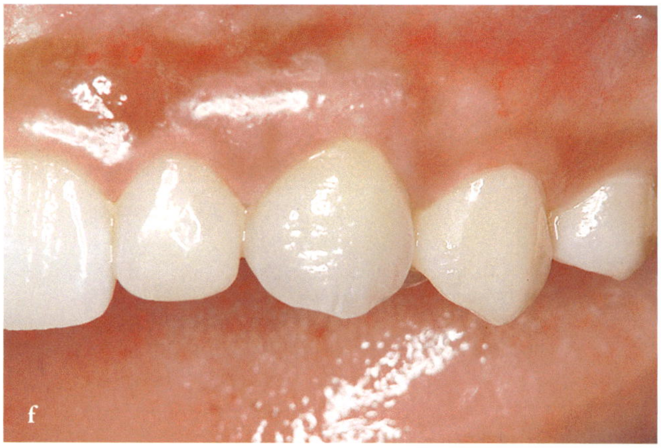

Fig 3-13f Clinical view 5 years after implant placement (2 years after CTG).

Class 3: Acceptable results

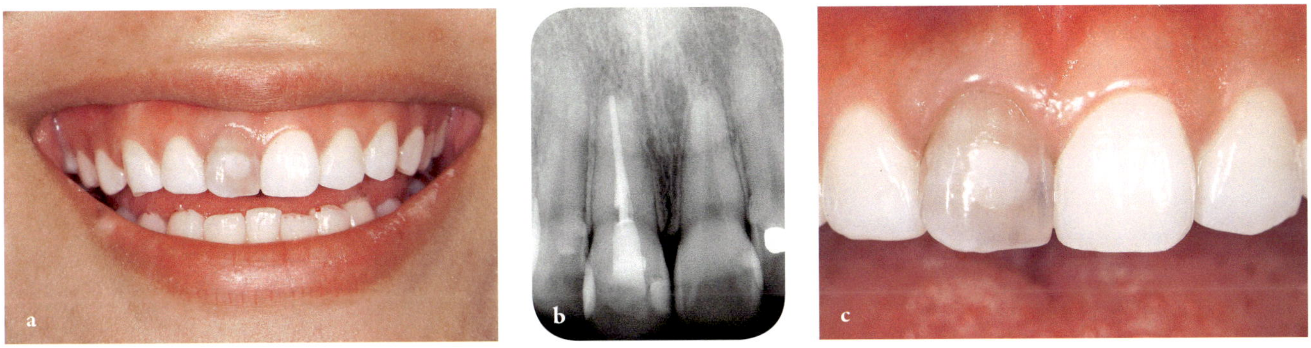

Figs 3-14a to 3-14c Facial view at initial examination. The patient presented with pain and a fractured central incisor.

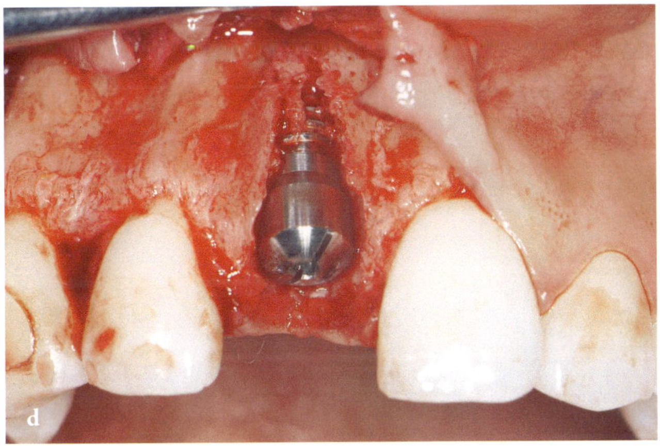

Fig 3-14d Placement of an immediate implant after orthodontic extrusion. Despite deficient buccal bone, the implant was positioned within the extraction socket.

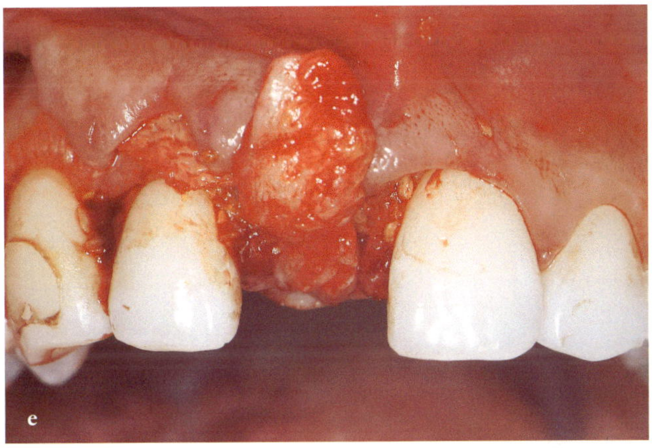

Fig 3-14e Guided bone regeneration with bone graft, resorbable membrane, and simultaneous connective tissue grafting.

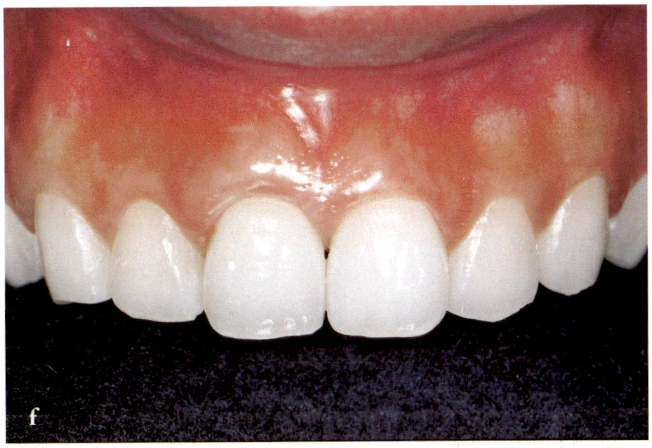

Fig 3-14f Facial view of definitive restoration. Slight loss of soft tissue volume was observed.

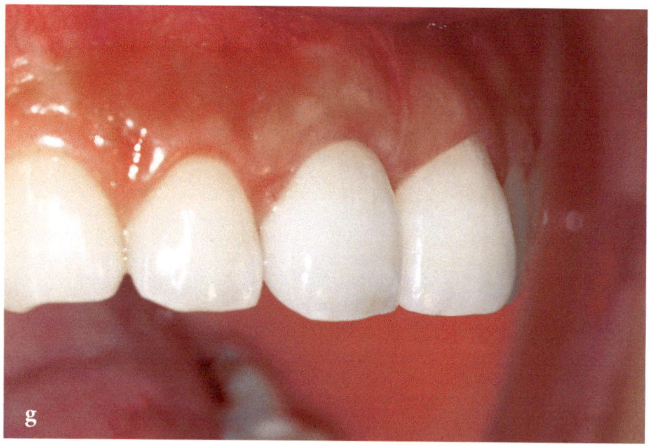
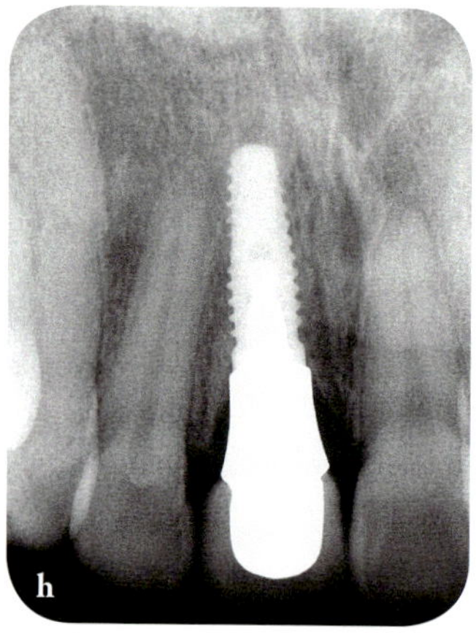

Figs 3-14g and 3-14h At the 2-year followed up, buccal tissue seems stable.

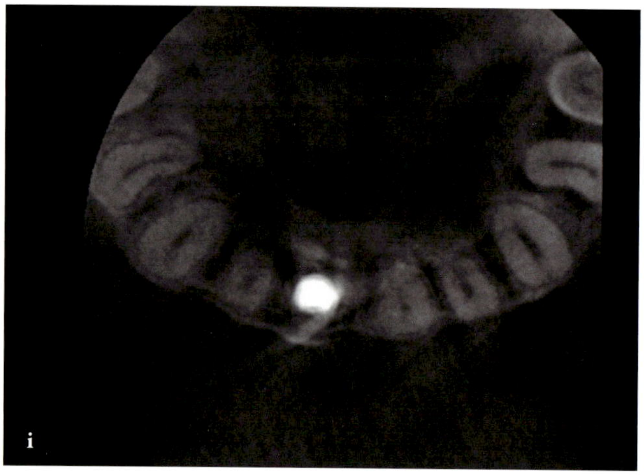
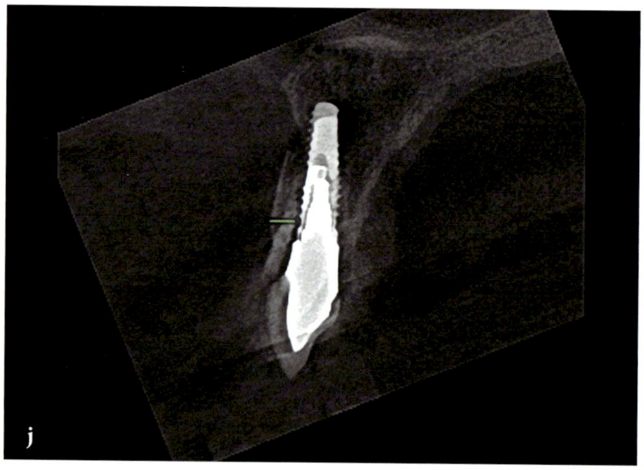

Figs 3-14i and 3-14j At the 2-year computed tomographic evaluation, buccal bone was maintained.

Class 4: Poor or unaccetable results

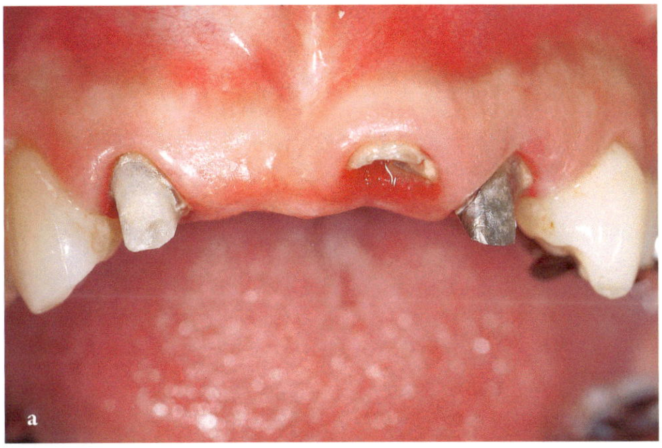
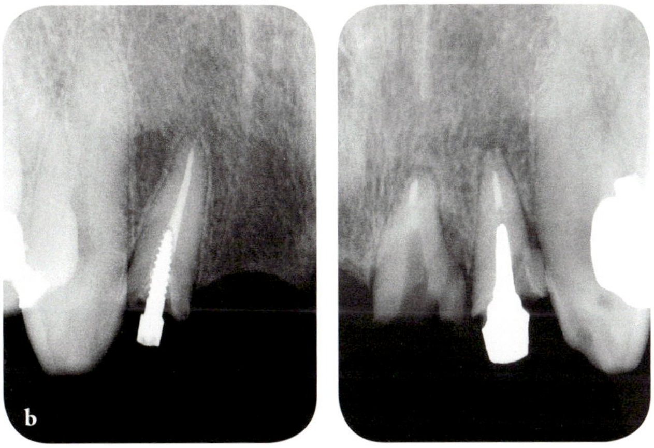

Figs 3-15a and 3-15b Facial view at initial examination. The remaining maxillary incisors are hopeless.

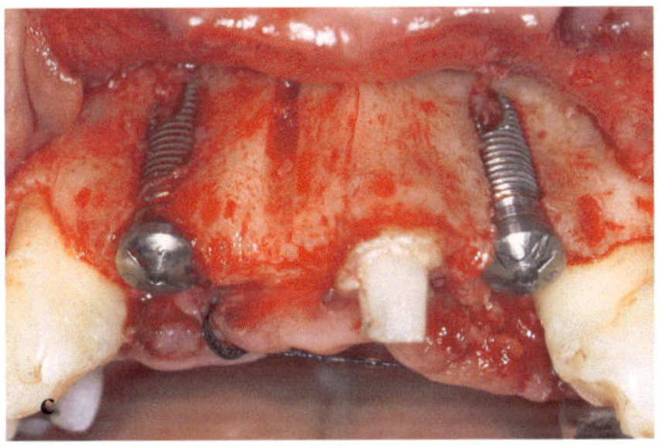
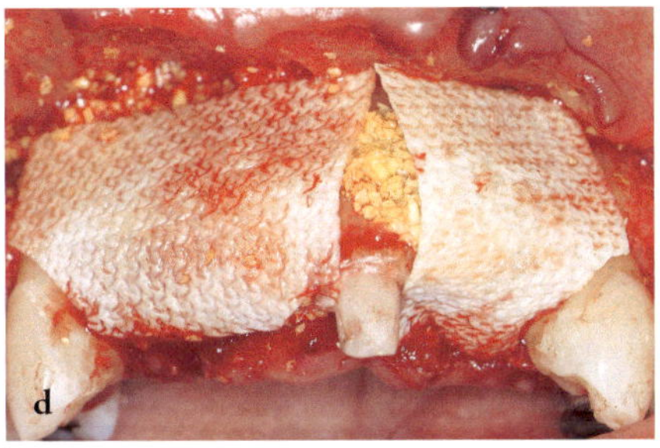

Figs 3-15c and 3-15d Facially inclined implant placement due to the existing atrophic bone anatomy.

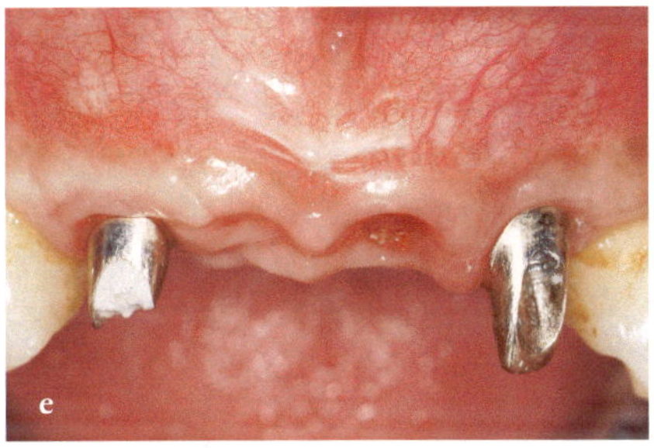

Fig 3-15e Facial view of definitive abutments.

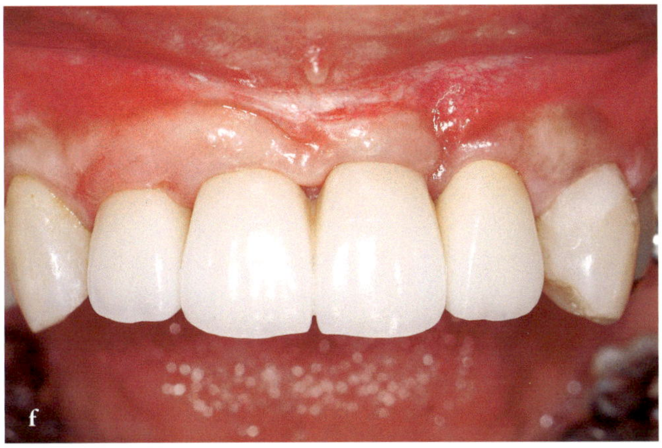
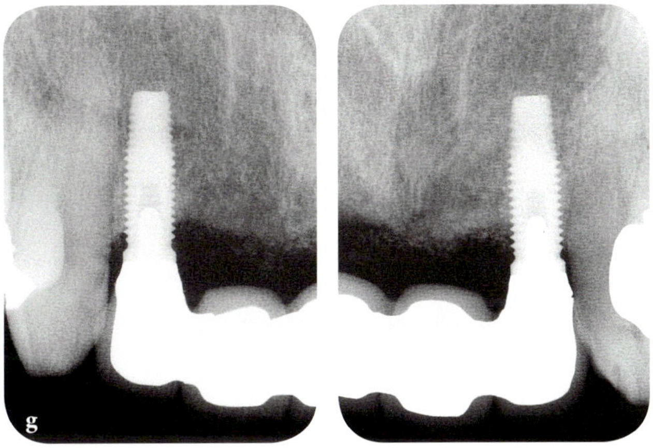

Figs 3-15f and 3-15g Facial view of definitive restorations. Uneven crown margins and inadequate soft tissue volume can be observed. Delayed implant placement is a better option for cases like this.

4D Concept in Complex Cases: Strategically Timed Serial Extractions and Immediate Implant Placement

In multiple-tooth implant cases associated with bone defects, application of the four-dimensional (4D) concept through the use of strategically timed serial extractions is exceedingly important to support a fixed provisional restoration during immediate implant placement treatment. In the case shown in Fig 3-16, there were three possible treatment options.

Option 1: Four implants in right central incisor–left canine area

The first option was to place four implants in both central incisor and the left lateral incisor and canine sites. With this option, the definitive restorations would be individual crowns, which is an advantage in terms of accessibility for hygiene. However, there are also many disadvantages. Mesiodistal positioning and depth control of the implant platform would be highly technique sensitive. Papilla height between adjoining implants would likely diminish, and the definitive restorations would require long contact points. Facial guided bone regeneration (GBR) may be necessary. Definitive restorations would not resemble natural dentition nor blend with the remaining dentition. In addition, treatment cost increases with the number of implants placed.

Option 2: Three implants in right central incisor–left canine area

The second option was to place three implants, either in the right central incisor and left lateral incisor and canine sites or in both central incisor sites and the left canine site. This may appear to be a realistic option; however, it is difficult to maintain a 3-mm distance between adjoining implants and therefore to create an adequate papilla height between them.

Option 3: Three implants in right lateral incisor–left canine area

The third option is to place three implants in the right lateral incisor and the left central incisor and canine sites. This patient's right lateral incisor is nonvital and requires a new restoration. If the tooth is strategically extracted and replaced by an implant, two pontics can be placed alternately with the three implants, thereby avoiding adjoining implants. The papilla height between implant and pontic is expected to be greater than that between adjoining implants. If the right lateral incisor were a vital tooth, this option would not be considered.

Decision

In this case, option 3 was selected with the patient's consent. Treatment was sequenced with strategically staged immediate implant placement. The provisional restoration was supported by remaining teeth while others were extracted and replaced using immediate implant placement. Once the implants were integrated, the teeth that supported the initial provisional restoration were extracted. Those sites were either replaced using immediate implant placement or preserved for a future pontic site. Following is the basic treatment sequence (see Fig 3-16):

1. After orthodontic extrusion, immediate implant placement was performed in the right lateral incisor and left central incisor sites.
2. A buccal flap was elevated, and the gap between the extraction socket and the implant was filled with bone graft material. The buccal flap was then advanced coronally. The right lateral incisor site was Class 1; the left central incisor site was Class 2.
3. Definitive abutments were connected to the implants 4 months later. At this time, orthodontic extrusion of the right central incisor and the left canine was initiated.
4. The right central incisor was extracted, and the socket was preserved with an ovate pontic and bone graft material.
5. The left canine was diagnosed as Class 3; therefore, GBR and connective tissue grafting (CTG) were done simultaneously with immediate implant placement.
6. To augment buccal soft tissue thickness, CTG was performed in the right canine and left central incisor to canine areas.
7. For the left canine, tissue sculpting with a provisional restoration was initiated 3 months after implant placement.
8. A final impression was taken with a custom impression coping, and then a definitive gold UCLA abutment was fabricated for the left canine.

Application of the 4D concept in a complex case: Strategically timed serial extractions and immediate implant placement

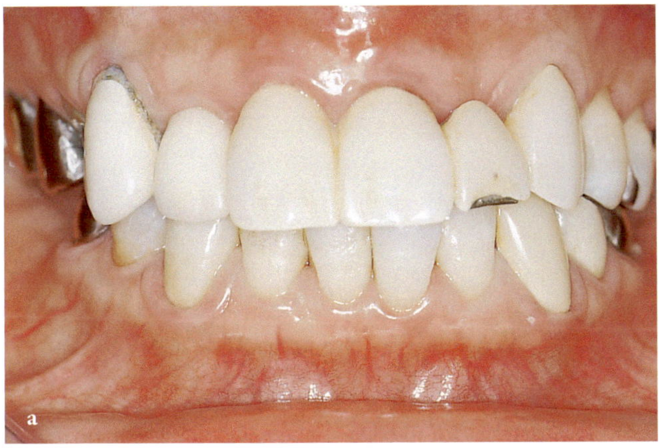

Fig 3-16a Facial view at initial examination. A thin periodontal biotype was observed.

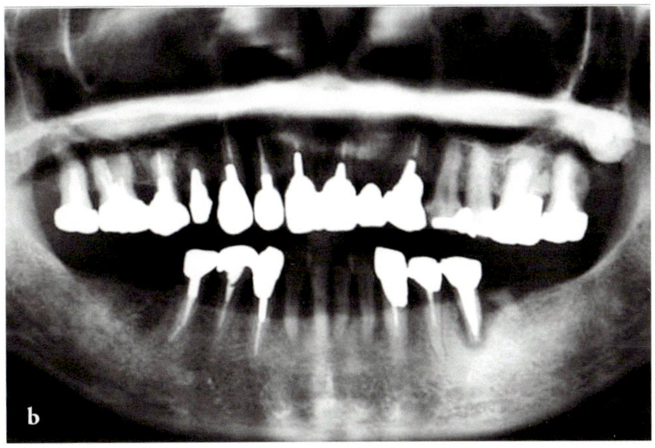

Fig 3-16b Panoramic radiograph at initial examination. The first step was to restore function and posterior support with implant treatment in the posterior mandible.

Fig 3-16c Periapical radiographs of the maxilla at the initial exam. The left canine had deep subgingival decay. Mobility of the bridge was noted. The left central incisor had internal decay.

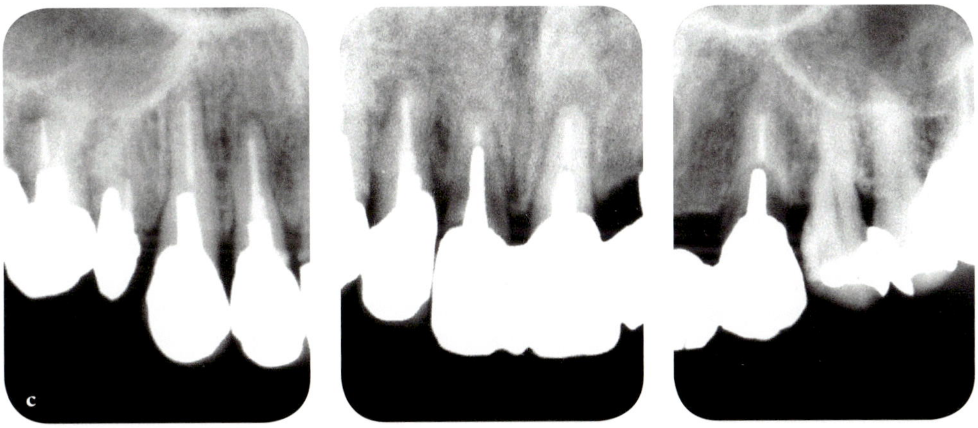

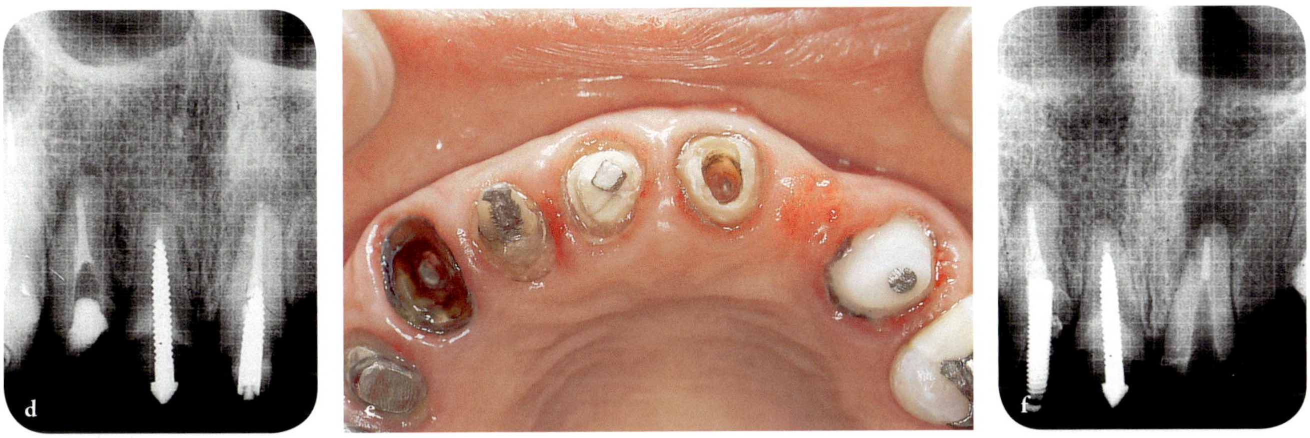

Figs 3-16d to 3-16f Periapical radiographs *(d and f)* and occlusal view *(e)* after removal of the existing restorations. Resin core buildup was performed on the left canine to support the provisional restoration. The right central incisor presented with a fracture, and the left central incisor presented with a perforation. Both were diagnosed as hopeless.

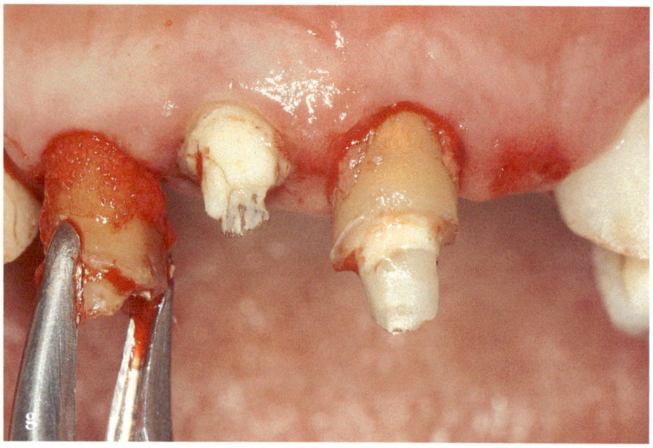

Fig 3-16g Situation following orthodontic extrusion of the right lateral incisor and left central incisor, during which a fixed provisional restoration was placed in the area from the right canine to the left canine.

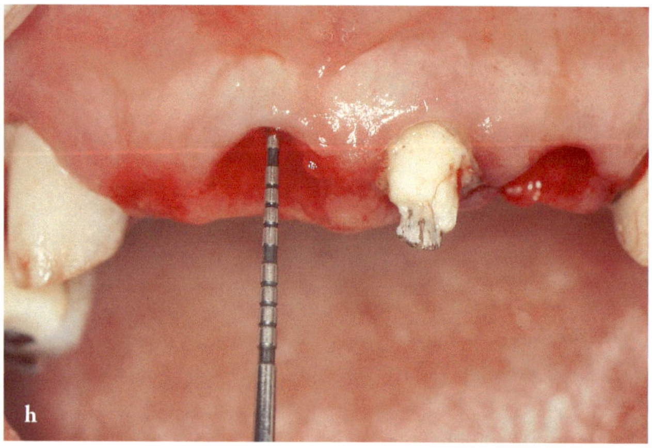

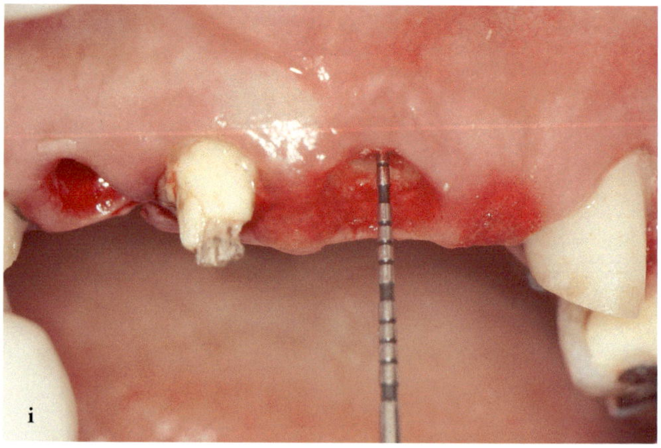

Figs 3-16h and 3-16i The right lateral incisor and left central incisor have been extracted and the buccal bone level confirmed in each site.

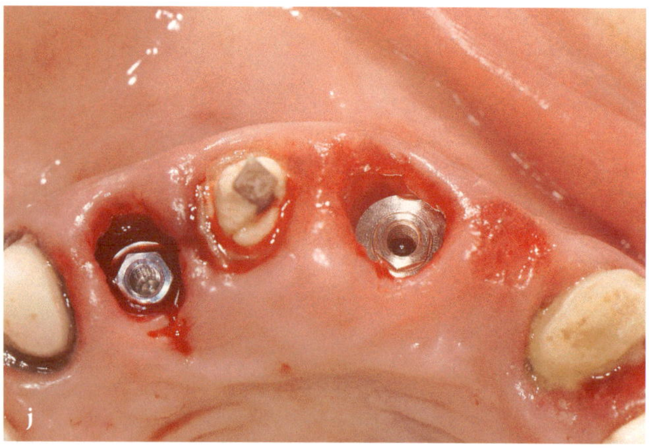

Fig 3-16j Occlusal view of implant placement. A gap between the implants and the buccal bone was maintained.

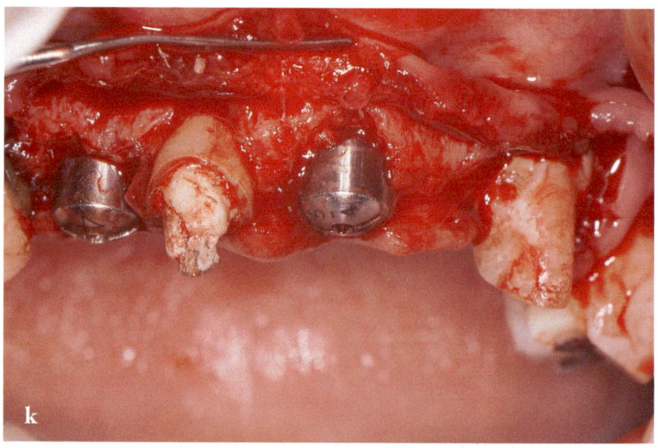

Fig 3-16k A flap was elevated, and buccal bone thickness was determined to be adequate at the right lateral incisor and thin at the left central incisor.

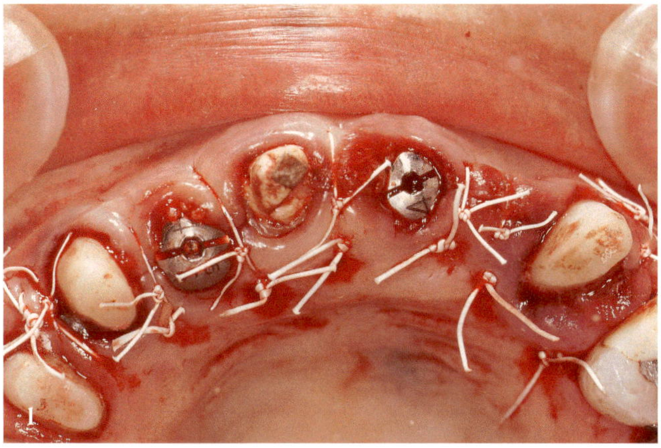

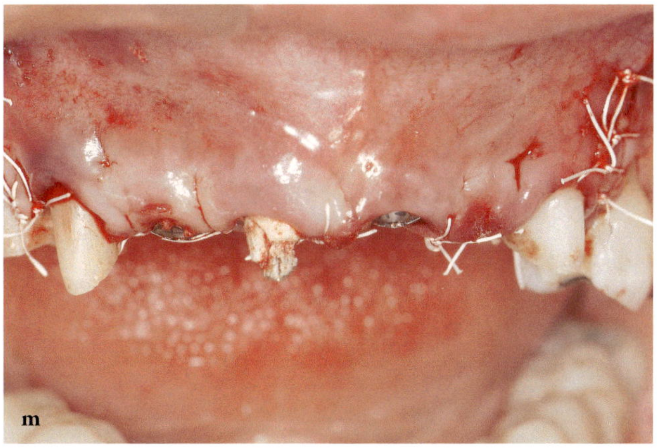

Figs 3-16l and 3-16m The gap between the implant and the buccal bone was grafted with bone at each site and then the buccal flap was coronally advanced and sutured.

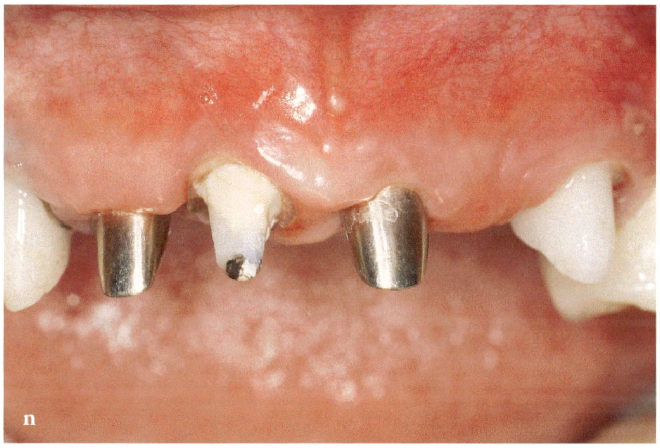

Fig 3-16n Definitive abutments were placed 4 months after implant placement.

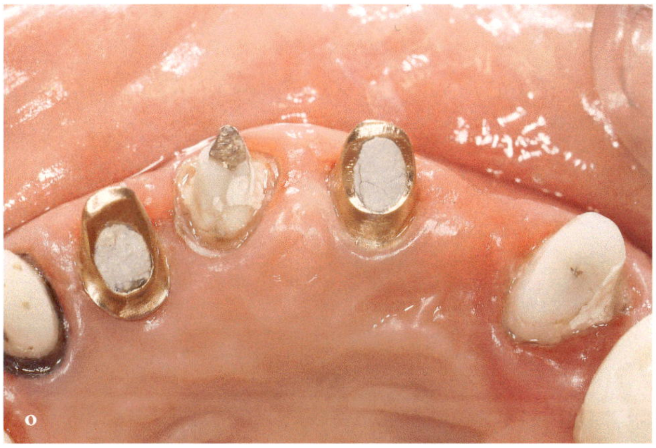

Fig 3-16o Occlusal view of abutments. The access holes of the abutments confirmed ideal implant positioning.

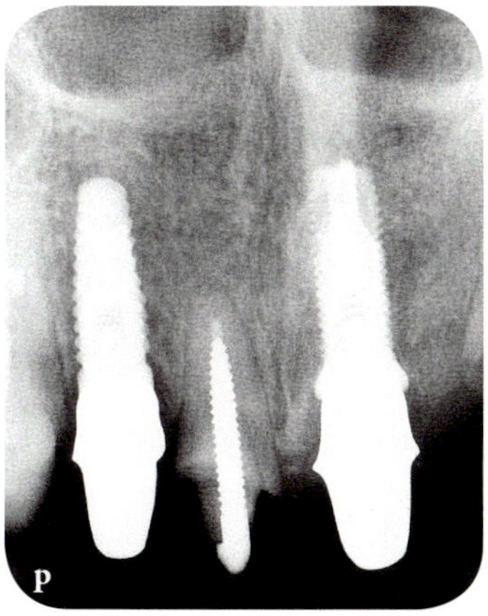

Fig 3-16p Periapical radiograph following placement of definitive abutments.

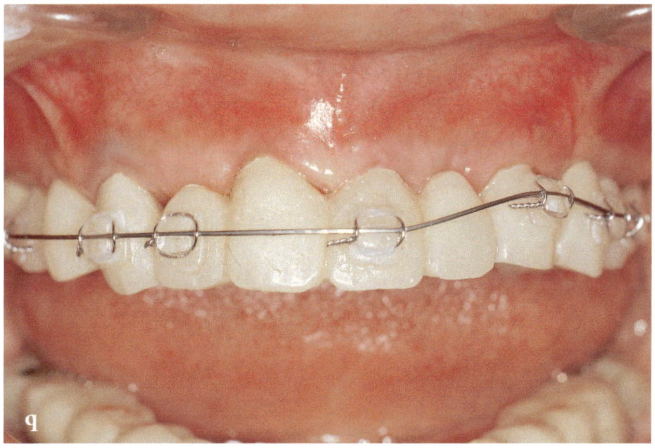

Fig 3-16q Orthodontic extrusion of the right central incisor and the left canine was performed.

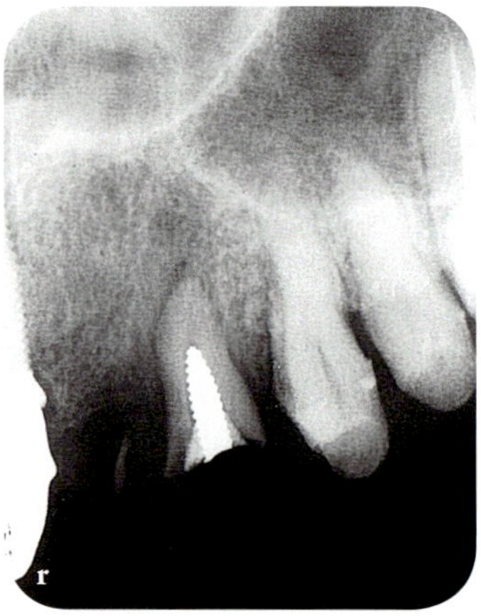

Fig 3-16r Periapical radiograph after 3 months of orthodontic extrusion.

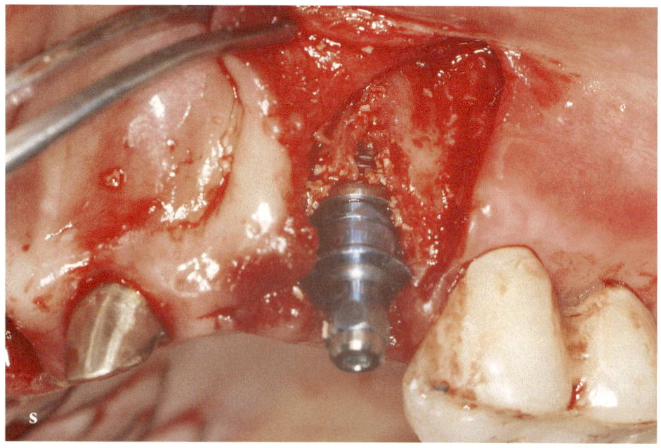

Fig 3-16s Immediate implant placement and simultaneous guided bone regeneration in the left canine site.

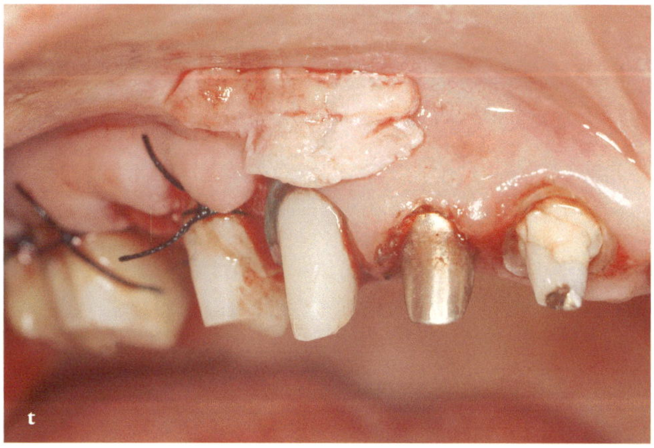

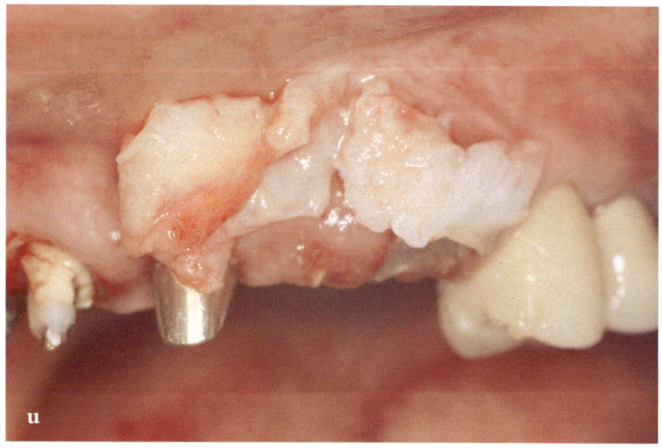

Figs 3-16t and 3-16u A connective tissue graft was harvested during periodontal surgery and placed at the right canine and the left central incisor to canine areas.

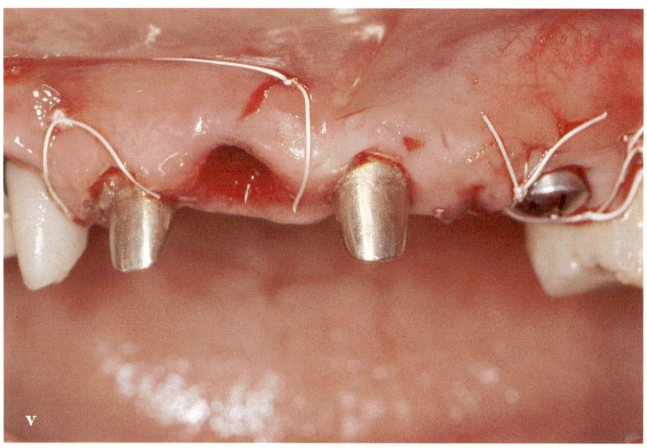

Fig 3-16v Clinical situation immediately following extraction of the right central incisor and CTG.

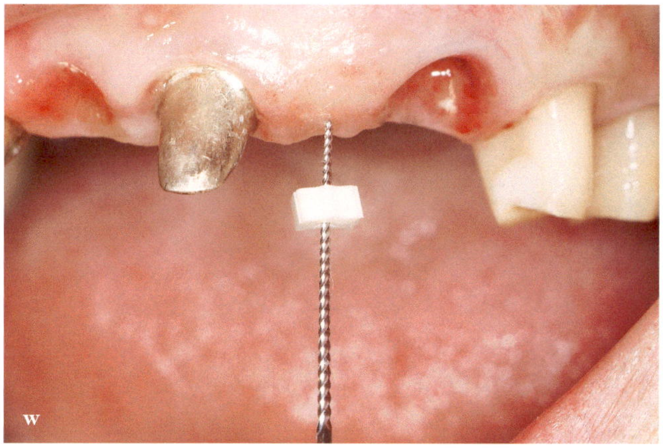

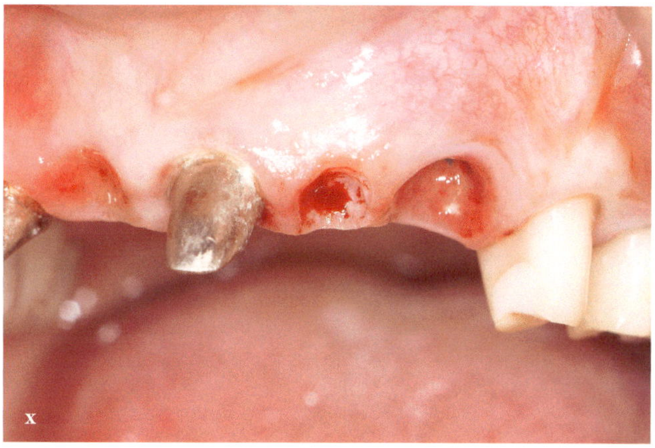

Figs 3-16w and 3-16x Gingivoplasty is performed on the left lateral incisor site to create an ovate pontic site. The results of tissue sculpting with a provisional restoration, which was initiated 3 months after implant placement, can be observed at the left canine site.

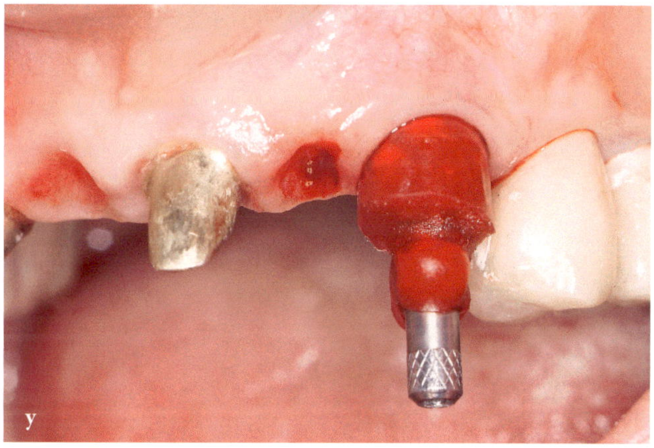

Fig 3-16y Final impression with a custom impression coping on the left canine.

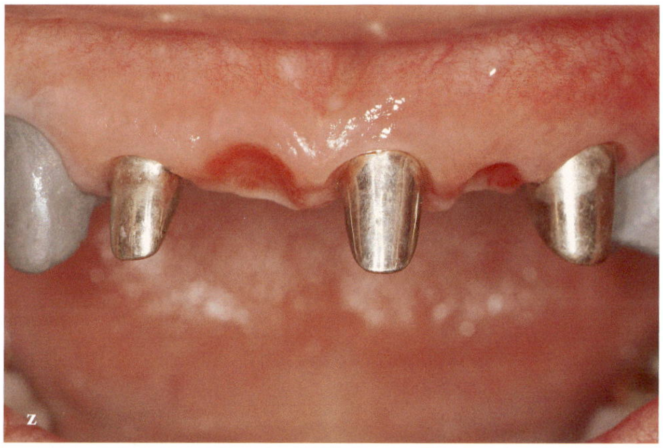

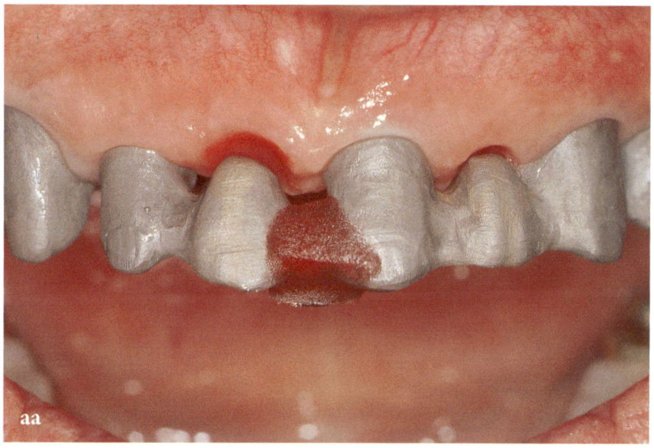

Figs 3-16z and 3-16aa Metal framework try-in.

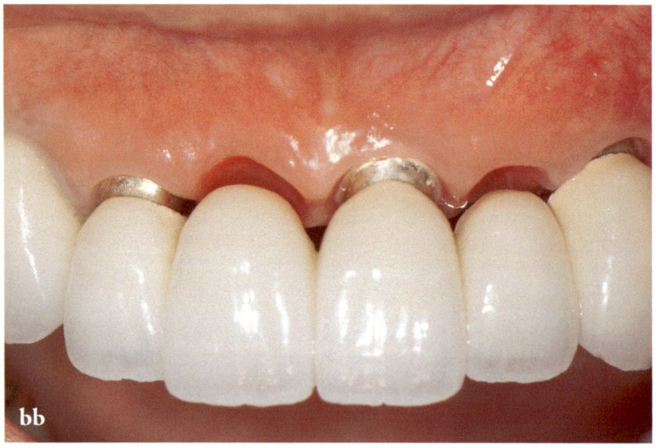

Fig 3-16bb Facial view of definitive restorations being placed.

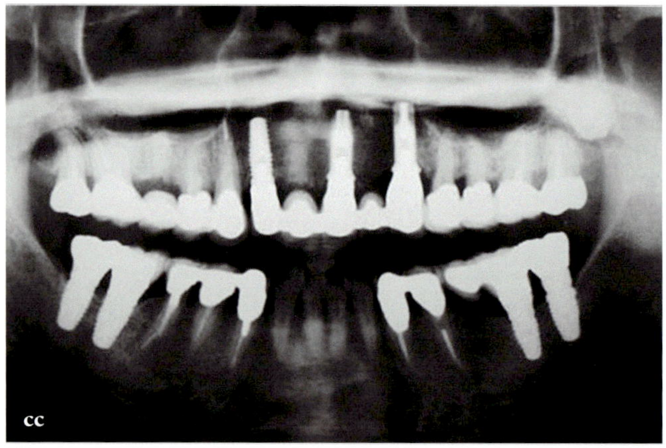

Fig 3-16cc Panoramic radiograph with definitive restorations in place.

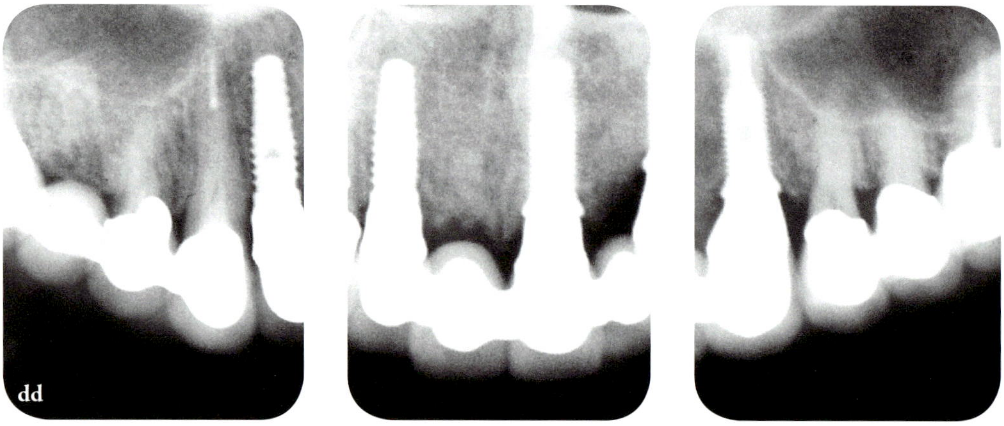

Fig 3-16dd Periapical radiographs of definitive restorations.

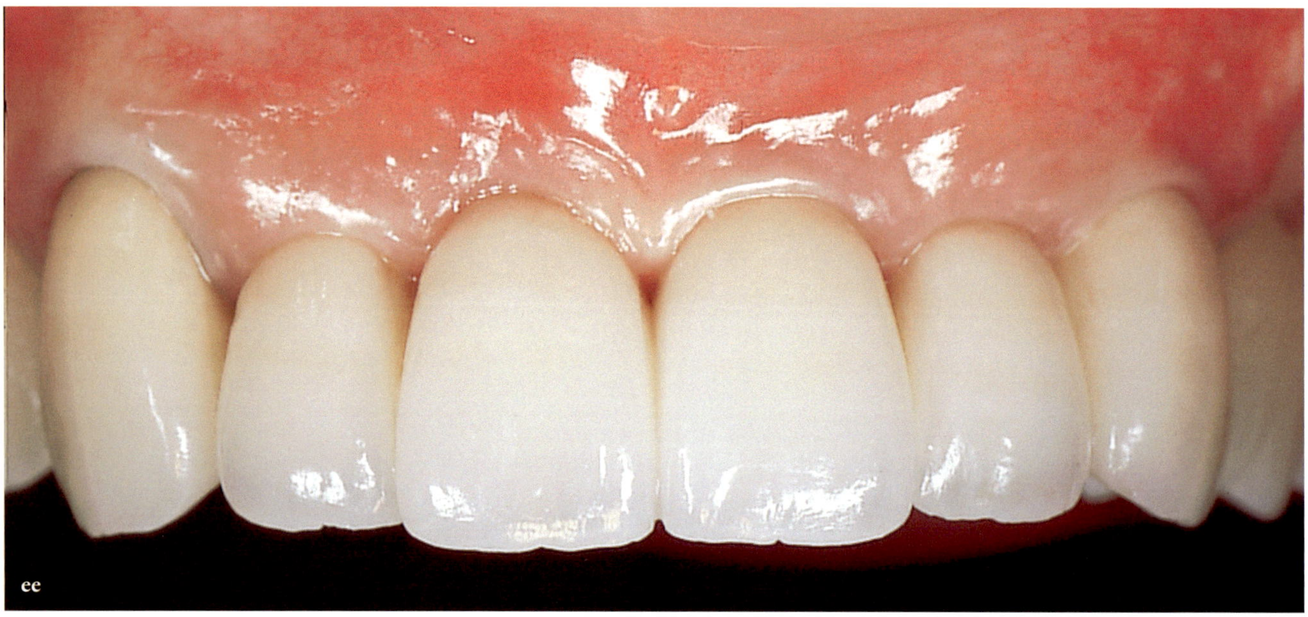

Fig 3-16ee Clinical view of definitive restorations.

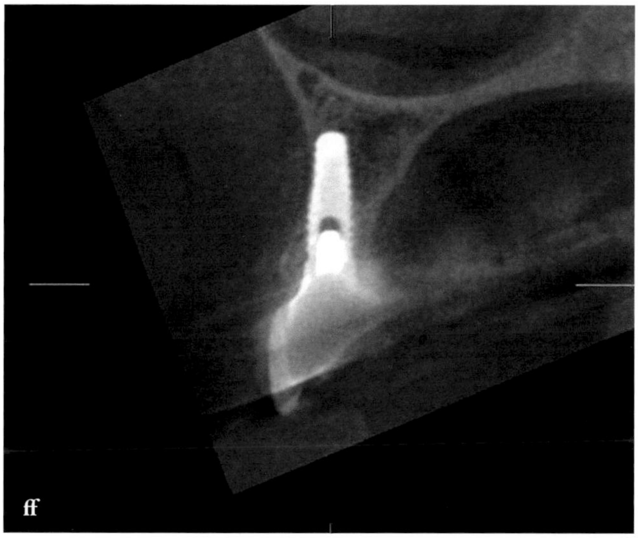

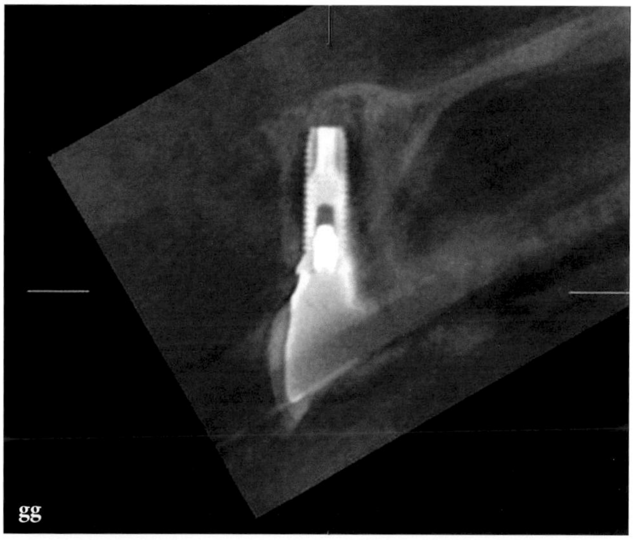

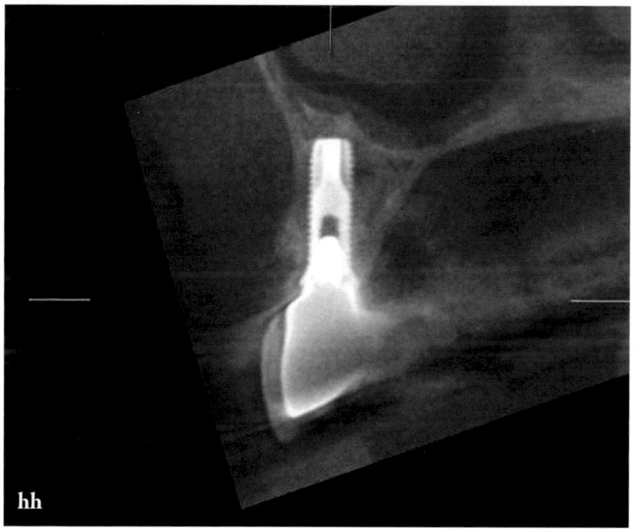

Figs 3-16ff to 3-16hh The 2-year computed tomographic evaluation shows maintenance of adequate buccal bone following immediate implant placement in the right lateral incisor *(ff)*, left central incisor *(gg)*, and left canine *(hh)* sites.

A Final Word of Caution

The importance of taking proper care in the evaluation and planning stages of extraction and immediate implant treatment cannot be overemphasized (Figs 3-17 and 3-18). The treatment plan must compensate for the inevitable buccal bone resorption that follows extraction—whether through orthodontic extrusion or GBR or both—even if the buccal bone is intact (Fig 3-19).

Learning from failure: Facial gingival recession

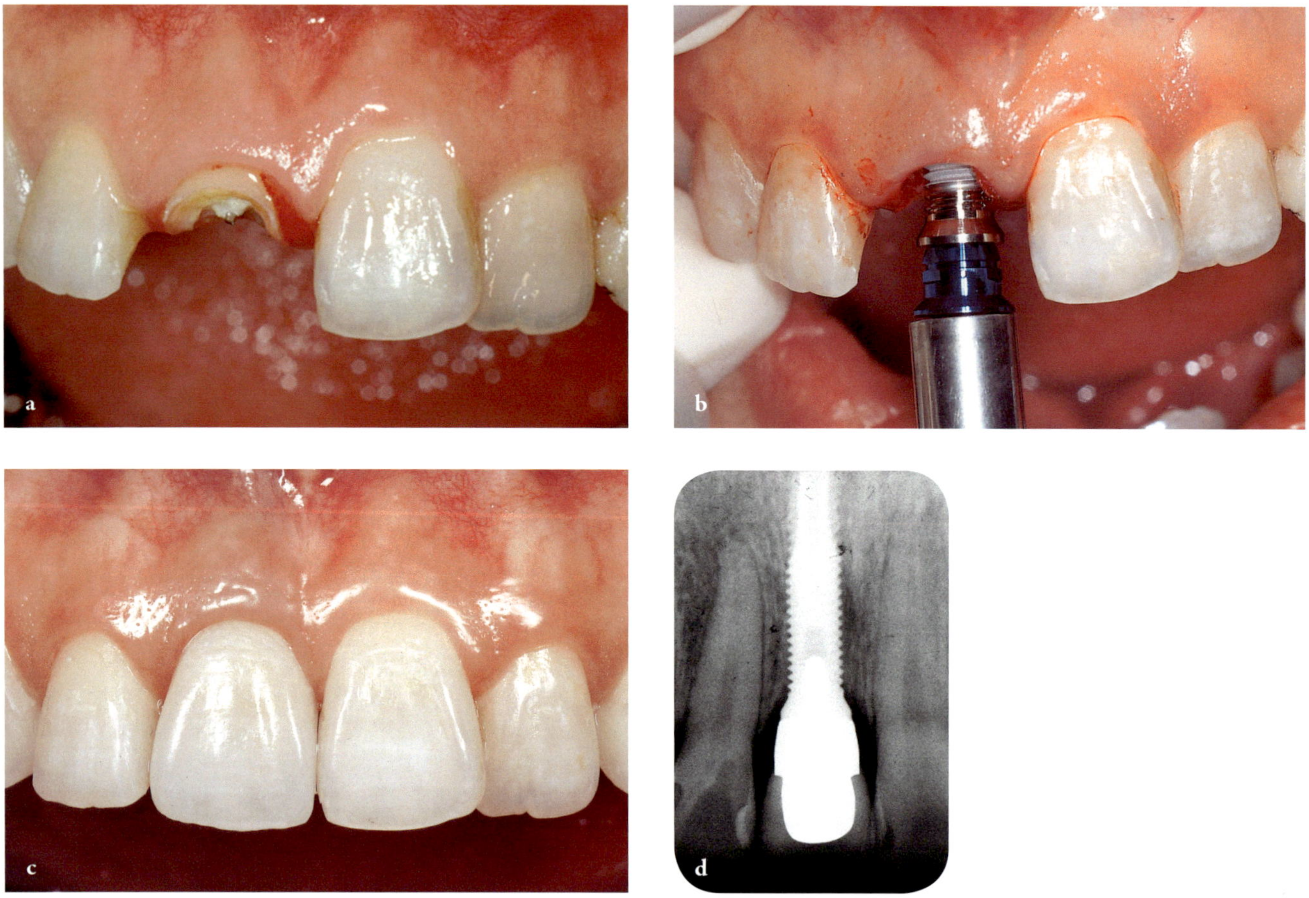

Figs 3-17a to 3-17d The right central incisor was diagnosed as hopeless due to the deep subgingival fracture in the palatal aspect. Following orthodontic extrusion, the implant was placed into the extraction socket immediately without flap elevation. An esthetic final result was achieved. This was the author's (AF) first immediate implant case.

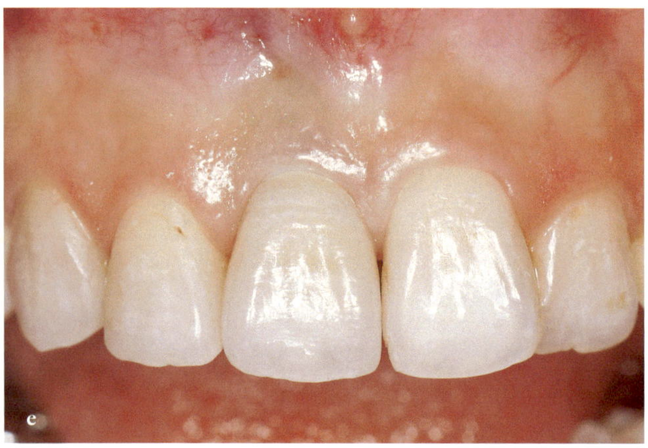

Fig 3-17e Lack of experience and a failure to understand immediate implant indications and appropriate treatment planning and sequencing led to facial gingival recession. Today, a tapered implant used with the platform switching technique would be selected in this case.

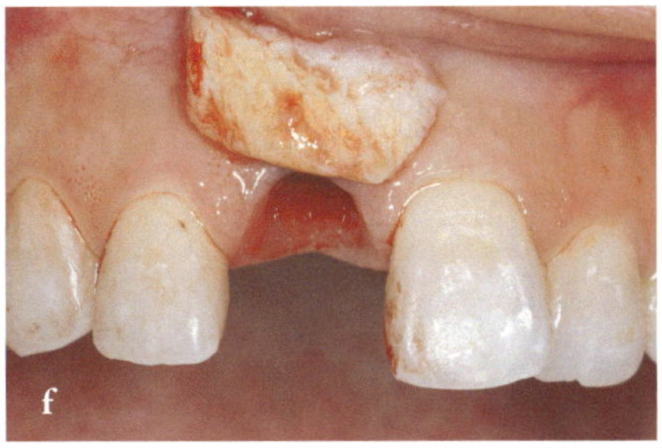

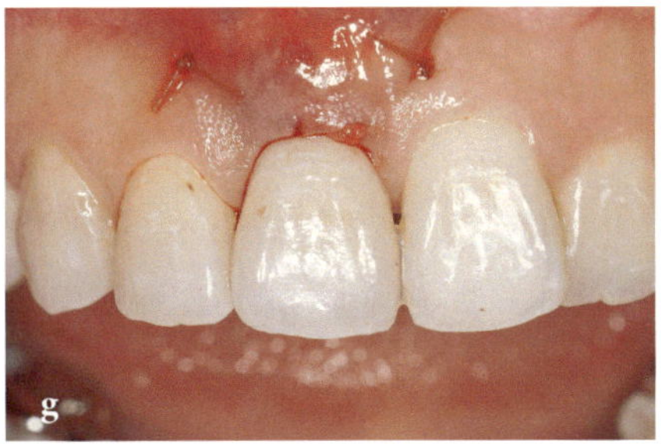

Figs 3-17f and 3-17g CTG was performed to correct the gingival recession.

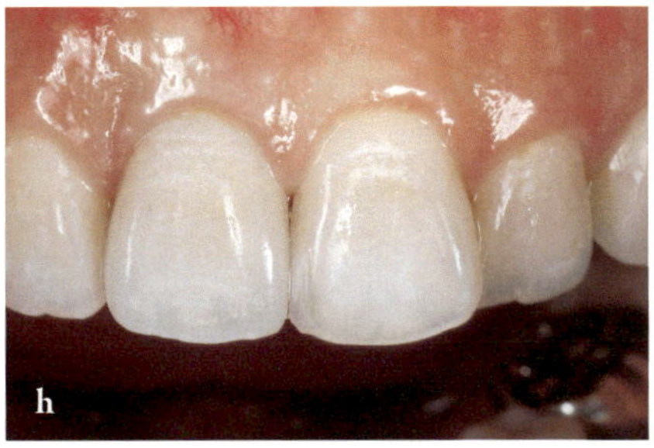

Fig 3-17h Clinical view at the 2.5-year follow-up (1 year after CTG).

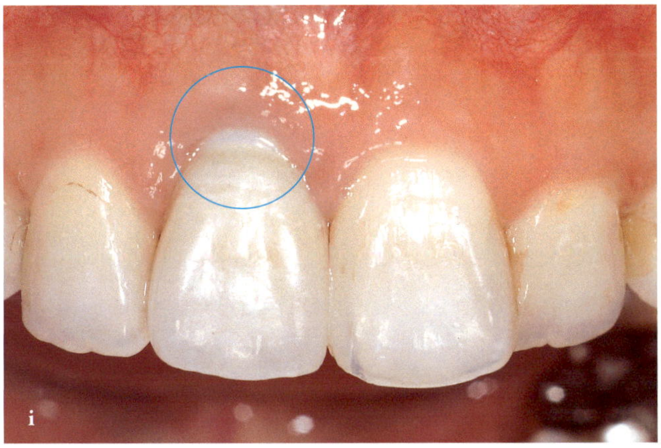

Fig 3-17i Gingival recession *(blue circle)* was once again observed 5 years later; however, the patient was pleased that the discoloration of the gingiva was corrected after CTG.

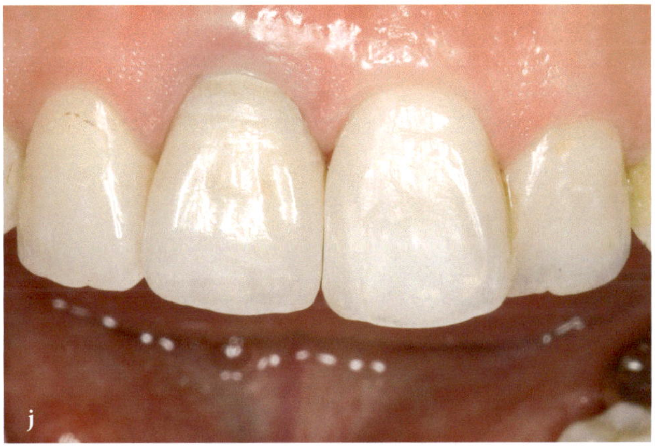

Fig 3-17j CTG was performed 1 year later.

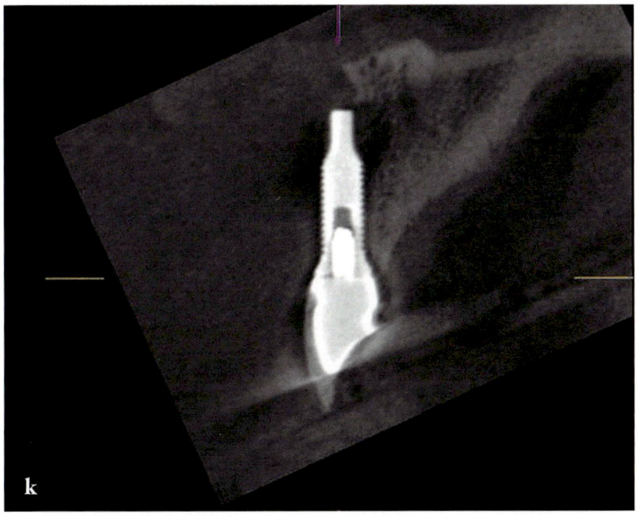

Fig 3-17k The 7-year computed tomographic evaluation reveals that the buccal bone is completely missing. Clinicians must understand the indications for immediate implant placement and principles for ideal implant positioning to avoid this situation.

☞ Clinical tips

- Use orthodontic extrusion whenever possible
- In principle, immediate implant placement. should only be performed in a four-wall socket.
- Anticipate that most four-wall sockets will be Class 2, ie, consider CTG with immediate implant placement.
- The implant must engage the palatal wall of the extraction socket; however, the platform should not be positioned too palatally.
- Avoid wide-diameter or flare-shaped implants.
- When in doubt, socket preservation or GBR should be considered.
- Do not rush!

Learning from failure: Deficient buccal tissue

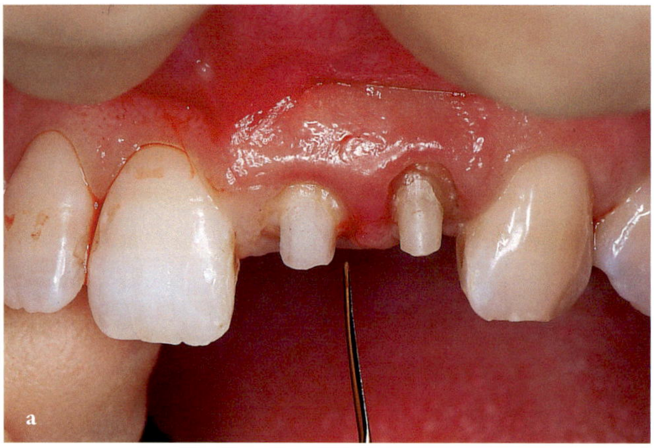
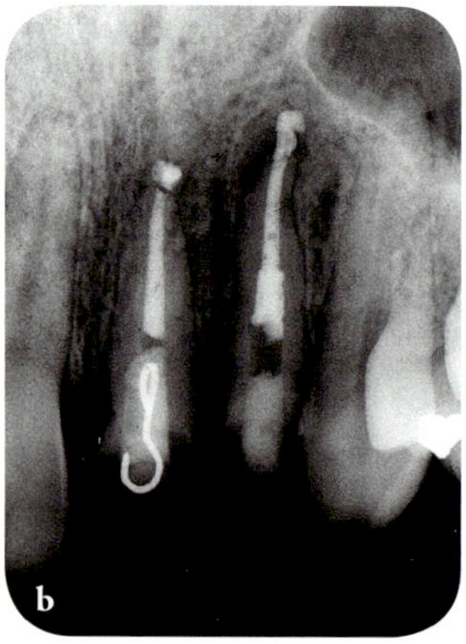

Figs 3-18a and 3-18b Extraction of the left central incisor of a 35-year-old woman was planned because of perforation. The tooth was extruded 3 mm and retained for 3 months prior to the extraction.

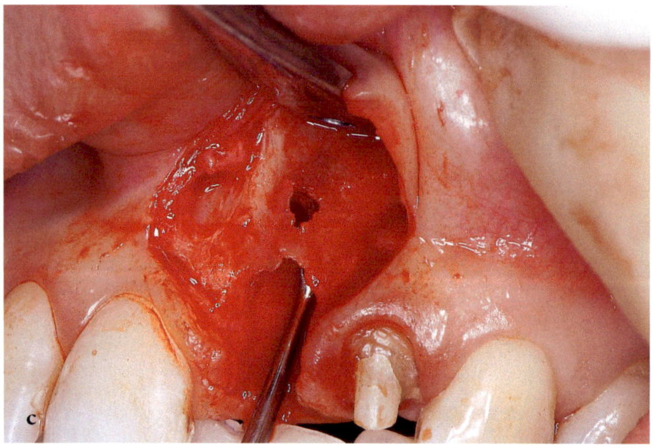

Fig 3-18c A small buccal flap was elevated after confirming a buccal bone defect.

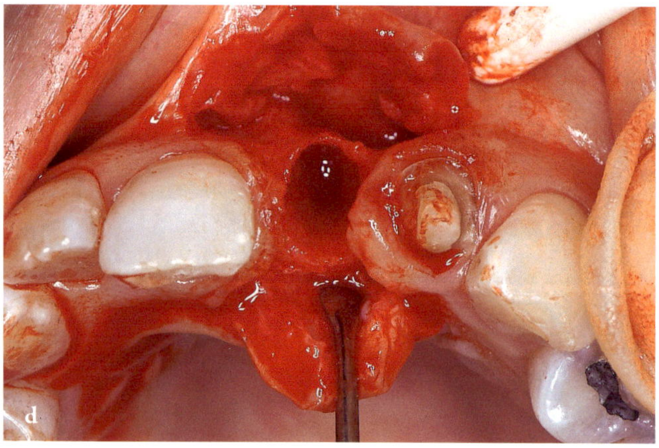

Fig 3-18d Occlusal view revealed thin buccal bone.

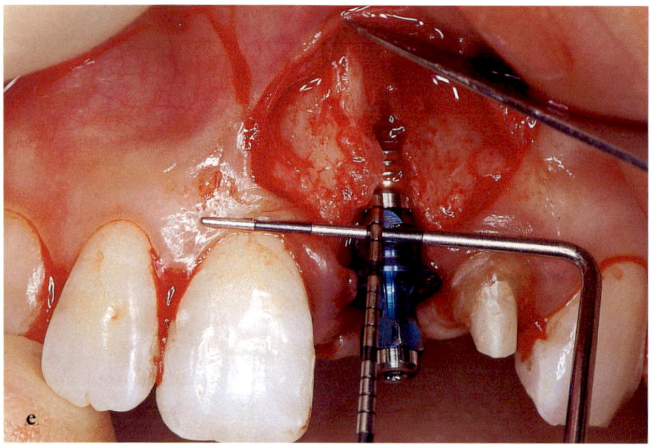
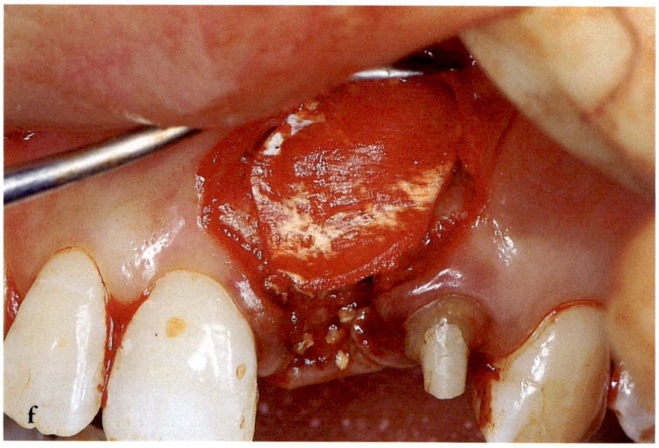

Figs 3-18e and 3-18f Xenograft was placed inside the extraction socket, then covered with a collagen membrane.

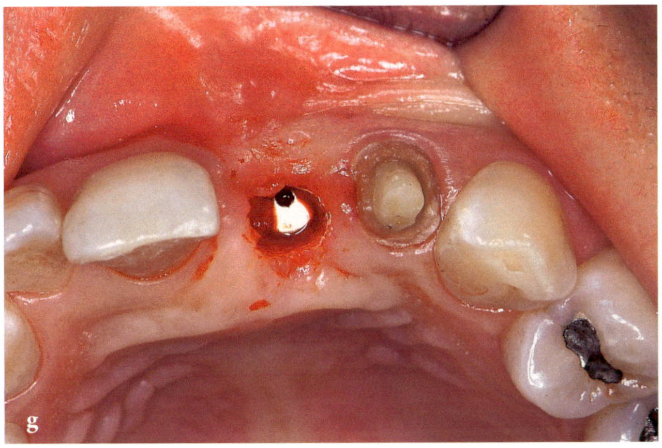

Fig 3-18g Stage-two surgery was performed with a tissue punch technique. The buccal tissue volume was deficient.

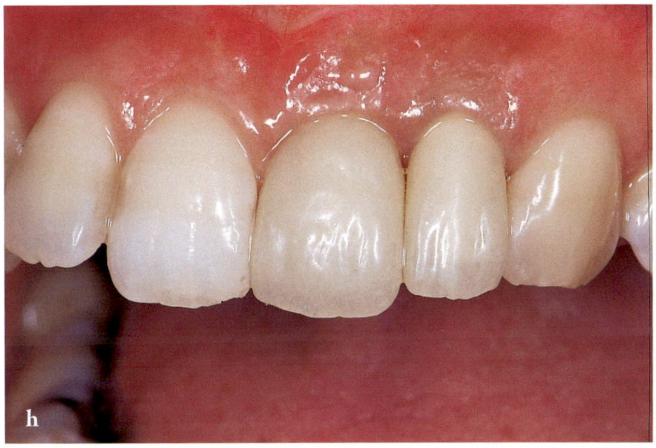

Fig 3-18h Clinical view at 6 months with provisional restorations in place.

Fig 3-18i A platform was positioned 3 mm apical of the free gingival margin.

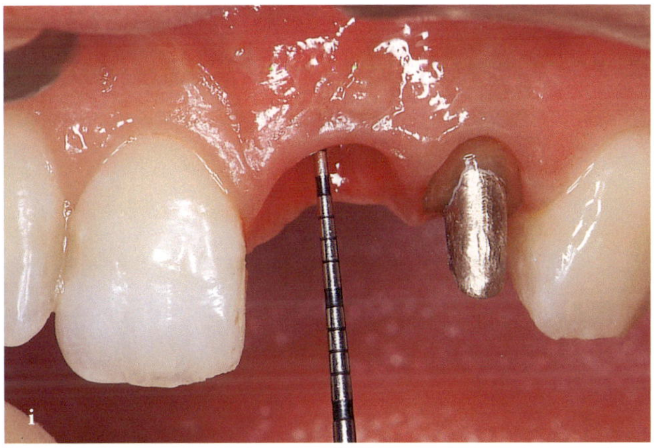

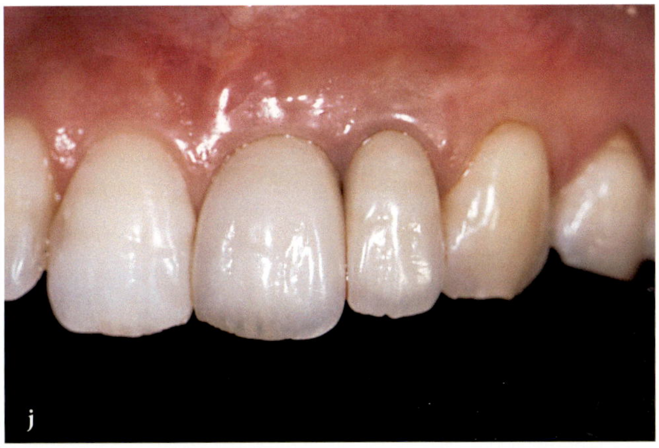

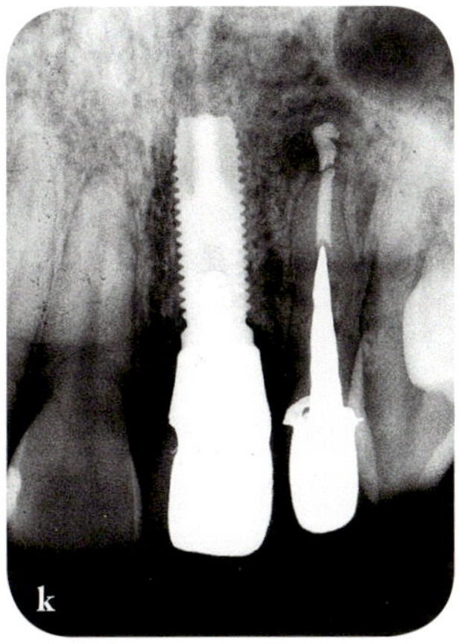

Figs 3-18j and 3-18k A definitive restoration was placed about 1 year after implant placement.

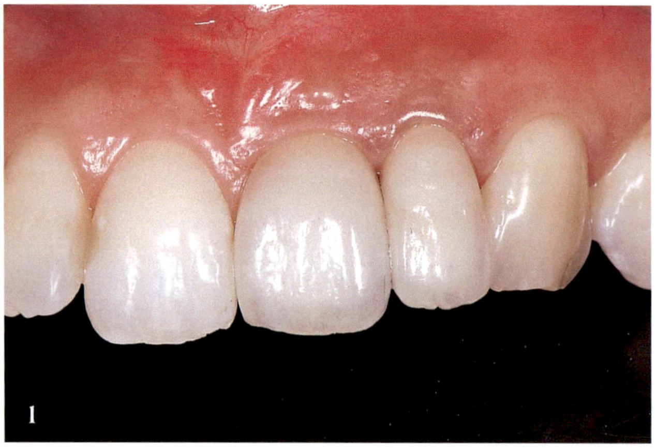

Fig 3-18l Clinical view at the 3-year follow-up. The distal papilla was regenerated.

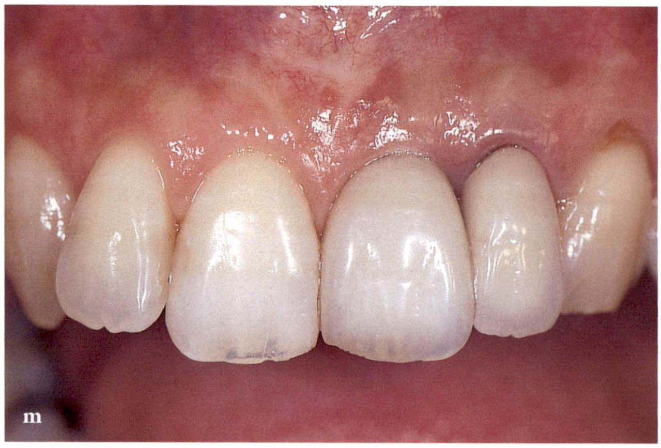

Fig 3-18m Clinical view at the 5-year follow-up. Gingival recession was observed at the left central and lateral incisors.

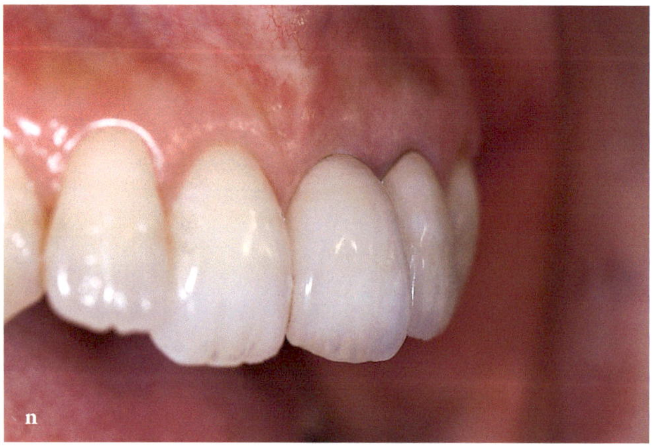

Fig 3-18n Buccal tissue volume is deficient.

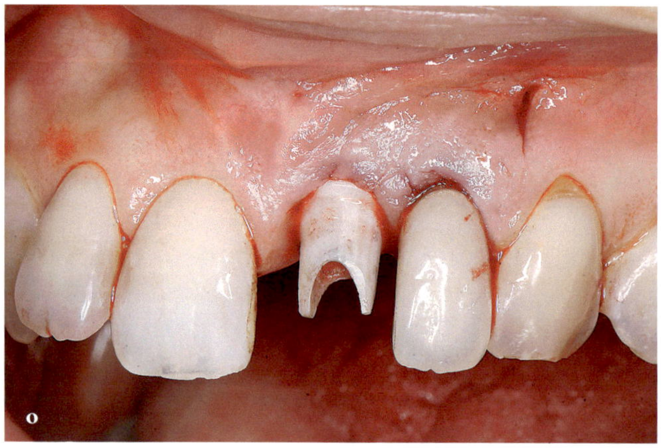

Fig 3-18o The CTG recipient site was prepared with a lateral envelope technique from distal of the left lateral incisor to preserve the papilla between the left central and lateral incisors.

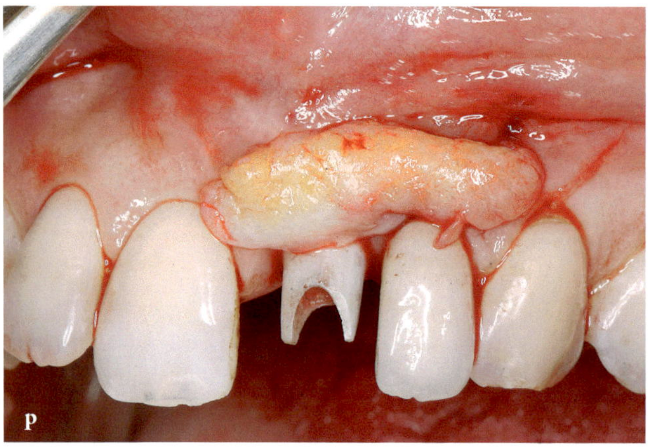

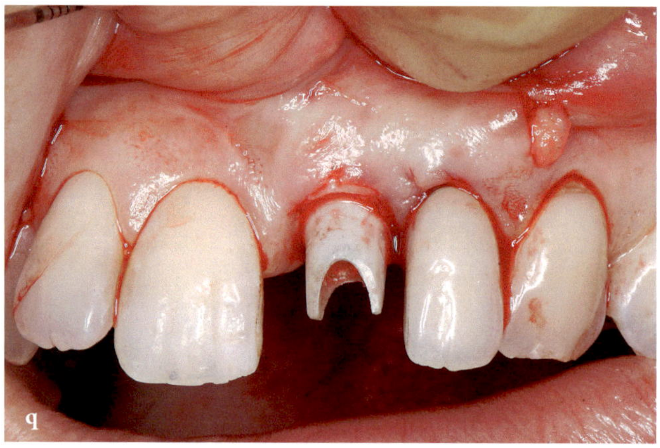

Figs 3-18p and 3-18q The CTG was harvested from the palate and placed into the recipient site.

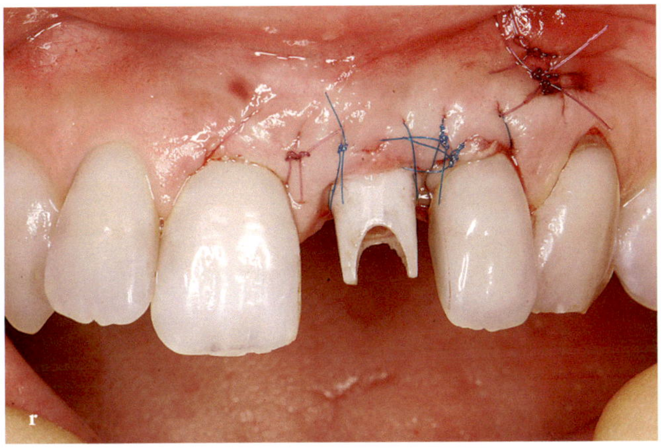

Fig 3-18r The CTG was stabilized with a suspension suture.

☞ Clinical tips

The GBR protocol used in this case was not adequate for a patient with a thin periodontal biotype and missing buccal bone. This may be the reason for the gingival recession within 5 years. The lateral envelope technique allows the clinician to preserve interproximal tissue and is effective in correcting soft tissue problems after definitive restorations are in place.

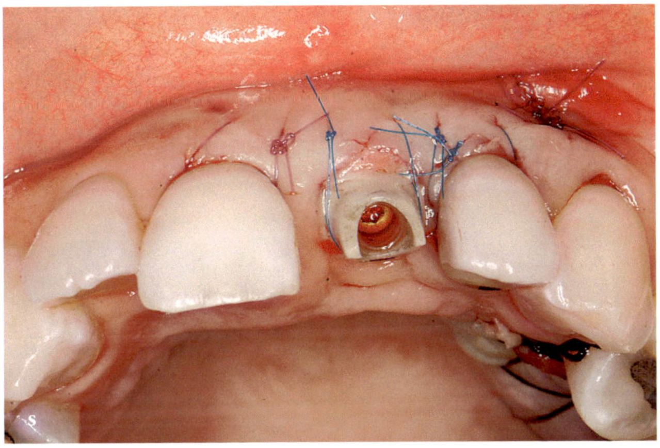

Fig 3-18s From the occlusal, increased buccal tissue volume was observed.

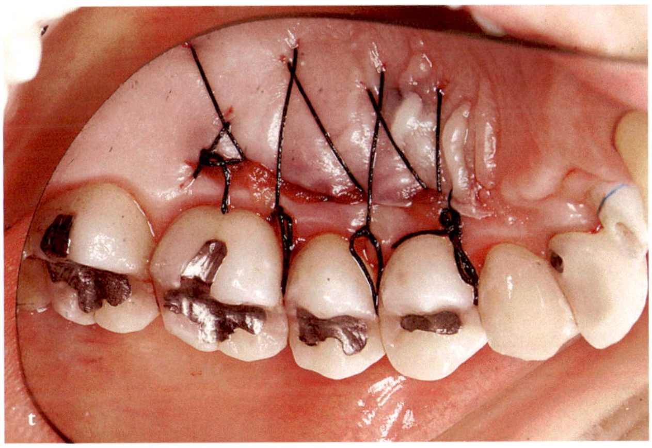

Fig 3-18t Palatal donor site.

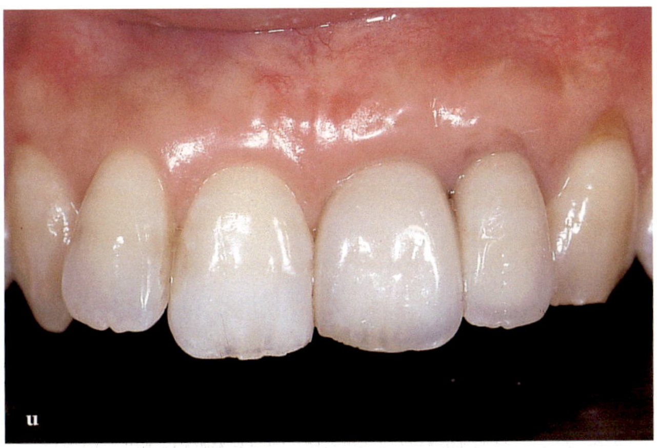

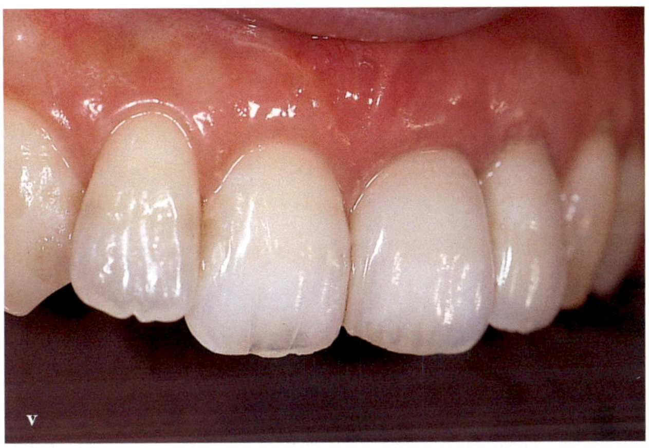

Figs 3-18u and 3-18v At 1 year following CTG, increased buccal volume was maintained, and gingival recession was corrected.

Immediate implant placement with orthodontic extrusion and GBR to compensate for buccal bone resorption

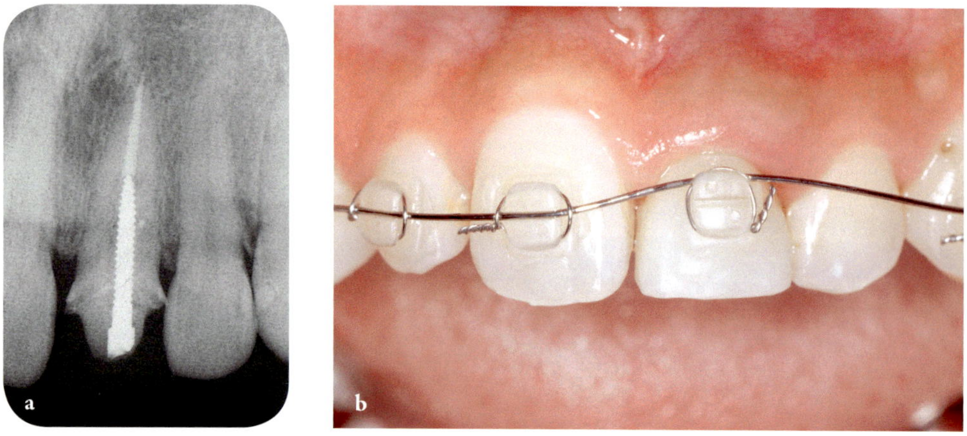

Figs 3-19a and 3-19b The left central incisor was hopeless because of a perforation. Orthodontic extrusion was initiated.

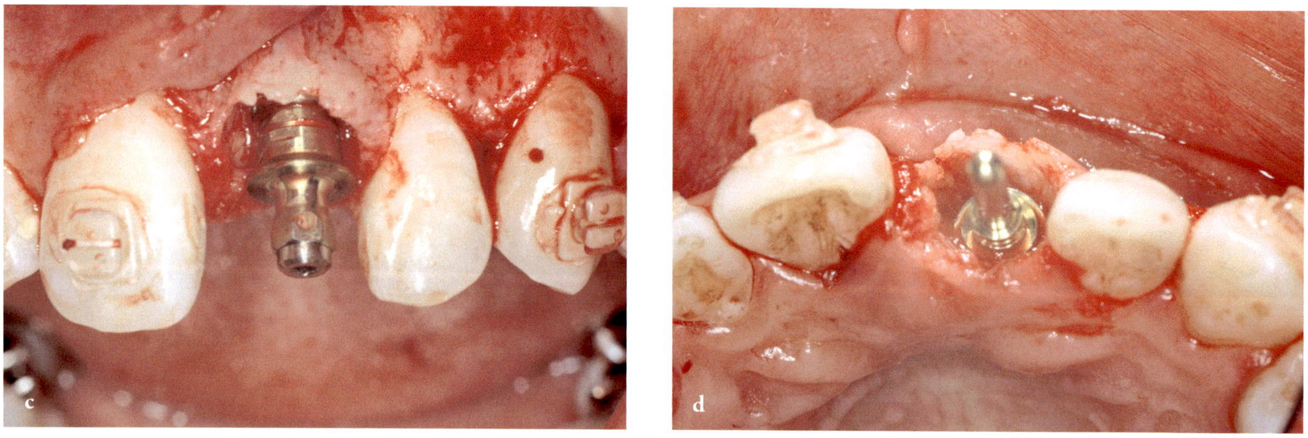

Figs 3-19c and 3-19d Immediate implant placement after orthodontic extrusion. Sufficient primary stability of the implant was obtained, and thin but intact buccal bone was observed.

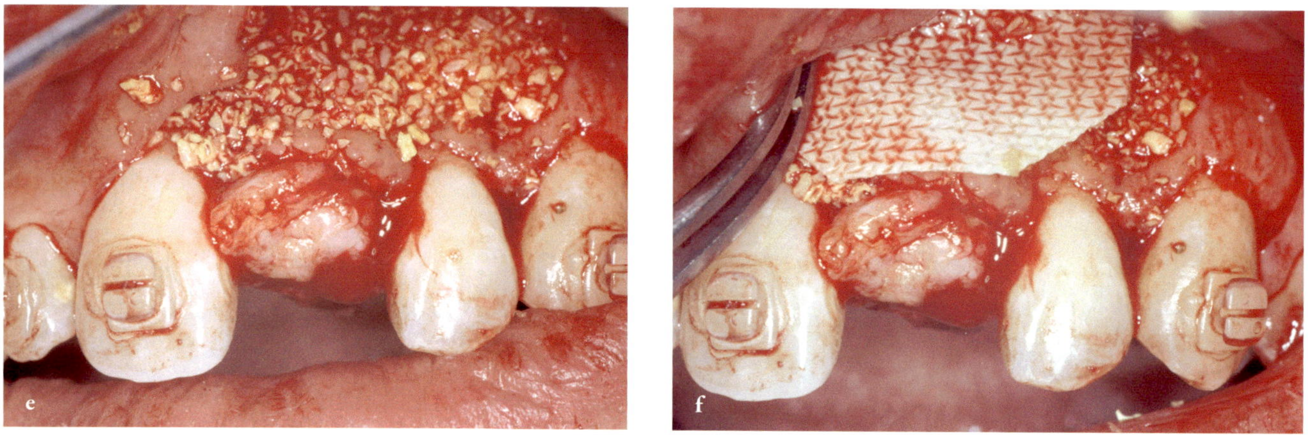

Figs 3-19e and 3-19f Bone graft and pedicle CTG were placed outside the extraction socket to compensate for buccal bone resorption. A pedicle CTG closed the extraction socket completely.

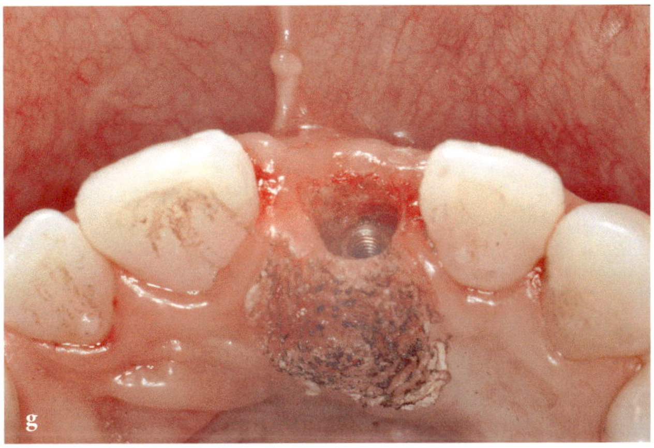

Fig 3-19g Four months later, the tissue punch technique was carried out with a CO_2 laser, and tissue sculpting was initiated with a screw-retained provisional restoration.

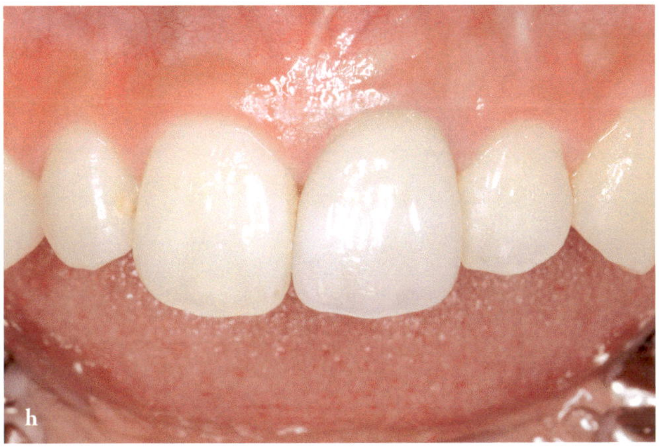

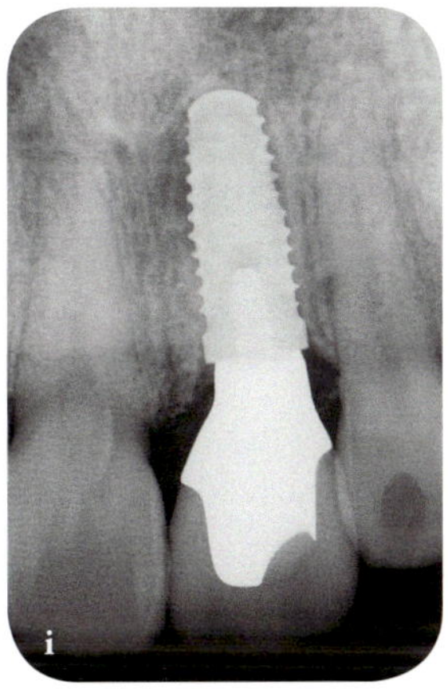

Figs 3-19h and 3-19i Facial view *(h)* and a periapical radiograph *(i)* at the 2-year follow-up.

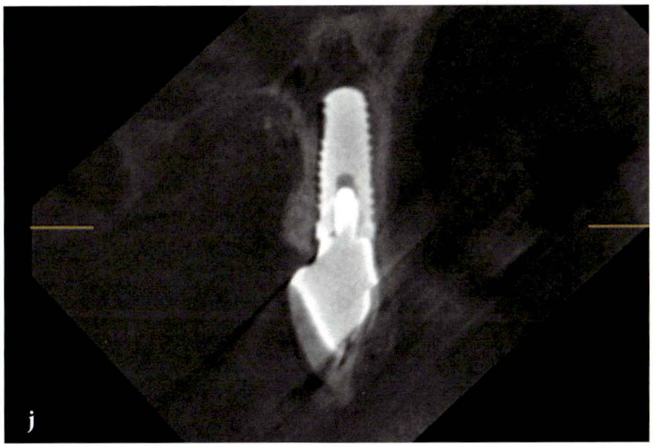

Fig 3-19j The 2-year computed tomographic evaluation showed that the buccal bone had been maintained.

References

1. Hämmerle CH, Chen ST, Wilson TG Jr. Consensus statements and recommended clinical procedures regarding the placement of implants in extraction sockets. Int J Oral Maxillofac Implants 2004; 19(suppl):26–28.
2. Becker W, Dahlin C, Lekholm U, et al. Five-year evaluation of implants placed at extraction and with dehiscences and fenestration defects augmented with ePTFE membranes: Results from a prospective multicenter study. Clin Implant Dent Relat Res 1999;1:27–32.
3. Lazzara RJ. Immediate implant placement into extraction sites: Surgical and restorative advantages. Int J Periodontics Restorative Dent 1989;9:332–343.
4. Paolantonio M, Dolci M, Scarano A, et al. Immediate implantation in fresh extraction sockets. A controlled clinical and histological study in man. J Periodontol 2001;72:1560–1571.
5. Becker BE, Becker W, Ricci A, Geurs N. A prospective clinical trial of endosseous screw-shaped implants paced at the time of tooth extraction without augmentation. J Periodontol 1998;69:920–926.
6. Becker W, Becker BE, Handelsman M, Ochsenbein C, Albrektsson T. Guided tissue regeneration for implants placed into extraction sockets: A study in dogs. J Periodontol 1991;62:703–709.
7. Chen ST, Darby IB, Adams GG, Reynolds EC. A prospective clinical study of bone augmentation techniques at immediate implants. Clin Oral Implants Res 2005;16:176–184.
8. Chen ST, Wilson TG Jr, Hämmerle CH. Immediate or early placement of implants following tooth extraction: Review of biologic basis, clinical procedures, and outcomes. Int J Oral Maxillofac Implants 2004;19:12–25.
9. Kan JYK, Rungcharassaeng K, Lozada J. Immediate placement and provisionalization of maxillary anterior single implants: 1-year prospective study. Int J Oral Maxillofac Implants 2003;18:31–39.
10. Araújo MG, Lindhe J. Dimensional ridge alterations following tooth extraction. An experimental study in the dog. J Clin Periodontol 2005;32:212–218.
11. Botticelli D, Persson LG, Lindhe J, Berglundh T. Bone tissue formation adjacent to implants placed in fresh extraction sockets: An experimental study in dogs. Clin Oral Implants Res 2006;17:351–358.
12. Evans CD, Chen ST. Esthetic outcomes of immediate implant placements. Clin Oral Implants Res 2008;19:73–80.
13. Chen ST, Darby IB, Reynolds EC. A prospective clinical study of nonsubmerged immediate implants: Clinical outcomes and esthetic results. Clin Oral Implants Res 2007;18:552–562.
14. Salama H, Salama M. The role of orthodontic extrusive remodeling in the enhancement of soft and hard tissue profiles prior to implant placement: A systematic approach to the management of extraction site defects. Int J Periodontics Restorative Dent 1993;13:312–333.
15. Small PN, Tarnow DP. Gingival recession around implants: A 1-year longitudinal prospective study. Int J Oral Maxillofac Implants 2000;15:527–532.
16. Wilson TG Jr, Schenk R, Buser D, Cochran D. Implants placed in immediate extraction sites: A report of histologic and histometric analyses of human biopsies. Int J Oral Maxillofac Implants 1998;13:333–341.
17. Botticelli D, Berglundh T, Buser D, Lindhe J. The jumping distance revisited: An experimental study in the dog. Clin Oral Implants Res 2003;14:35–42.
18. Funato A, Salama MA, Ishikawa T, Garber DA, Salama H. Timing, positioning, and sequential staging in esthetic implant therapy: A four-dimensional perspective. Int J Periodontics Restorative Dent 2007;27:313–323.
19. Maynard JG Jr, Wilson RD. Physiologic dimensions of the periodontium significant to the restorative dentist. J Periodontol 1979;50(4):170–174.
20. Kan JY, Rungcharassaeng K, Umezu K, Kois JC. Dimensions of peri-implant mucosa: An evaluation of maxillary anterior single implants in humans. J Periodontol 2003;74:557–562.
21. Kois JC. Predictable single tooth peri-implant esthetics: Five diagnostic keys. Compend Contin Educ Dent 2001;22(3):199–206.

Chapter 4

Extraction Socket Preservation and Root Submergence

in the Esthetic Region

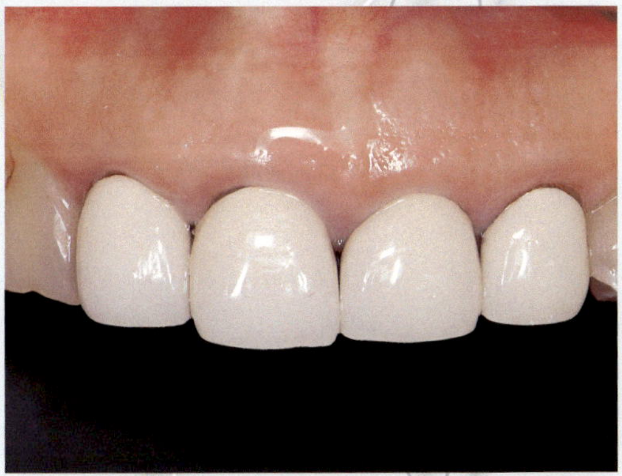

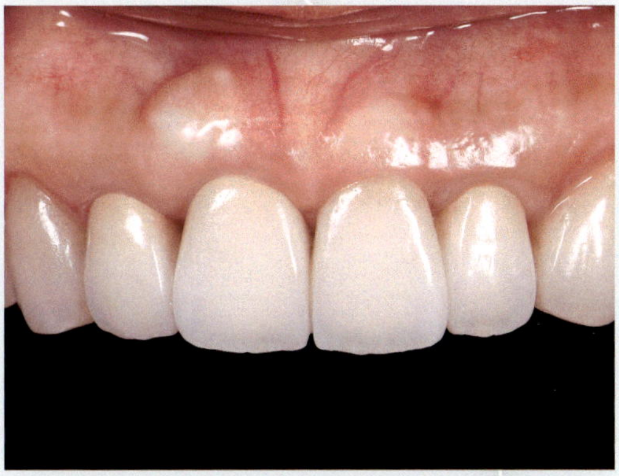

This chapter discusses the application of the extraction socket preservation technique. According to the classification of immediate implant sites presented in chapter 3 (see Fig 3-10), in a Class 3 situation, a staged approach using a socket preservation technique prior to implant placement provides a more predictable outcome and fewer, if any, complications. Even in a Class 1 situation, the staged approach may be more appropriate for inexperienced clinicians.

The advantages of using the root submergence technique to preserve the alveolar bone frame in pontic sites are also discussed in this chapter.

Extraction Socket Preservation

Literature review

Schropp et al[1] reported that tooth extraction triggers resorption of the surrounding tissue and the alveolar ridge by up to 30% in 3 months and up to 50% in 1 year. Lekovic et al[2,3] used nonresorbable and resorbable membranes to cover extraction sockets and found that both outperformed the untreated control extraction sockets in terms of alveolar process preservation. Nevins et al[4] compared extraction sockets grafted with Bio-Oss (Geistlich) and a control group of nongrafted sockets. All sites were completely covered with a coronally advanced buccal flap at the conclusion of surgery. This approach can reduce alveolar ridge resorption to some degree, but rarely can such procedures completely preserve the alveolar ridge frame. However, the soft tissue management protocol of this approach could result in an adverse soft tissue profile, ie, a coronally advanced mucogingival junction. Wang et al[5] introduced a socket preservation technique without soft tissue closure of the socket (Fig 4-1):

1. Atraumatic extraction to preserve thin buccal bone
2. Thorough debridement of the socket and intramarrow penetration to stimulate bleeding
3. Placement of bone graft materials in socket
4. Closure of the socket with collagen sponge
5. Creation of ovate pontic to preserve papillae form

Iasella et al[6] studied a socket preservation technique using freeze-dried bone allograft (FDBA) and a collagen membrane but without complete closure of the socket. They compared this technique with a nongrafted control site. Results showed that socket preservation successfully reduced loss of ridge width and height. Some clinicians have questioned whether there may be problems of increased soft tissue migration at the crestal area with implant treatment,[7] but this approach decreased alveolar ridge resorption without soft tissue profile alteration.

Techniques in the posterior region

In a posterior region without esthetic concerns, bone grafting only in the extraction socket may preserve sufficient alveolar ridge dimensions for implant placement (Fig 4-2).

Extraction socket preservation technique introduced by Wang et al[5]

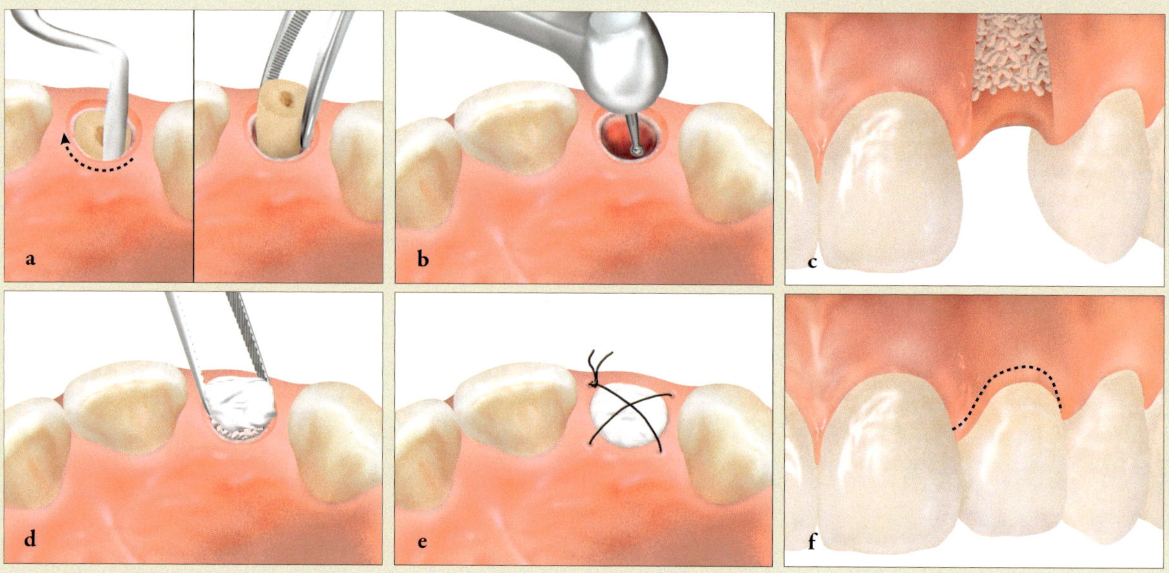

Fig 4-1 *(a)* Atraumatic extraction with periotome. *(b)* Intramarrow penetration to stimulate bleeding into the socket. *(c)* Filling of the socket with bone graft material. *(d)* Sealing of the socket with a collagen sponge. *(e)* Mattress suture over the socket. *(f)* Ovate pontic to maintain papilla shape.

Socket preservation with bone grafting only in the posterior region prior to the implant placement

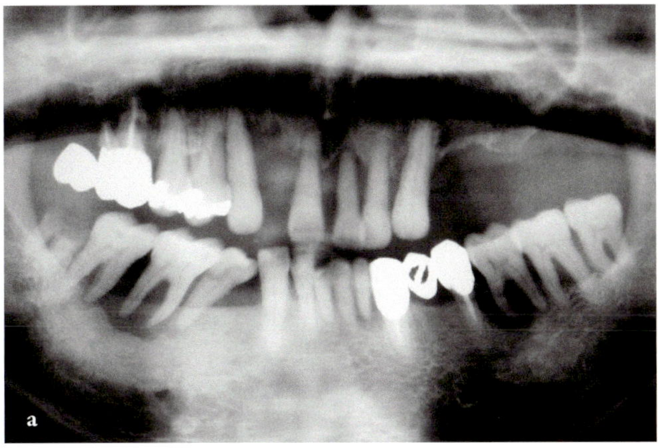
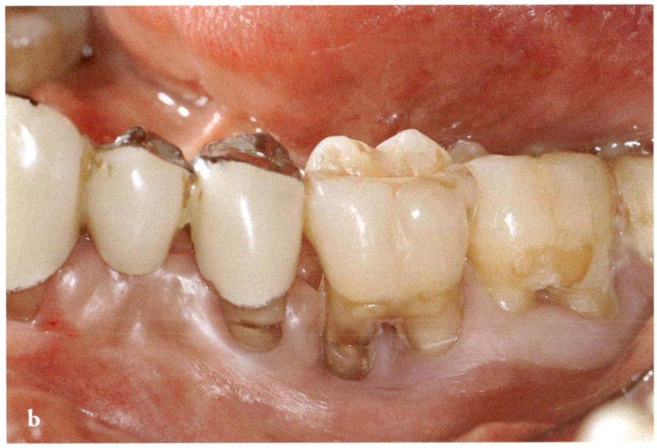

Figs 4-2a and 4-2b Panoramic radiograph *(a)* and lateral clinical view *(b)* at initial examination. Immediate implant placement was not considered because of bone loss in the molar region. Socket preservation was selected to preserve the alveolus and to shorten the treatment period.

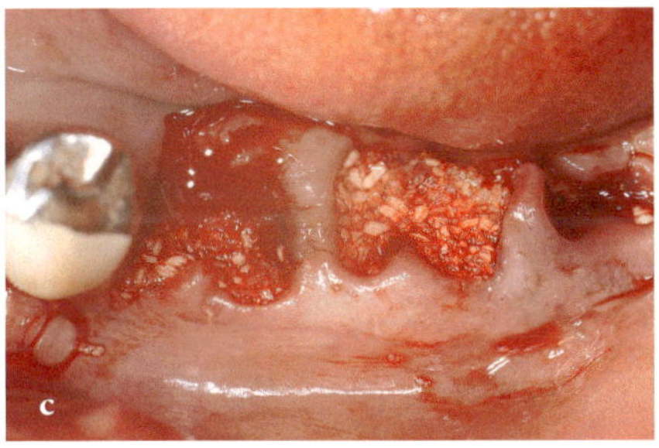

Fig 4-2c Following the extractions, the sockets were filled with bone graft materials.

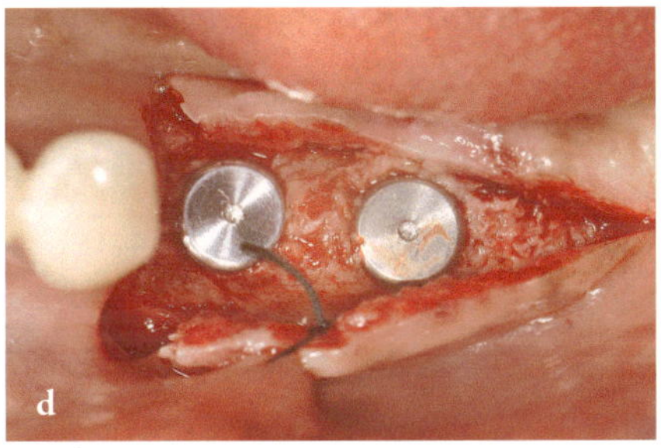

Fig 4-2d Wide-diameter implants were placed into the preserved ridge 4 months later.

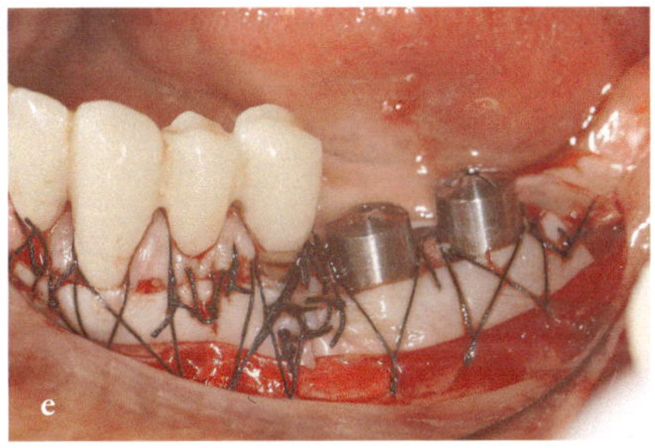

Fig 4-2e Stage-two surgery with a free gingival graft was performed 3 months after implant placement.

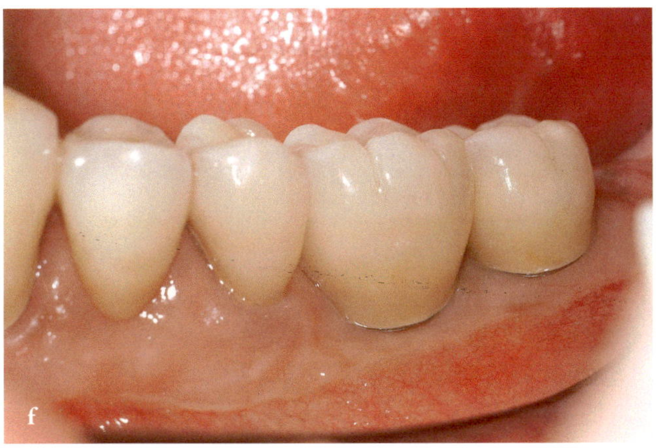

Fig 4-2f Lateral view of definitive restorations. The right mandibular molar region was treated in the same manner.

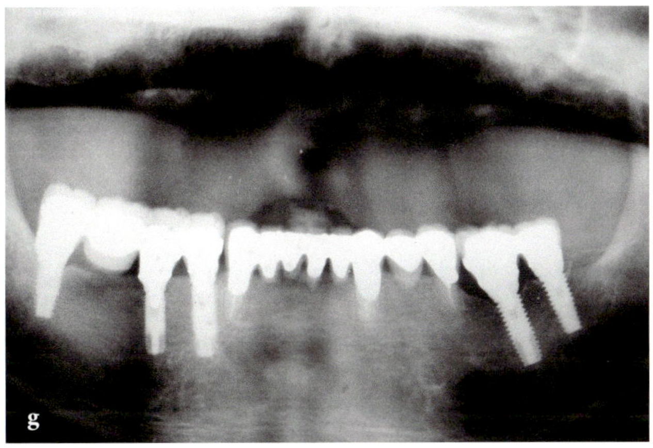

Fig 4-2g Panoramic radiograph obtained at the 5-year follow-up.

Techniques in the esthetic region

As described in chapter 3, orthodontic extrusion of the tooth targeted for immediate implant placement is recommended to compensate for the inevitable buccal bone resorption following extraction (Fig 4-3); however, many patients will not accept this option. An alternative for Class 3 sites is a staged approach using a socket preservation technique and subsequent implant placement.

The bone surrounding the teeth targeted for extraction must be thoroughly examined by computed tomographic (CT) scans, radiographs, and bone soundings. The lingual bone wall must be intact for immediate implant placement and socket preservation in the esthetic region. Even if all bone walls are intact, socket preservation without preliminary orthodontic extrusion will result in buccal bone resorption. Therefore, it may be appropriate to overcorrect buccally by up to 20% to compensate for this (Figs 4-4 and 4-5).

Fickl et al[8] reported that treating the extraction socket by filling it with xenograft and closing it with a free gingival graft seemed beneficial in limiting the resorption process after tooth extraction. In addition, bone grafting outside of the extraction socket buccally and subsequent primary closure with a free gingival graft, a pedicle connective tissue graft, or a resorbable membrane help to reduce alveolar ridge resorption following extraction.

Socket preservation following orthodontic extrusion

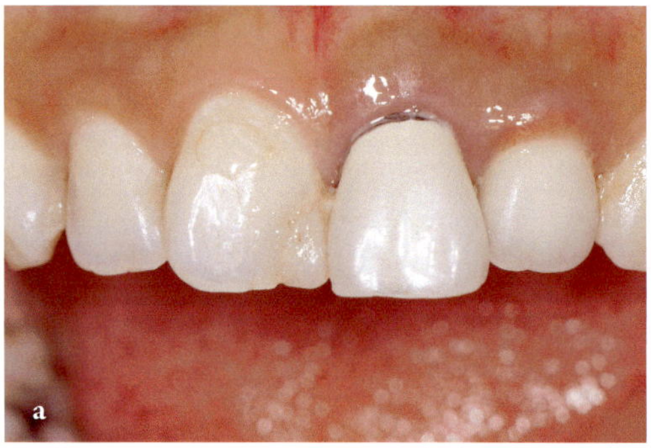

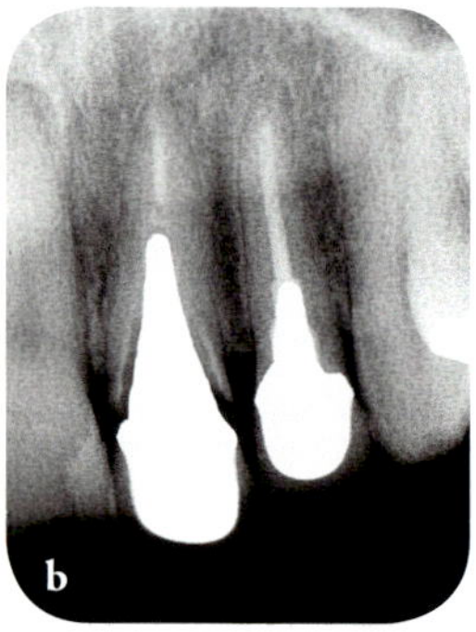

Figs 4-3a and 4-3b Fracture of the left central incisor.

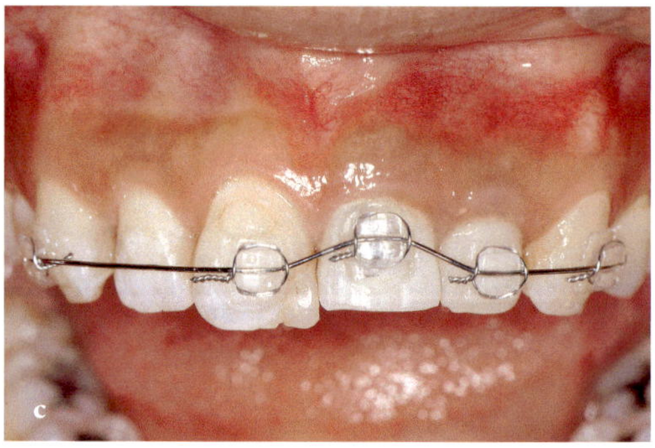

Fig 4-3c A deficient buccal socket wall was anticipated after orthodontic extrusion, ie, the site was Class 3 (see Fig 3-10). Therefore, a staged approach with socket preservation was selected over immediate implant placement.

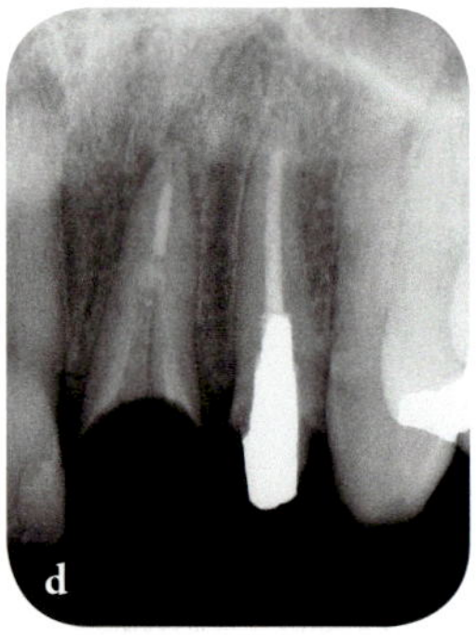

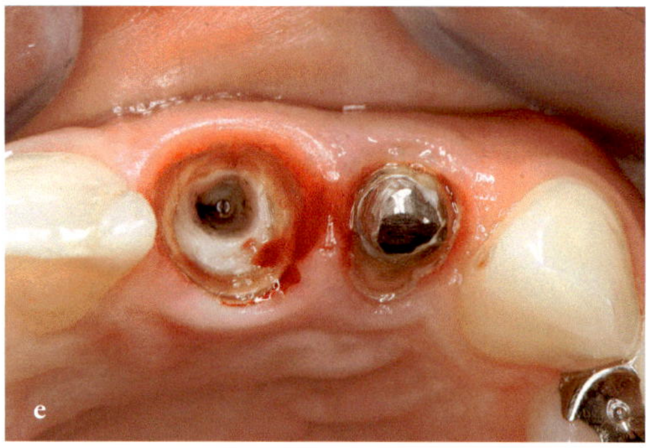

Figs 4-3d and 4-3e Periapical radiograph *(d)* and occlusal view *(e)* following orthodontic extrusion.

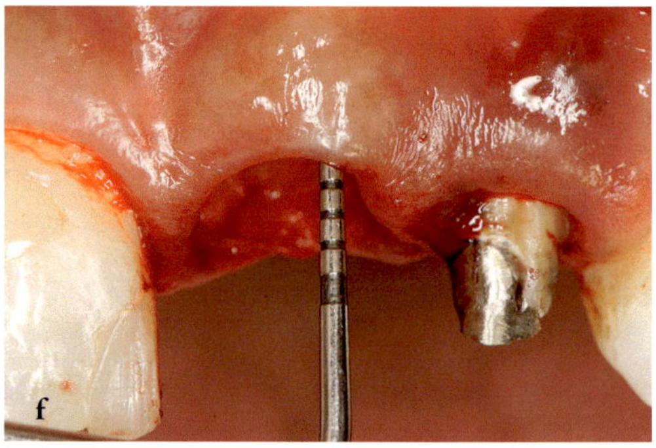

Fig 4-3f Following extraction, an intrasulcular incision was made around the adjacent teeth. The buccal gingiva was elevated to create space for a bone graft.

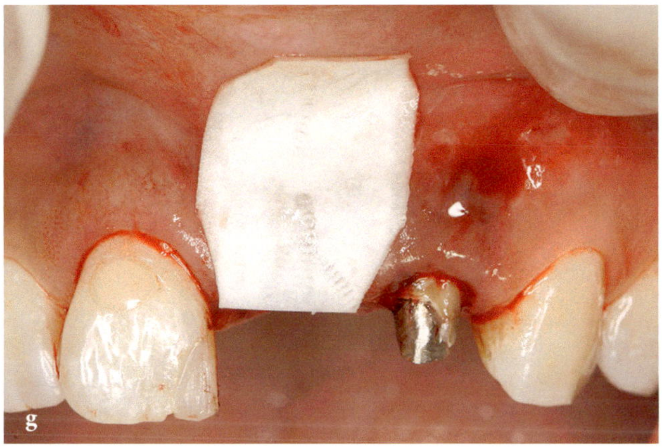

Fig 4-3g After confirming deficient buccal bone, a resorbable membrane was placed.

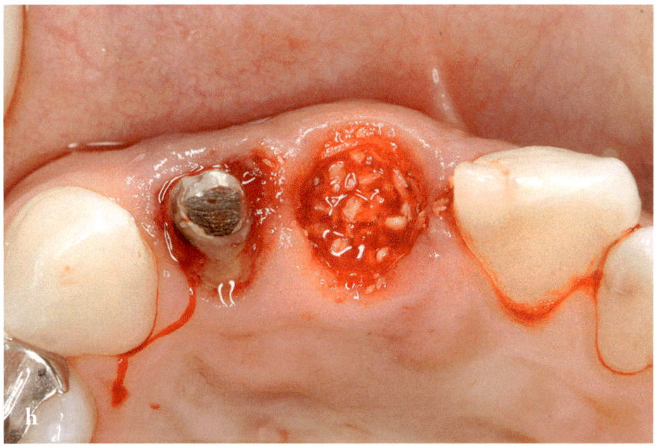

Fig 4-3h The socket was filled with bone graft material. Note the overcorrection in the buccal area.

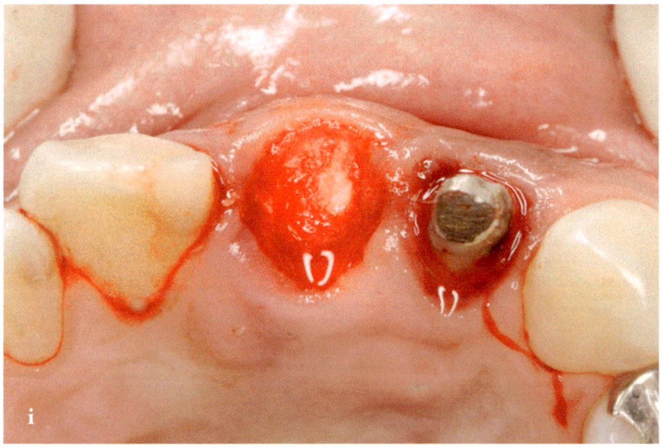

Fig 4-3i The socket was sealed with a collagen sponge and an ovate pontic.

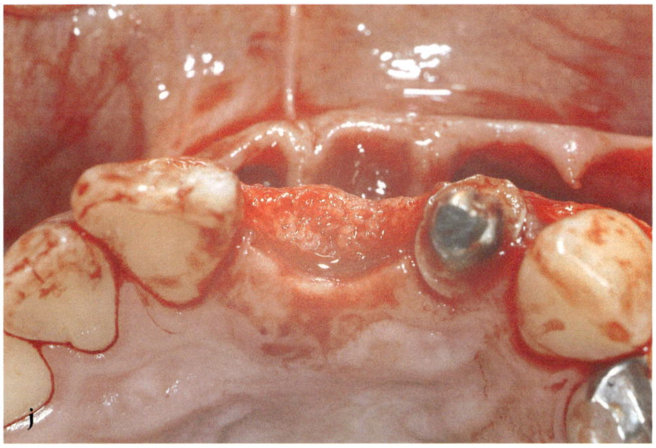

Fig 4-3j The extraction socket was well preserved.

Flapless implant placement following socket preservation

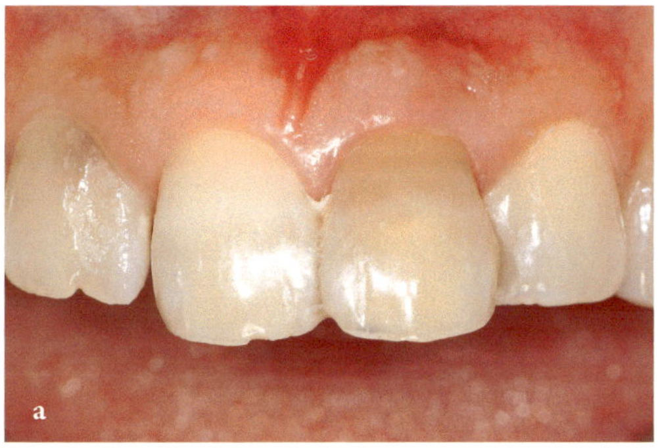

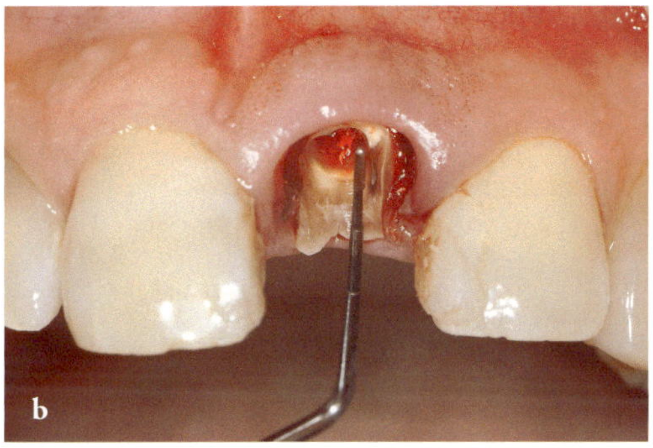

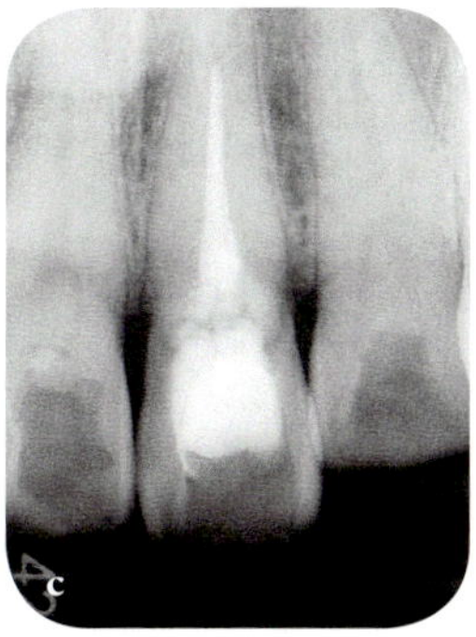

Figs 4-4a to 4-4c Fractured left central incisor.

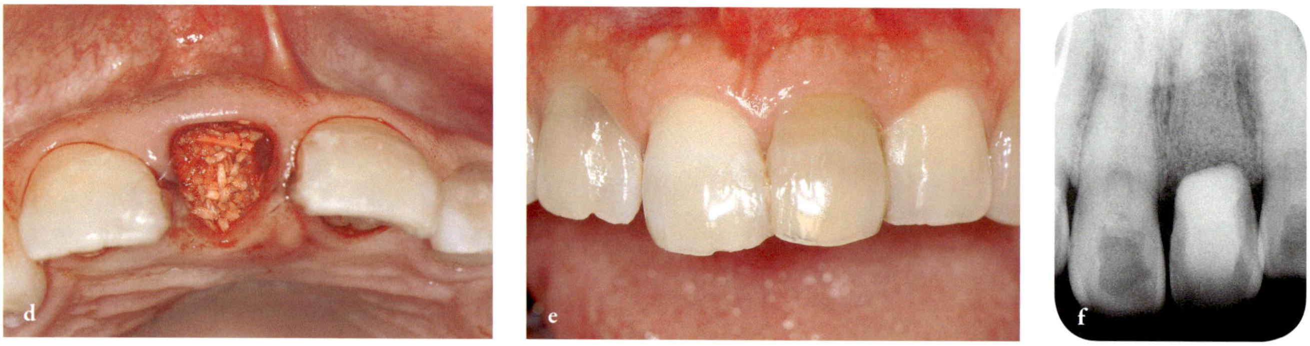

Figs 4-4d to 4-4f Following extraction, the socket was filled with bone graft and sealed with a collagen plug and ovate pontic (the reshaped extracted tooth).

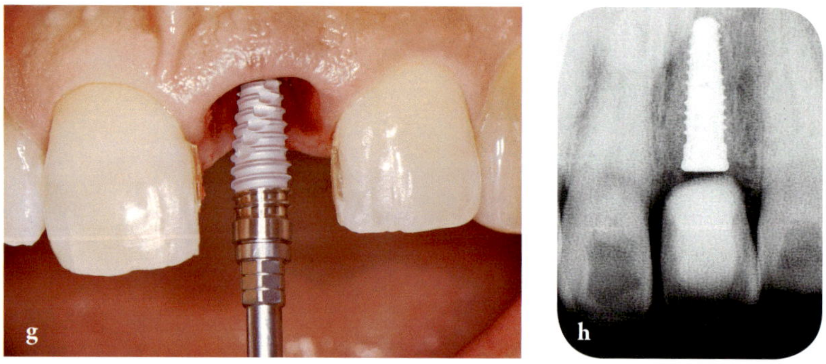

Figs 4-4g and 4-4h Flapless implant placement with the tissue punch technique was carried out 4 months later.

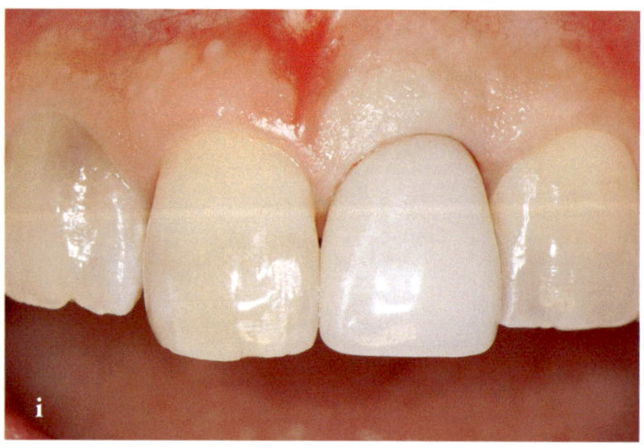

Fig 4-4i Four months following implant placement, stage-two surgery was performed with a laser tissue punch technique. Tissue sculpting was accomplished with a provisional restoration.

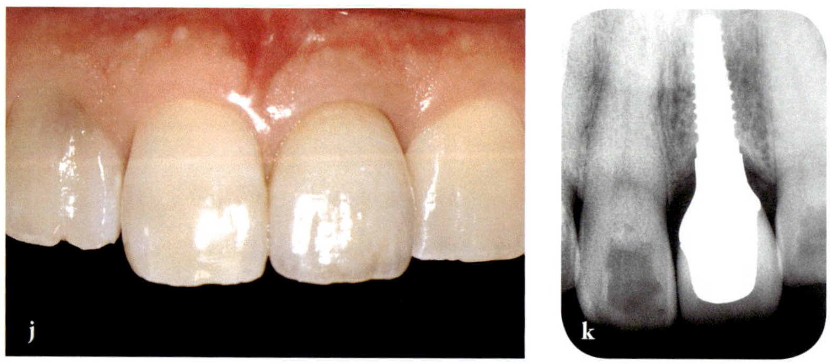

Figs 4-4j and 4-4k Facial view and periapical radiograph of the definitive restoration.

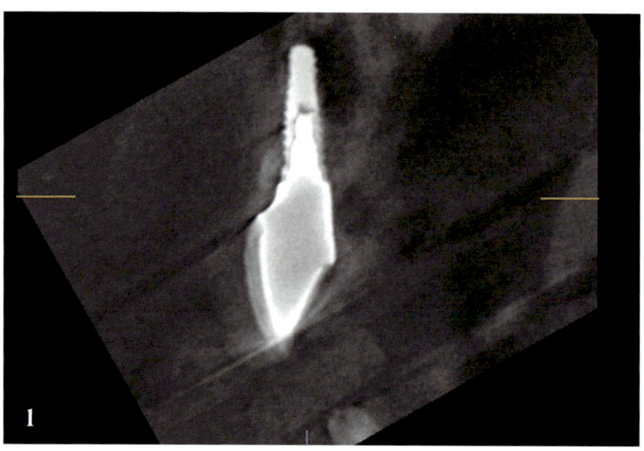

Fig 4-4l The 2-year CT evaluation showed that buccal bone thickness was maintained.

New approaches to socket preservation: Using rhPDGF

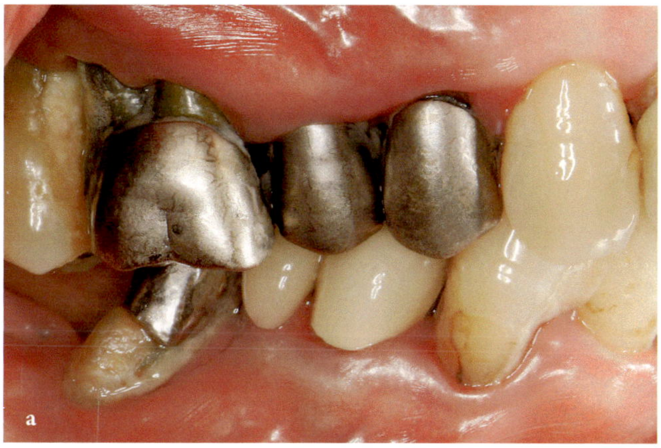

Fig 4-5a Pretreatment lateral view.

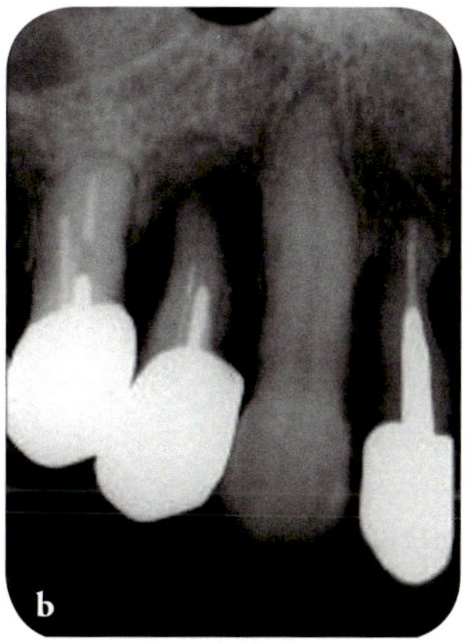

Fig 4-5b An extended periapical lesion was noted. Severe alveolar ridge resorption was anticipated following extraction.

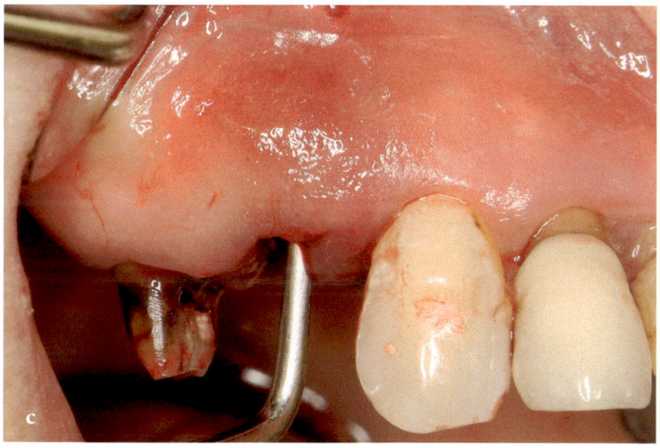

Fig 4-5c Total loss of buccal bone was confirmed following extraction.

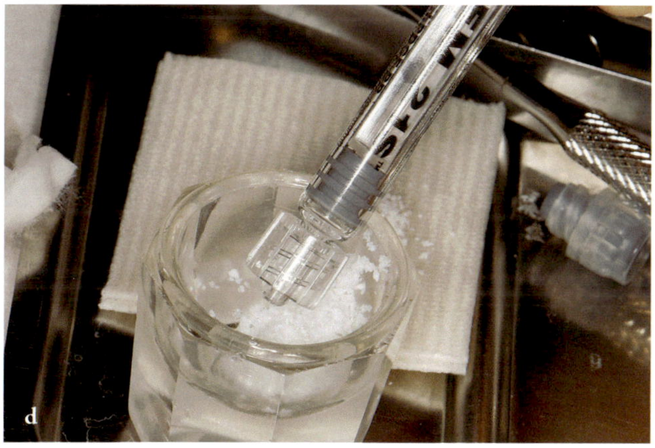

Fig 4-5d Xenograft was mixed with recombinant human platelet-derived growth factor (rhPDGF).

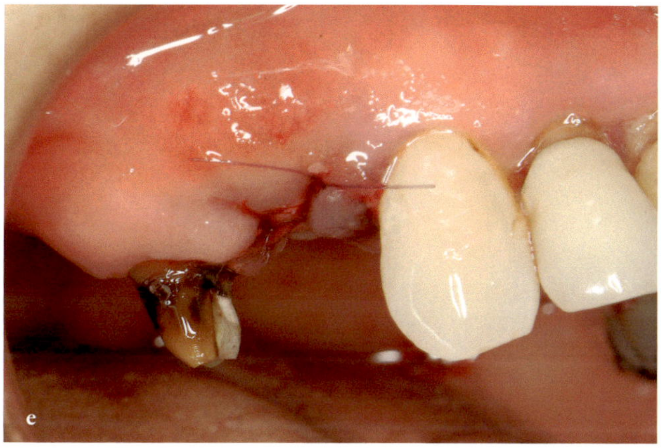

Fig 4-5e Following thorough debridement, the extraction socket was filled with the xenograft-rhPDGF mixture and sealed with a collagen plug.

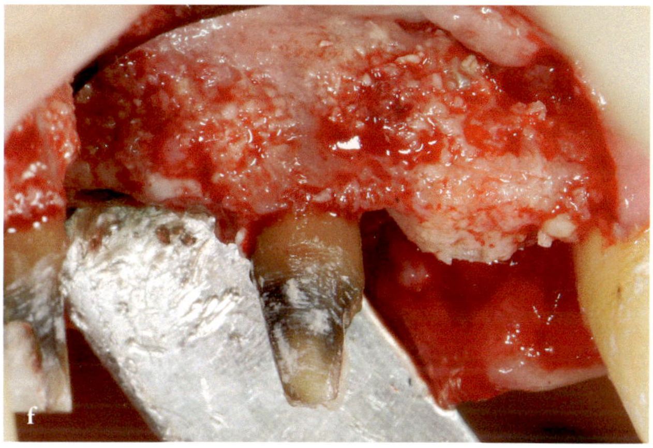

Fig 4-5f At implant placement 16 months later, bone regeneration beyond the adjacent osseous crest was observed.

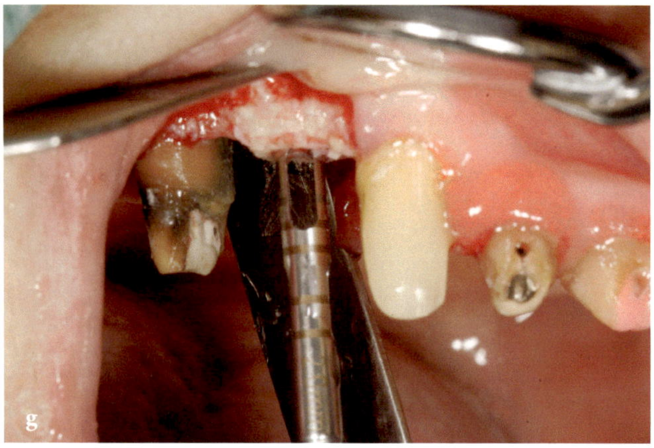

Fig 4-5g Implant site osteotomy was performed with a trephine bur.

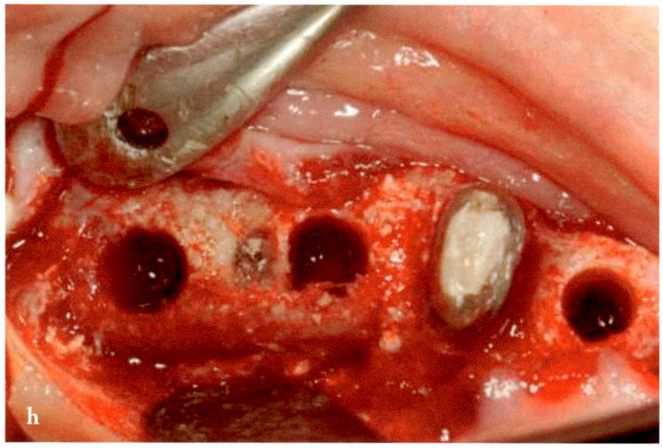

Fig 4-5h Occlusal view of implant osteotomy site. Adequate buccal bone width was observed.

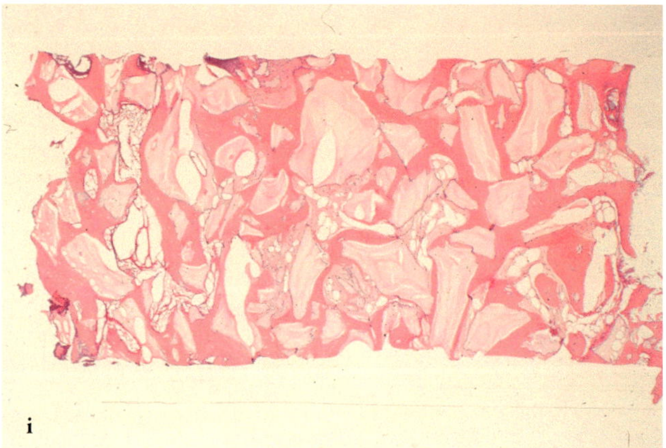

Fig 4-5i Histologic evaluation of the core sample from the implant site osteotomy. The xenograft was completely surrounded by newly formed bone. (Courtesy of Dr Takeshi Ishida.)

Before guided bone regeneration

In multiple-tooth implant cases associated with extractions, three-dimensional alveolar ridge augmentation with guided bone regeneration (GBR) is often necessary at the targeted extraction site and in the adjacent edentulous area. Delayed GBR after extraction with appropriate soft tissue healing may potentially decrease complications. However, bone and soft tissue alteration following extraction could compromise treatment predictability. Performing socket preservation before GBR would resolve that issue and increase the safety and predictability of the procedure by maintaining the soft tissue profile. An 8-week healing period is required between socket preservation and GBR to allow soft tissue coverage of the extraction site (Fig 4-6).

Socket preservation prior to GBR

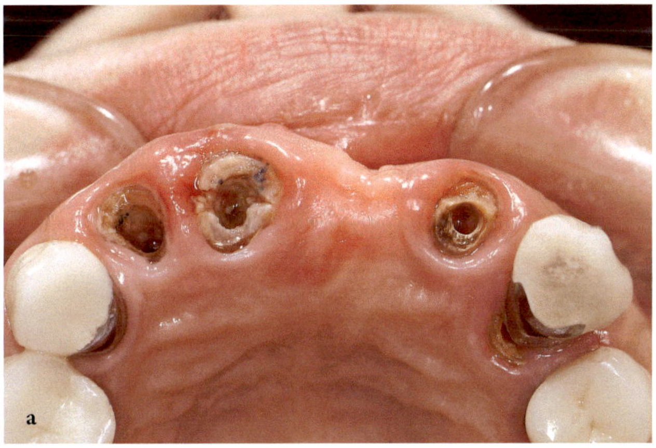

Fig 4-6a Occlusal view of teeth targeted for extraction. The ridge in the area of the left central incisor presented with a buccal concavity.

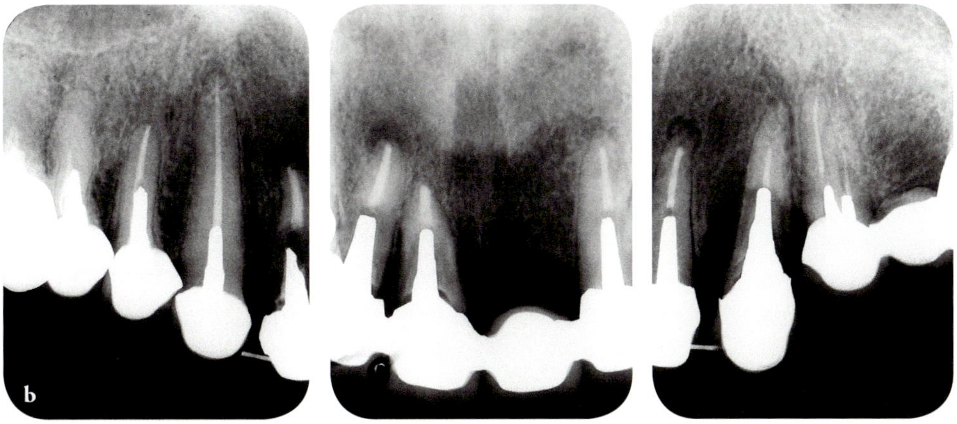

Fig 4-6b The area from the distal side of the right central incisor to the mesial side of the left canine presented with advanced bone loss. Severe ridge resorption following extraction was anticipated.

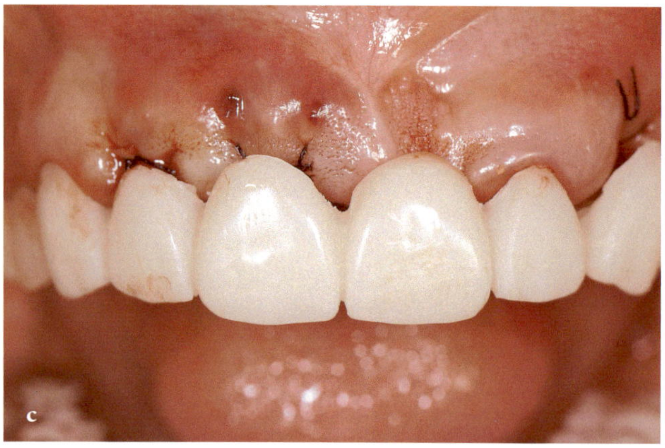

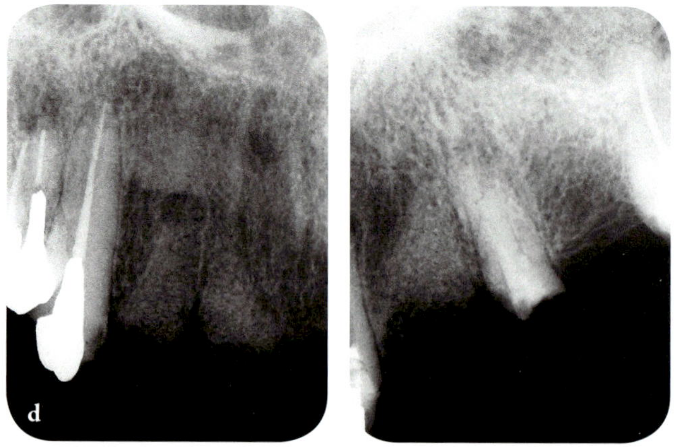

Figs 4-6c and 4-6d Following extraction and thorough debridement, the sockets were filled with bone graft materials.

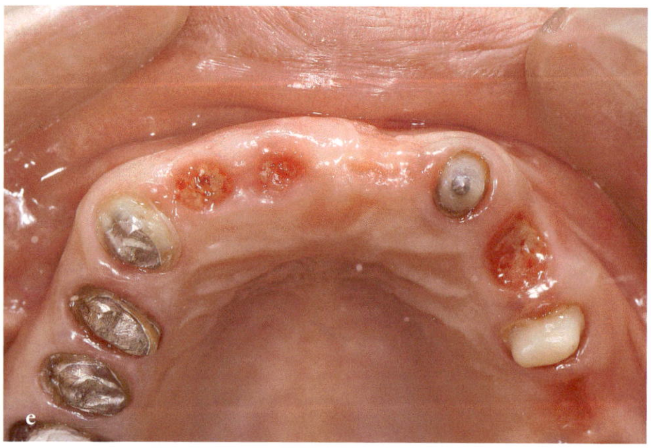

Fig 4-6e Two months later, the alveolar ridge seemed to maintain its shape, but the soft tissue healing was incomplete. Soft tissue healing over the extraction sockets would have been better without the placement of bone graft materials.

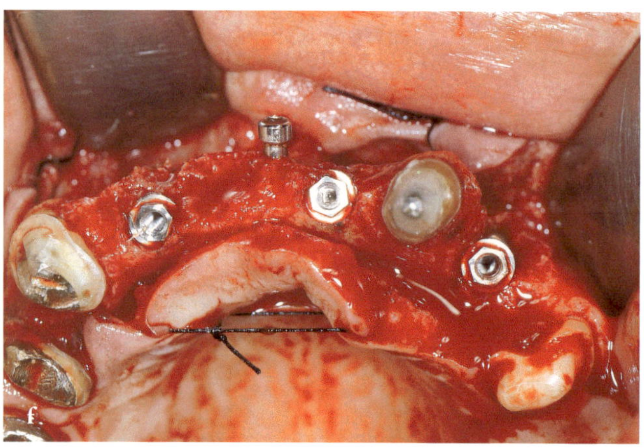

Fig 4-6f Grafted bone was completely removed from the site of the left canine.

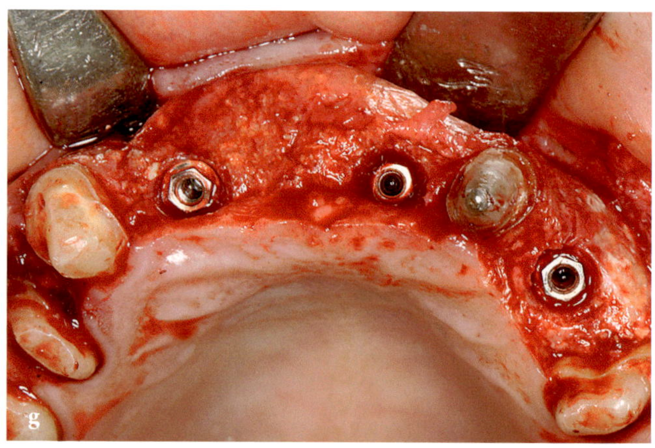

Fig 4-6g The buccal bone was augmented using GBR.

Limitations

Bone graft materials in the extraction socket may not be completely incorporated into the bone tissue. In such cases, bone graft materials and the surrounding tissue must be removed prior to a simultaneous implant placement and bone graft (GBR) in the same area. Socket preservation cannot entirely prevent alveolar bone resorption, but it is beneficial for reducing gingival recession and increasing subsequent GBR volume, especially in the esthetic region. With the socket preservation technique, residual soft tissue, insufficient bleeding in the extraction socket, and/or improper use of a resorbable membrane could result in less bone formation (Figs 4-7 and 4-8).

Learning from failure: Unsuccessful preservation of the alveolar ridge

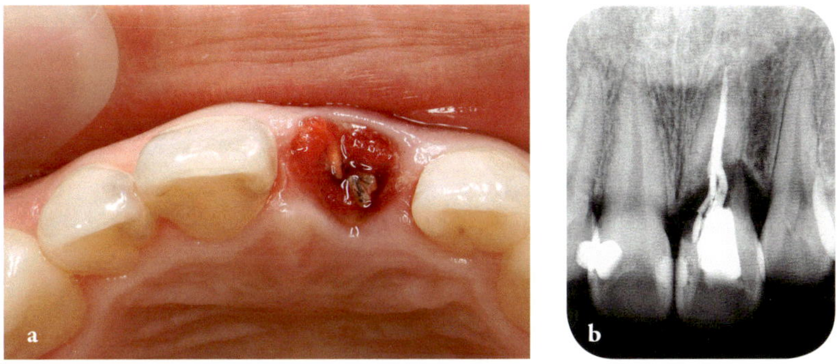

Figs 4-7a and 4-7b Occlusal view *(a)* and periapical radiograph *(b)* at initial examination of the left central incisor, which presented with fracture and decay.

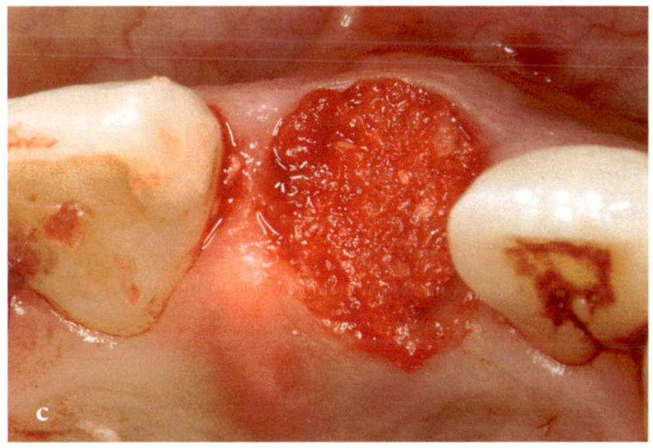

Fig 4-7c Following extraction, thorough debridement was performed, a resorbable membrane was placed buccally, and the extraction socket was filled with bone graft.

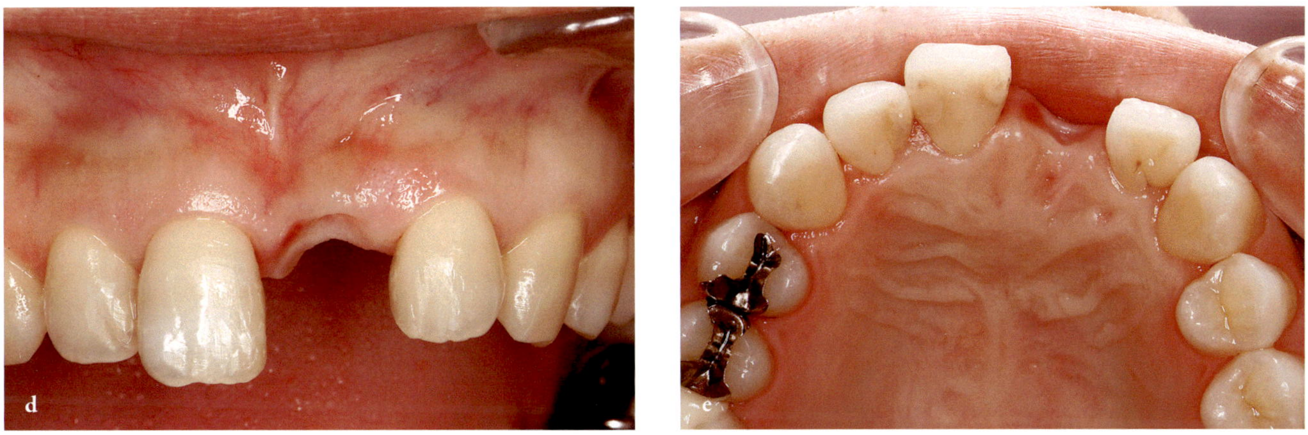

Figs 4-7d and 4-7e Four months later, clinical evaluation showed that the alveolar ridge was not preserved as intended.

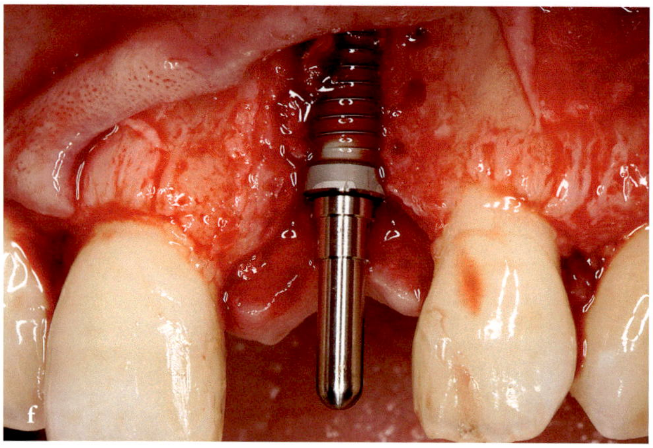

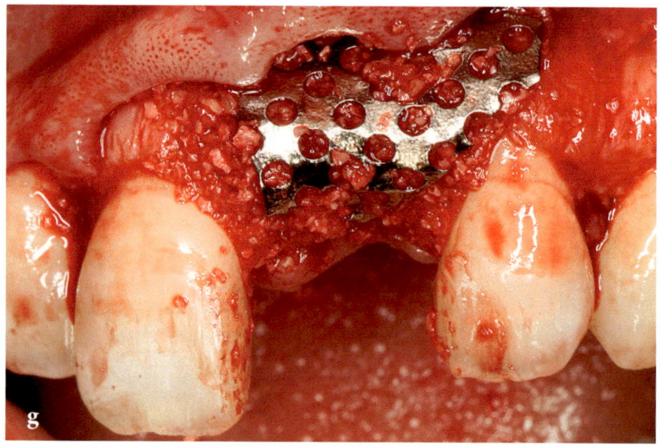

Figs 4-7f and 4-7g Implant placement with simultaneous GBR using titanium mesh.

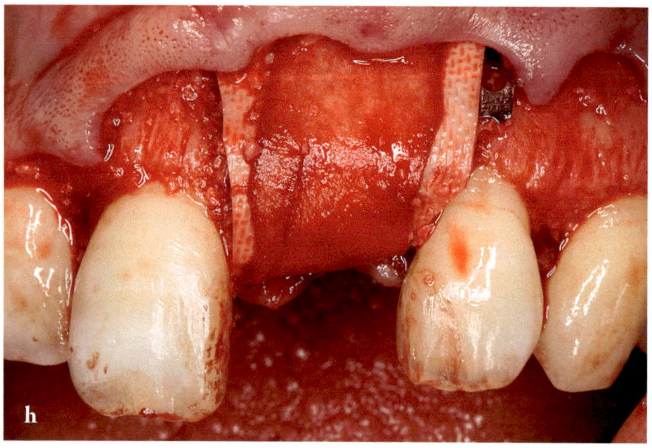

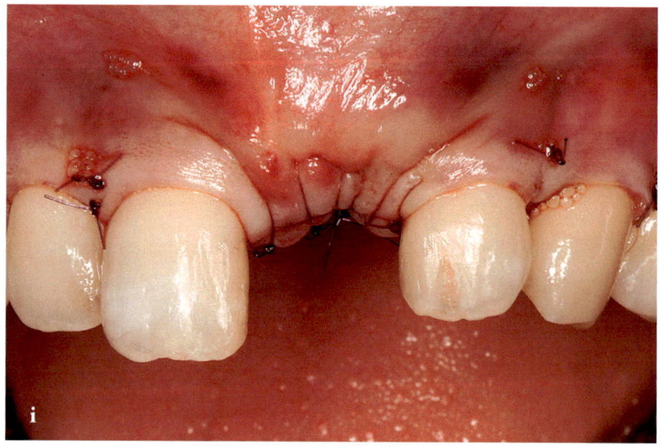

Figs 4-7h and 4-7i A resorbable membrane was placed over the titanium mesh and sutured.

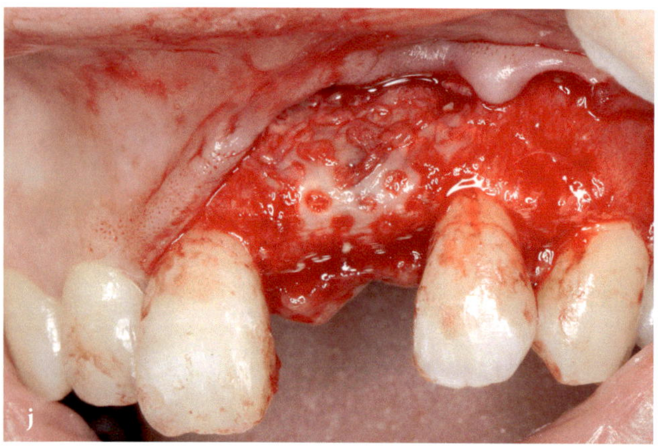

Fig 4-7j Six months later, bone regeneration was confirmed.

☞ Clinical tips

The disadvantages of socket preservation include difficult membrane positioning, unpredictable ridge resorption, and soft tissue migration into the extraction socket. The protocol must be refined to reduce these disadvantages.

Learning from failure: Unsuccessful soft tissue healing

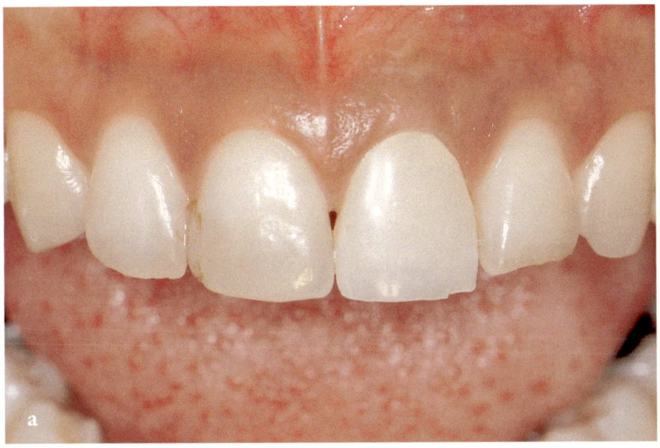

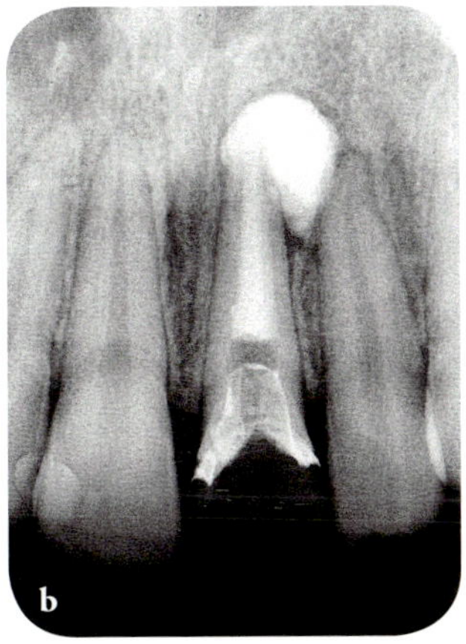

Figs 4-8a and 4-8b Facial view *(a)* and periapical radiograph *(b)* at initial examination. The left central incisor presented with a gingival abscess and fracture and was diagnosed as hopeless.

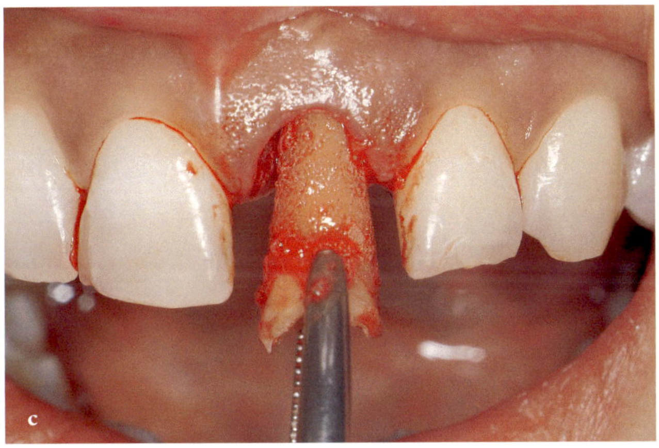

Fig 4-8c Thorough debridement was performed following extraction, and the socket was filled with bone graft.

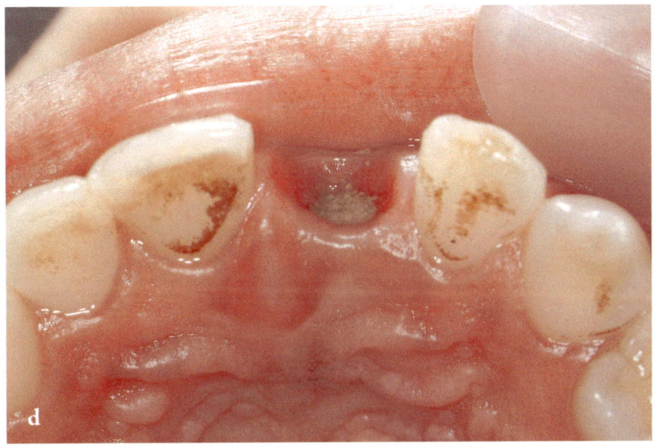

Fig 4-8d Two months later, the soft tissue had not healed over the extraction socket.

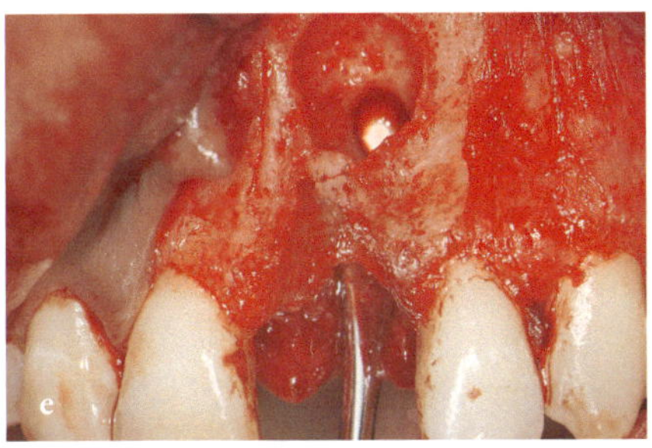

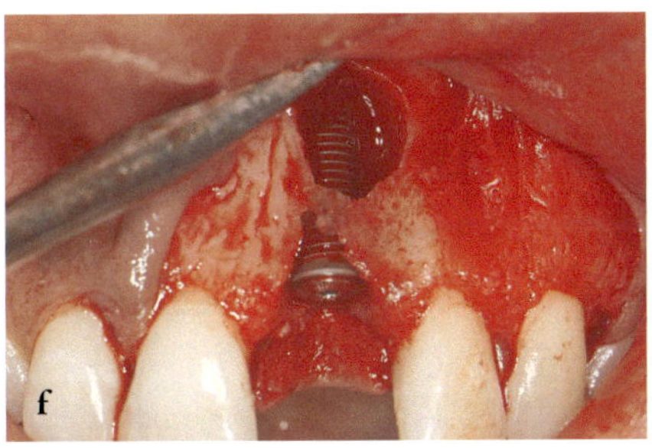

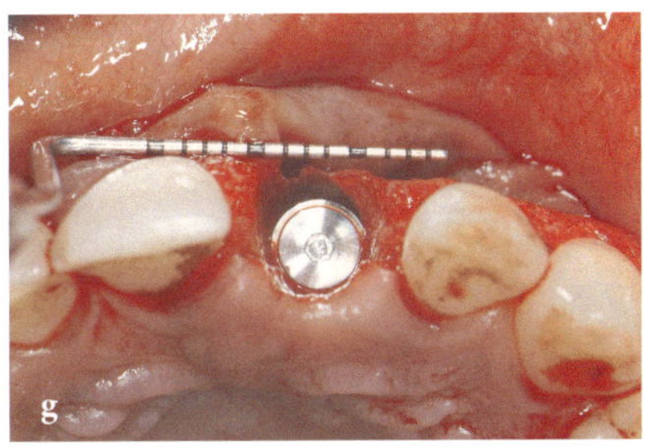

Figs 4-8e to 4-8g The buccal flap was elevated, the bone graft material was completely removed, and the area was thoroughly debrided. Bleeding was stimulated from surrounding bone. Implant placement was performed with simultaneous GBR using titanium mesh.

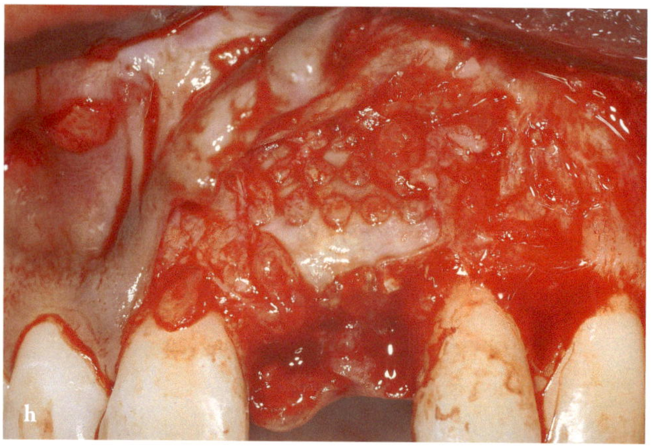
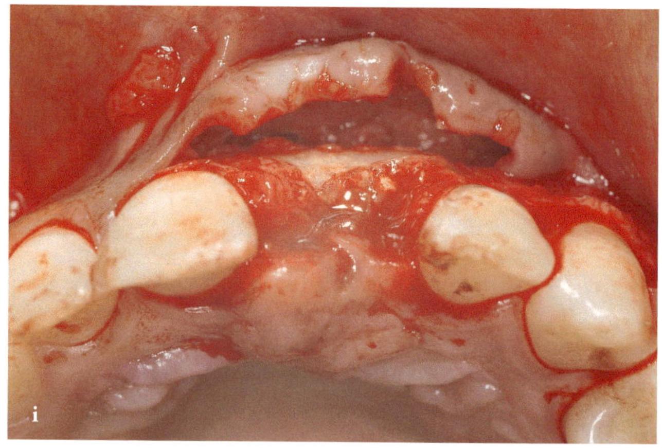

Figs 4-8h and 4-8i Six months later, an adequate amount of bone was regenerated on the buccal aspect of the implant.

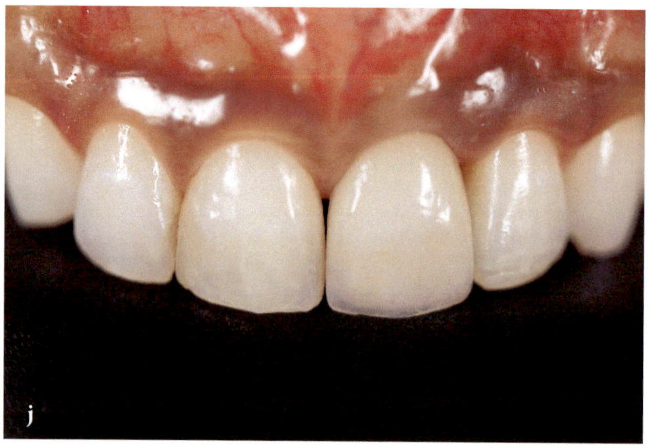
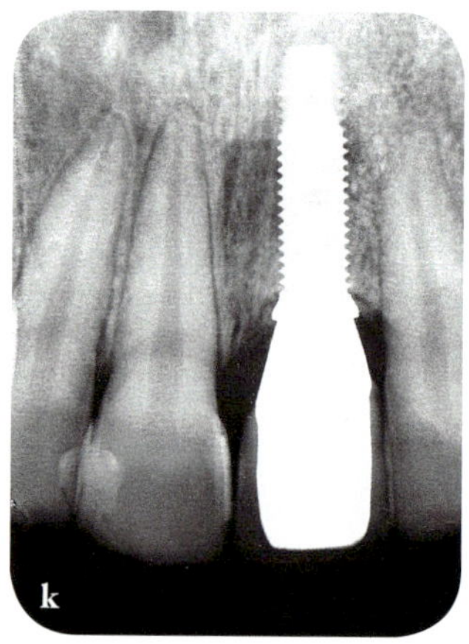

Figs 4-8j and 4-8k Facial view *(j)* and periapical radiograph *(k)* of the definitive restoration.

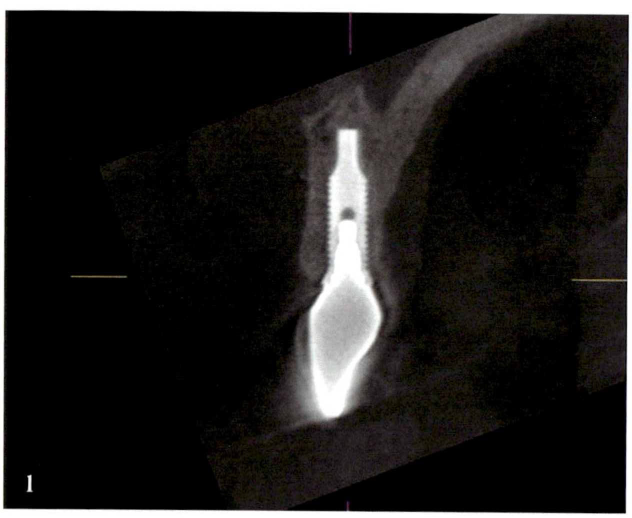

Fig 4-8l One-year CT evaluation.

☞ Clinical tips

Flap elevation during the socket preservation procedure would have aided debridement and the precise positioning of the membrane. Staged extraction and implant placement with GBR might be a better option in a case such as this.

Root Submergence Technique for Pontic Site Development

Pontics in the esthetic region in multiple implant cases

Today, a single-tooth implant in the esthetic region has good potential for success, but restoring multiple-tooth defects with implant-supported prostheses that resemble the natural dentition is still a challenge. Once an implant is placed in function, the biologic width is established around the implant-abutment interface. This triggers peri-implant bone remodeling and resorption. The creation of papillae between adjoining implants becomes difficult because of this potential bone remodeling and resorption and because of compromised blood supply in the peri-implant tissue. The ultimate height of the soft tissue around adjoining implants is lower than that around and adjacent to the natural tooth or pontic. A body of current evidence suggests that inserting a pontic to avoid adjacent implants helps to maintain the bone and soft tissue around the implant, creating a more esthetic result.

Using the root submergence technique (RST) to maintain the natural tooth at the intended pontic site can preserve a much greater amount of surrounding tissue than using the socket preservation technique, which almost always leads to some crestal bone resorption. RST maintains the natural attachment apparatus of the tooth in the pontic site, which allows for better preservation of the alveolar bone frame and an esthetic final result. In some cases, orthodontic extrusion is necessary to create underlying bone support for the ideal pontic form (Figs 4-9 and 4-10).

Root submergence technique: Case 1

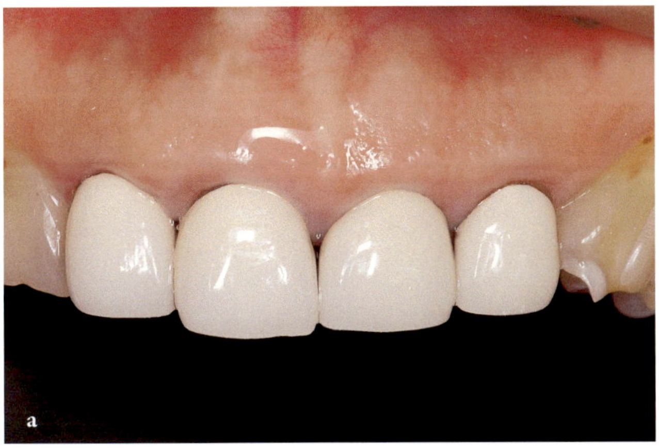

Fig 4-9a A 55-year-old woman presented with esthetic and functional problems.

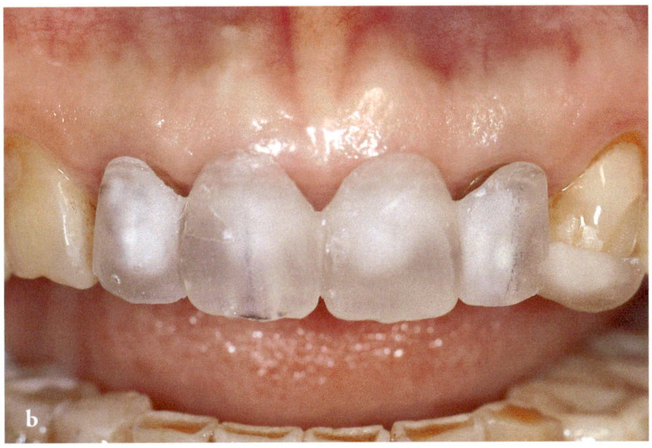

Fig 4-9b A surgical stent was created to represent the treatment goal.

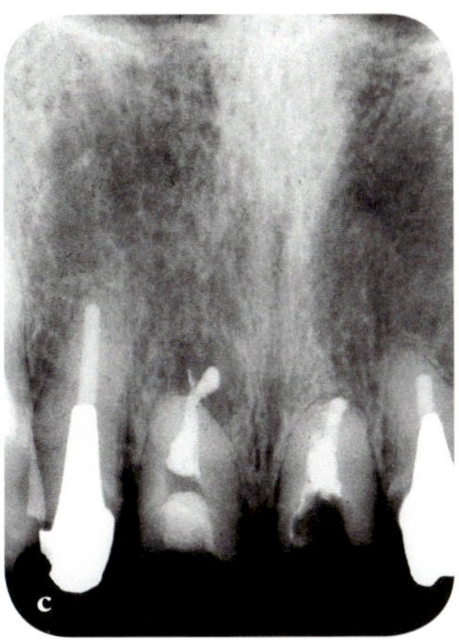

Fig 4-9c The central incisors and the left lateral incisor will be replaced by two implants and a pontic.

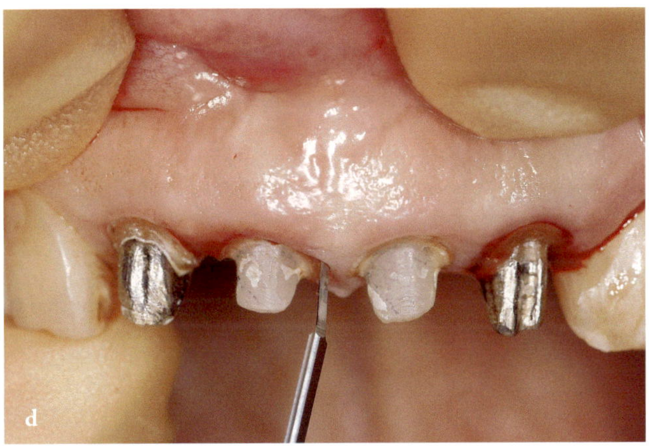

Fig 4-9d Facial view before surgery.

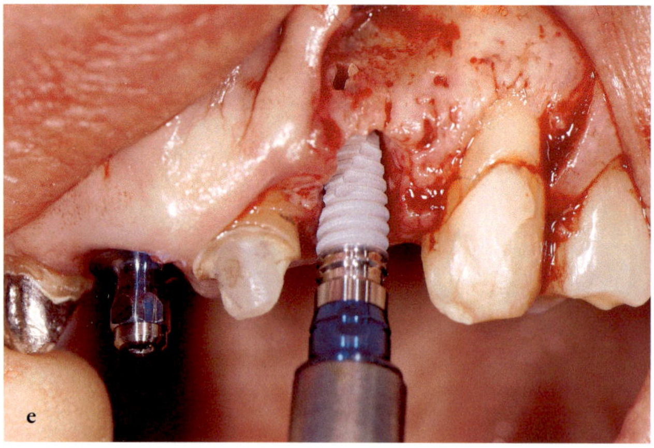

Fig 4-9e Flapless immediate implant placement was performed at the right central incisor site, which was Class 1 (see Fig 3-10), and immediate implant placement and simultaneous GBR were performed at the left lateral incisor site, which was Class 3.

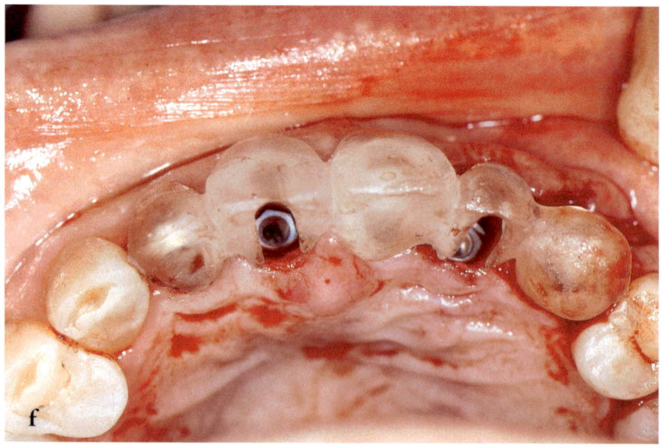

Fig 4-9f The implants were ideally positioned.

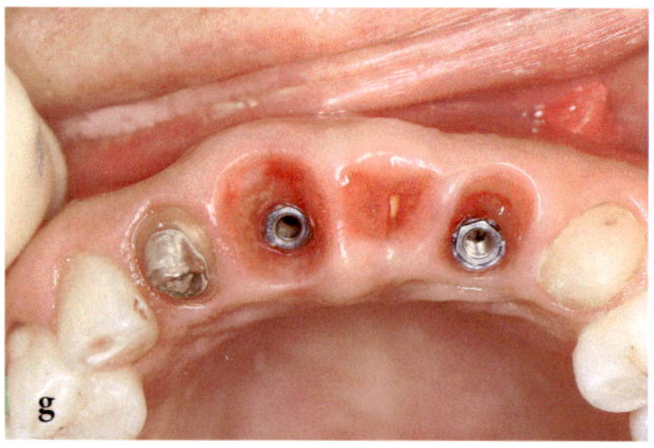

Fig 4-9g Occlusal view 2 months following the reduction of remaining root of the left central incisor to the alveolar crest level.

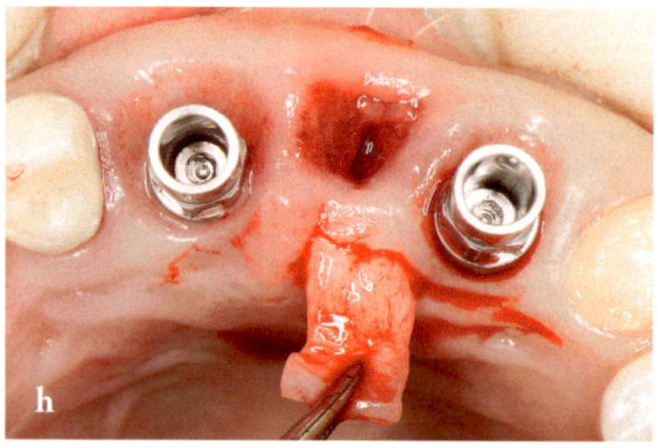

Fig 4-9h After thorough debridement of the root surface of the left central incisor, a connective tissue graft was inserted palatally.

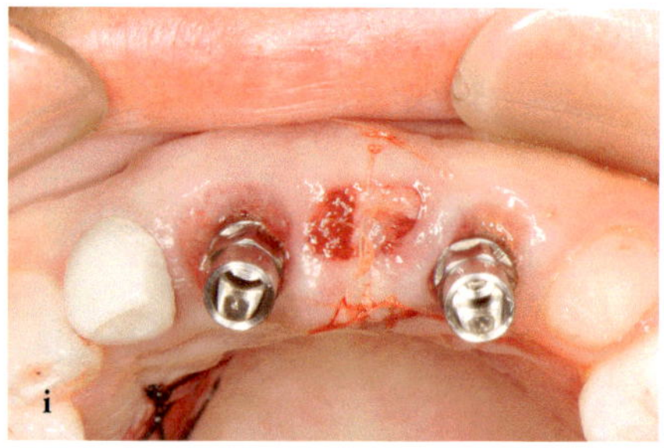

Fig 4-9i Occlusal view after suturing.

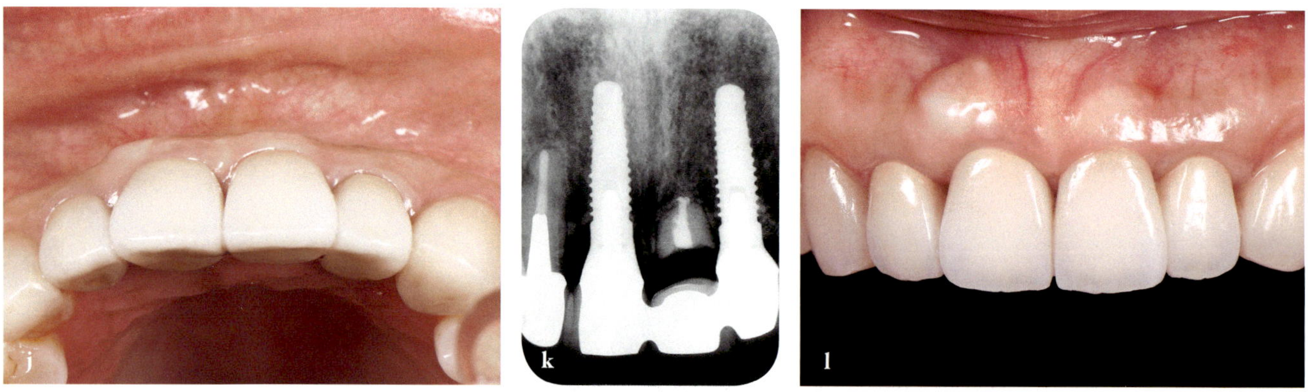

Figs 4-9j to 4-9l Results 3 years after immediate implant placement and 2 years 3 months following root submergence. A healthy and natural soft tissue profile was maintained at the implant and pontic sites.

Root submergence technique: Case 2

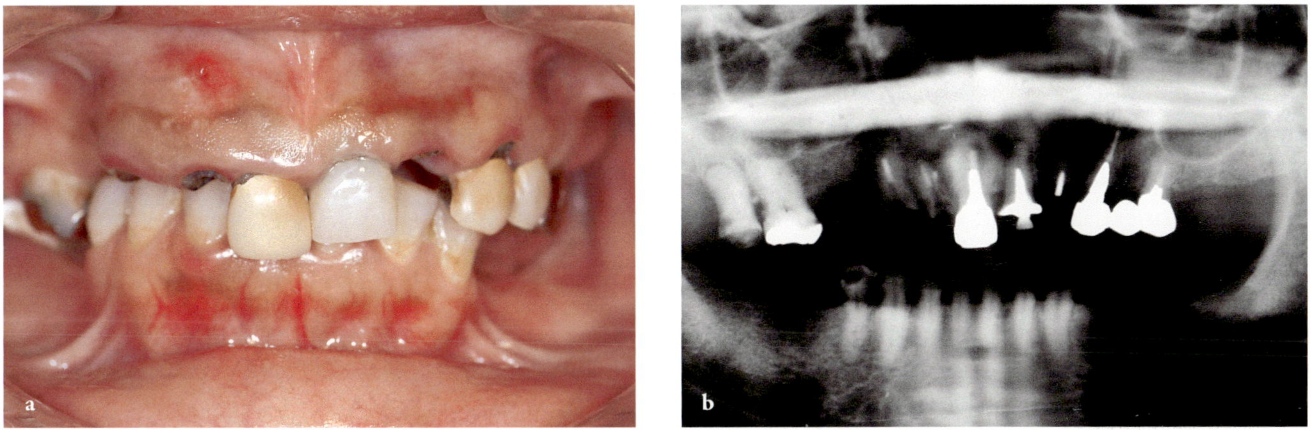

Figs 4-10a and 4-10b Facial view *(a)* and panoramic radiograph *(b)* at initial examination. The patient requested implant treatment.

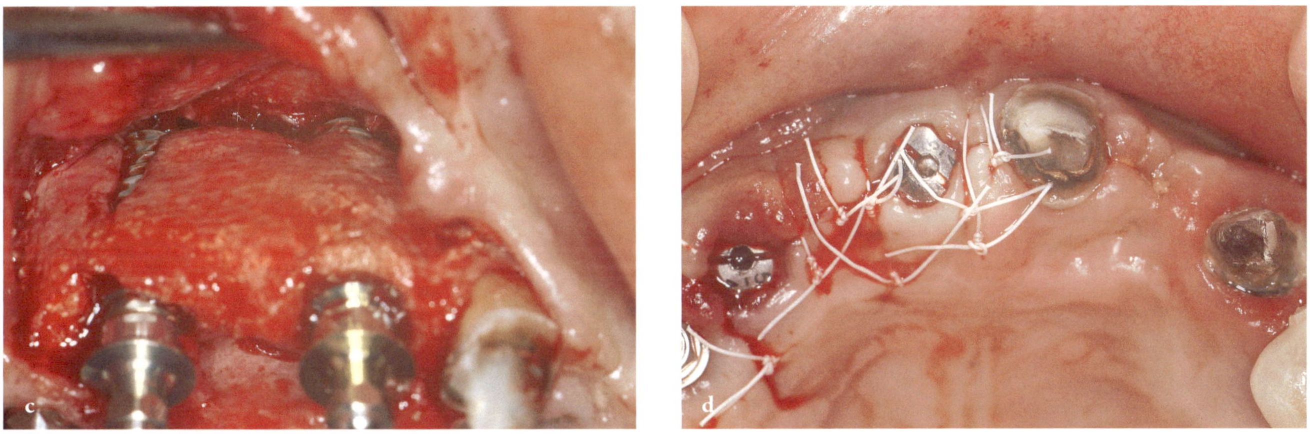

Figs 4-10c and 4-10d Following GBR, two implants were placed in the right central incisor to canine area using a single-stage protocol.

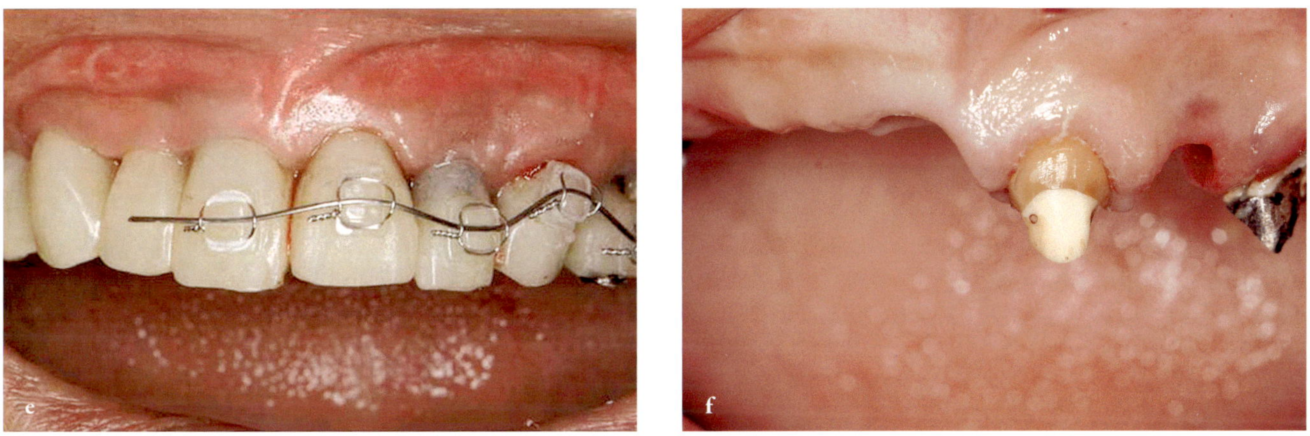

Figs 4-10e and 4-10f The left central incisor and canine were orthodontically extruded, using an implant as an anchor.

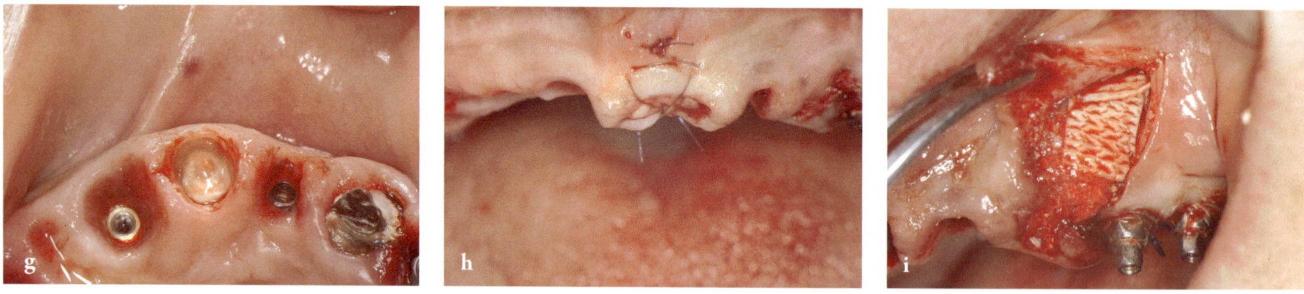

Figs 4-10g to 4-10i The left central incisor was reduced to the alveolar crest level and submerged with a connective tissue graft. Following extraction of the left canine, the extraction socket was augmented with bone graft and a resorbable membrane. An ovate pontic was placed to maintain the papillae form.

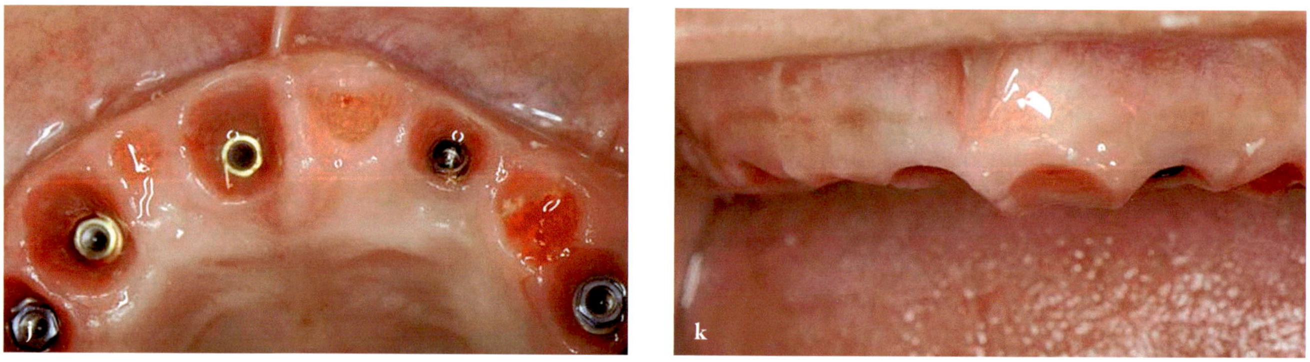

Figs 4-10j and 4-10k The alveolar ridge form and papillae were well maintained with the submergence of the left central incisor.

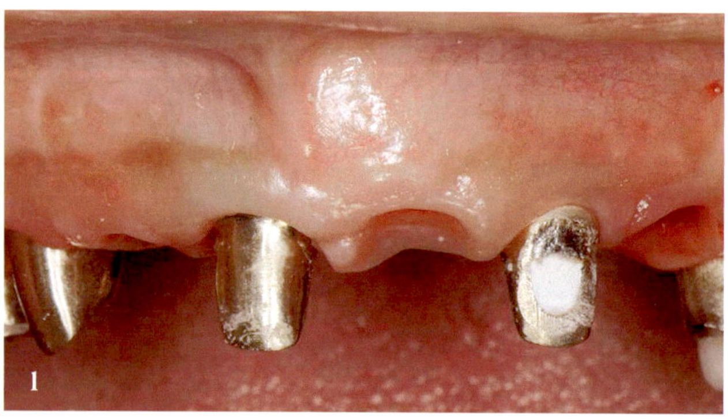

Fig 4-10l Facial view with definitive abutments.

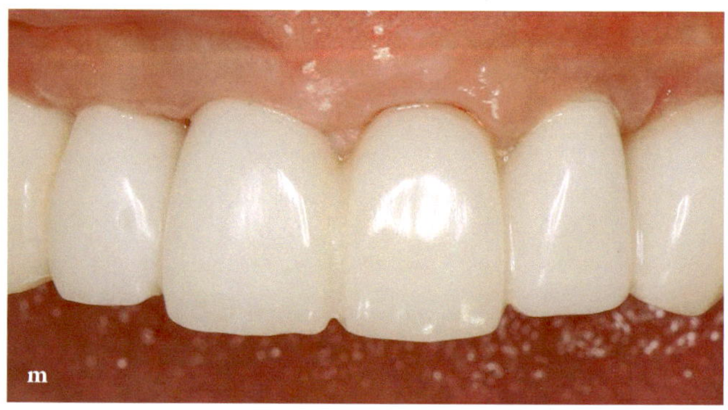

Fig 4-10m Facial view with definitive restorations.

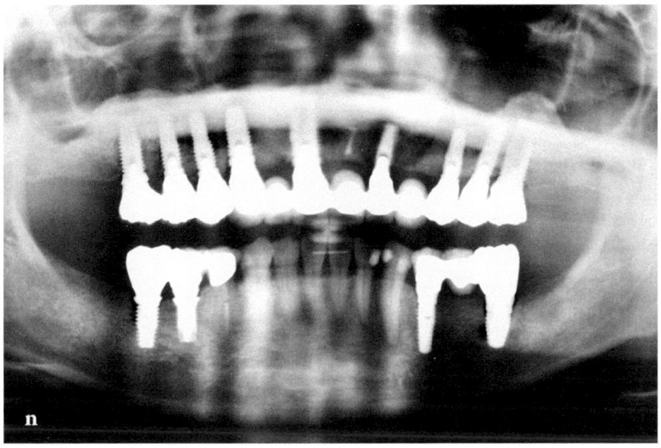

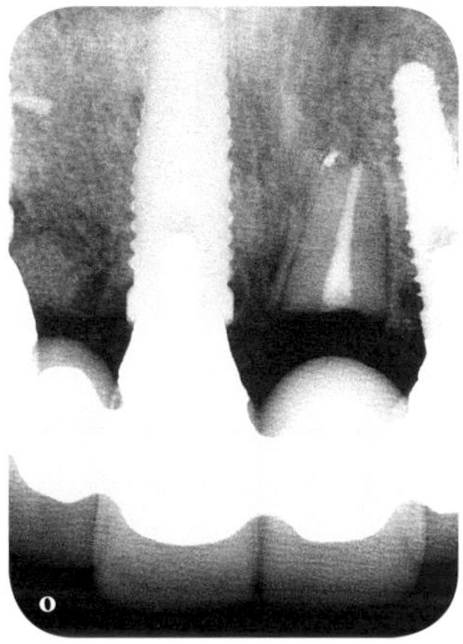

Figs 4-10n and 4-10o Panoramic *(n)* and periapical *(o)* radiographs with the definitive restorations in place.

Literature review

In the second half of the 1960s, clinicians documented use of a procedure in both animals and humans that involved resecting the crown of a tooth, covering it with a buccal or buccolingual flap, and submerging the root. This procedure was originally conceived as a way to prevent alveolar bone resorption following tooth extractions. In most cases, dental pulps were vitally preserved, or root canal treatments were performed before or during the procedure. The purpose was to prevent epithelial downgrowth in periodontal regeneration or to maintain the alveolar ridge height and frame for overdenture treatment. According to Casey and Lauciello,[9] there have been reports of more than 10 years' observation of submerged endodontically treated roots under complete dentures without resorption of alveolar bone.

O'Neal et al[10] performed a 30- to 120-day histologic examination of 16 endodontically treated submerged roots in dogs that were cut 2 mm below the surface of the bone. They reported that 62.5% of root specimens had more than half of their cut surface covered with bone and identified complete bone coverage on the cut surfaces of the 60-day specimens.

In 1975, Guyer[11] submerged vital roots for the first time in a human and reported that the two roots displayed radiographically normal conditions and that the alveolar ridge frames were clinically maintained for 27 months.

In 1976, Plata et al[12] performed a 12-week histologic evaluation of 12 vital submerged roots that were cut 2 mm below the surface of the bone. They reported that eight of the roots had complete bone coverage on the cut surfaces and all pulps were vitally retained.

Bowers et al[13] submerged vital teeth with infrabony defects from nine patients and created notches at regions on the root that had been covered with dental calculus. They performed vital RST on 30 regions with bone graft (demineralized FDBA) and on 13 regions without bone graft. After 6 months, all 43 regions were evaluated histologically. The volume and frequency of the formation of bone, cementum, and new attachment increased with the use of bone graft, and there was potential for the formation of a new attachment apparatus on the cut surface of the dentin. This study showed that epithelial exclusion with bone graft and root submergence could be used to treat infrabony defects with a high level of predictability. No root resorption, ankylosis, or pulp death was observed. Documented complications with RST include gingival tissue perforation and cyst formation, but necrotic and infected dental pulps have seldom been reported. To prevent perforation, the roots should be excised so that they are positioned slightly lower than the surface of the bone and then beveled to avoid exposed sharp edges.

von Wowern and Winther[14] published a 4-year follow-up study of 20 cases of crown-resected, endodontically treated roots. They reported that gingival tissue perforation occurred in 11 cases, which they designated as failures. If roots were submerged and dentures were placed, the alveolar ridge was often not preserved. There are no similar reports of gingival perforation or exposure associated with pontic sites where occlusal forces were not directly acting on the gingiva. Harper[15] submerged an endodontically treated root in the anterior maxilla, creating a "submerged root/pontic" site. Successful results were demonstrated over a 6-year follow-up period.

Although implant technology is constantly improving, it is safe to assume that implants will never surpass the natural tooth's ability to preserve the surrounding bone and soft tissue height. RST eliminates the risk of caries and periodontitis and, more importantly, allows for maximum preservation of the surrounding alveolar bone and soft tissue by retaining the natural tooth root.

In the 1960s, RST was introduced to preserve the alveolar ridge; later it was used to prevent downgrowth of the epithelium during the regeneration of periodontal tissue. Today, the concepts and techniques of osseointegration, periodontal plastic surgery, tissue regeneration, and esthetic restoration have dramatically advanced our field. RST should be recognized anew as an effective technique for maximum tissue preservation and for enhancing the esthetics of pontic sites in the esthetic zone (see Figs 4-9 and 4-10).

References

1. Schropp L, Wenzel A, Kostopoulos L, Karring T. Bone healing and soft tissue contour changes following single-tooth extraction: A clinical and radiographic 12-month prospective study. Int J Periodontics Restorative Dent 2003;23:313–323.
2. Lekovic V, Kenney EB, Weinlaender M, et al. A bone regenerative approach to alveolar ridge maintenance following tooth extraction. Report of 10 cases. J Periodontol 1997;68:563–570.
3. Lekovic V, Camargo PM, Klokkevold PR, et al. Preservation of alveolar bone in extraction sockets using bioabsorbable membranes. J Periodontol 1998;69:1044–1049.
4. Nevins M, Camelo M, De Paoli S, et al. A study of the fate of the buccal wall of extraction sockets of teeth with prominent roots. Int J Periodontics Restorative Dent 2006;26:19–29.
5. Wang HL, Kiyonobu K, Neiva RF. Socket augmentation: Rationale and technique. Implant Dent 2004;13:286–296.
6. Iasella JM, Greenwell H, Miller RL, et al. Ridge preservation with freeze-dried bone allograft and a collagen membrane compared to extraction alone for implant site development: A clinical and histologic study in humans. J Periodontol 2003;74:990–999.
7. Bartee BK. Evaluation of a new polytetrafluoroethylene guided tissue regeneration membrane in healing extraction sites. Compend Contin Educ Dent 1998;19:1256–1258, 1260, 1262–1264.
8. Fickl S, Zuhr O, Wachtel H, Bolz W, Huerzeler M. Tissue alterations after tooth extraction with and without surgical trauma: A volumetric study in the beagle dog. J Clin Periodontol 2008;35:356–363.
9. Casey DM, Lauciello FR. A review of the submerged-root concept. J Prosthet Dent 1980;43:128–132.
10. O'Neal RB, Gound T, Levin MP, del Rio CE. Submergence of roots for alveolar bone preservation. I. Endodontically treated roots. Oral Surg Oral Med Oral Pathol 1978;45:803–810.
11. Guyer SE. Selectively retained vital roots for partial support of overdentures: A patient report. J Prosthet Dent 1975;33:258–263.
12. Plata RL, Kelln EE, Linda L. Intentional retention of vital submerged roots in dogs. Oral Surg Oral Med Oral Pathol 1976;42:100–108.
13. Bowers GM, Chadroff B, Carnevale R, et al. Histologic evaluation of new attachment apparatus formation in humans. Part III. J Periodontol 1989;60:675–682.
14. von Wowern N, Winther S. Submergence of roots for alveolar ridge preservation. A failure (4-year follow-up study). Int J Oral Surg 1981;10:247–250.
15. Harper KA. Submerging an endodontically treated root to preserve the alveolar ridge under a bridge—A case report. Dent Update 2002;29:200–203.

Chapter 5

Ridge Augmentation

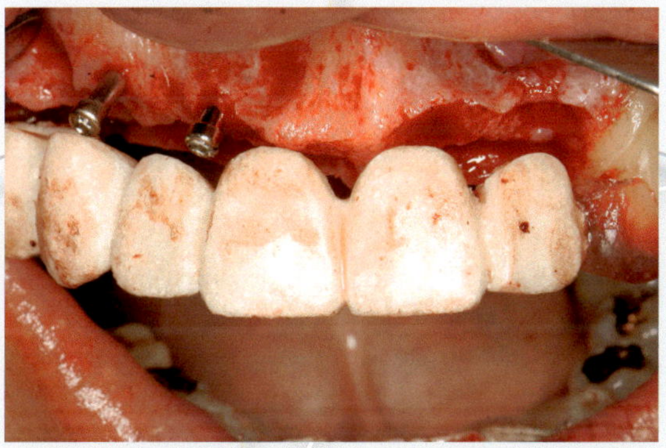

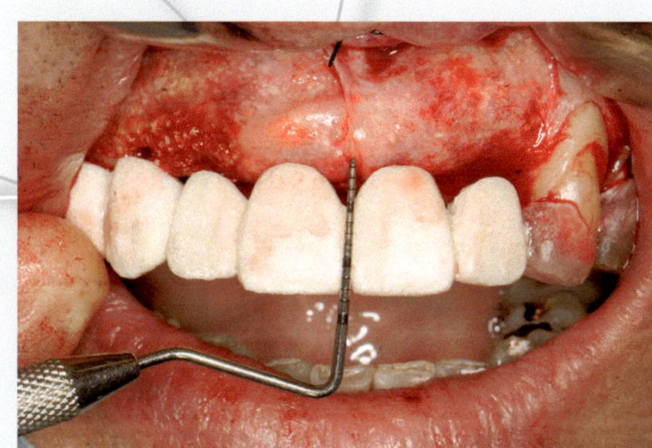

Ridge augmentation is now considered vital not only for facilitating implant placement in the atrophic alveolar ridge but, for creating esthetic final results with implant treatment. In this chapter, the goals, timing, and surgical techniques of ridge augmentation are discussed with an emphasis on achieving optimal esthetic results from implant treatment.

Necessity of Ridge Augmentation

Alveolar ridge remodeling and resorption are inevitable after tooth extraction, even if socket preservation techniques are used. Existing periodontal and periapical infections or denture use may increase bone resorption following extraction. Ridge augmentation is therefore necessary to support an esthetic soft tissue profile around the definitive restorations in most cases the authors treat today.

Options for Ridge Augmentation

Ridge augmentation can be accomplished through the following procedures:

- Guided bone regeneration (GBR)
- Block bone graft
- Distraction osteogenesis
- Orthodontic forced eruption

The alveolar ridge can be augmented three-dimensionally (3D) with GBR or a block bone graft. Primary closure of the soft tissue is one of the keys for successful augmentation with either GBR or the block bone graft.[1] GBR is used more often than the block bone graft because it is less invasive and less technique sensitive. Advantages and disadvantages of GBR are listed in Box 5-1. Studies have reported the range of augmentation to be 1.5 to 5.5 mm horizontally[2,3] and 3 to 8.5 mm vertically.[4–6] Actual results may vary based upon clinical skills, surgical protocol, the patient's healing potential, and the location of the targeted augmentation site. Implants placed in regenerated bone show similar success and long-term stability compared with those placed in native bone.[7,8]

Purpose of GBR in Implant Treatment

There are two major types of goals for ridge augmentation in implant treatment—functional and esthetic. Functional goals include *(1)* augmenting an atrophic alveolar ridge to enable implant placement, *(2)* allowing for optimal length and diameter of the implant for better biomechanics, and *(3)* creating a ridge and crown form that facilitates access for oral hygiene maintenance by the patient (Fig 5-1). In the molar region, functional goals should be kept in mind when planning ridge augmentation techniques and sequencing.

Simply placing an implant in existing alveolar bone does not guarantee an esthetic result or the implant's longevity. The implant must be placed in an ideal position in all three dimensions. Further, a sufficient amount of surrounding bone should be augmented to sustain adequate papilla height and to prevent gingival recession, thereby avoiding the common effects of implant-specific bone remodeling. In relation to tooth extraction and implant placement, the timing and sequencing of ridge augmentation during implant treatment is critical.

Box 5-1 Advantages and disadvantages of GBR

Advantages
- Can produce three-dimensional alveolar ridge augmentation
- Compatible with a variety of bone graft materials
- Can be performed simultaneously with implant placement
- Compatible with complex ridge defect anatomies

Disadvantages
- Has the potential to cause soft tissue complications
- Requires reentry surgery to remove barrier membranes
- May cause a coronal shift of the mucogingival junction

Functional goals of GBR

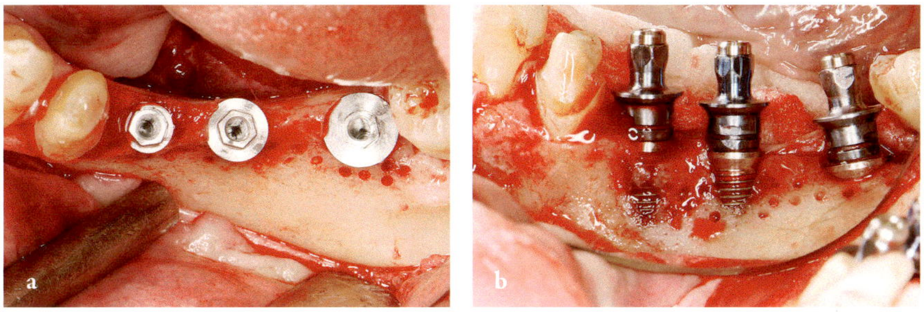

Figs 5-1a and 5-1b Implants were placed in the molar region of a narrow alveolar ridge, and buccal threads were exposed.

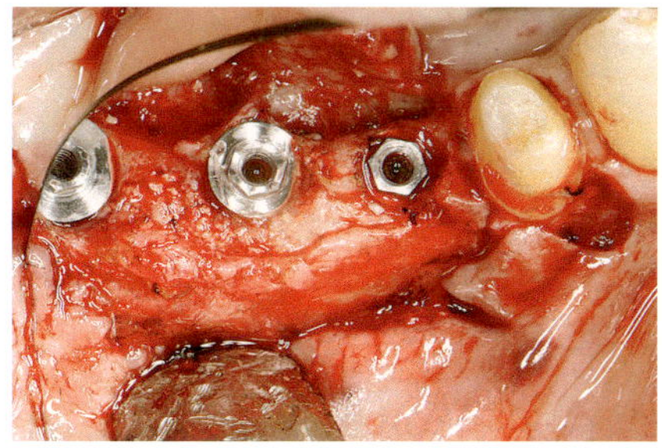

Fig 5-1c GBR was carried out with a collagen membrane. The exposed threads were covered with bone.

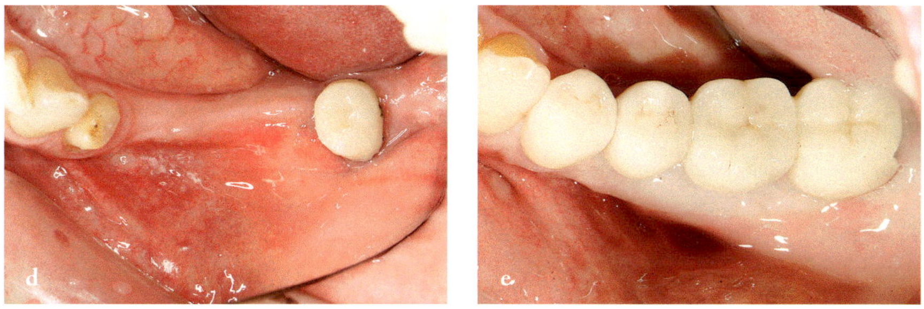

Figs 5-1d and 5-1e Occlusal views, before and after treatment. GBR enabled the final restorations to resemble the natural dentition.

Box 5-2 Timing of extraction and implant placement with GBR

1. Timing of extraction and GBR
   - Immediate GBR: Socket augmentation
   - Early GBR: Following 2 months of healing
   - Delayed GBR: Following 6 months or more of healing
2. Timing of implant placement and GBR
   - Simultaneous approach: Requires 4 to 6 months of healing
   - Staged approach
     a. Extraction: Requires 2 months of healing
     b. GBR: Requires 6 months of healing
     c. Implant placement: Requires 4 to 6 months of healing

Timing of Ridge Augmentation

In full-mouth reconstructions, restoring posterior occlusion and function must be given priority to protect the anterior region. The categorization of the timing of extraction and implant placement with GBR is summarized in Box 5-2.

Timing of extraction and GBR

Immediate GBR (socket augmentation)

The advantages of immediate GBR are that it reduces the number of surgical interventions while maximizing the preservation of existing tissue. Indications are:

- Severe bone loss but adequate soft tissue height around the tooth targeted for extraction (Fig 5-2).
- Bone augmentation outside of the extraction socket (In this circumstance, immediate GBR ensures esthetic results.).

GBR with a resorbable membrane

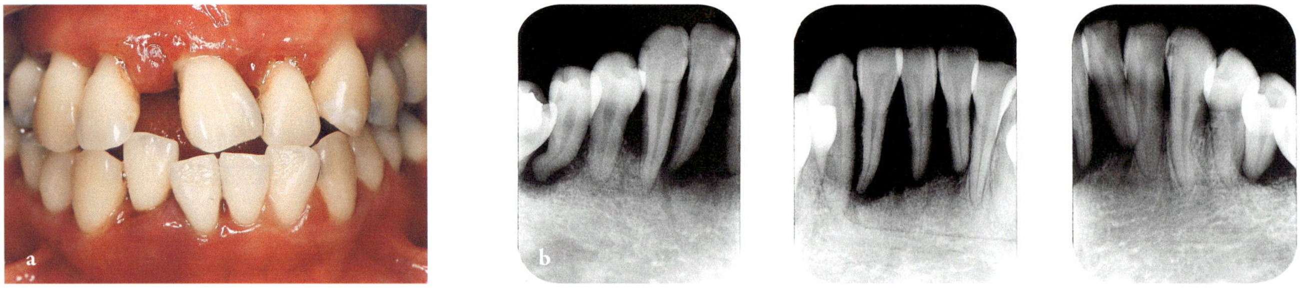

Figs 5-2a and 5-2b Facial view *(a)* and periapical radiographs *(b)* at initial examination. Advanced bone loss beyond the apex was observed.

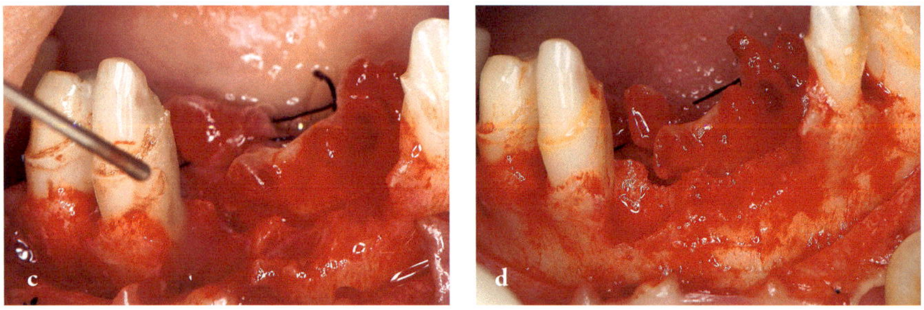

Figs 5-2c and 5-2d Extraction and immediate GBR were performed to prevent soft tissue shrinkage following extraction.

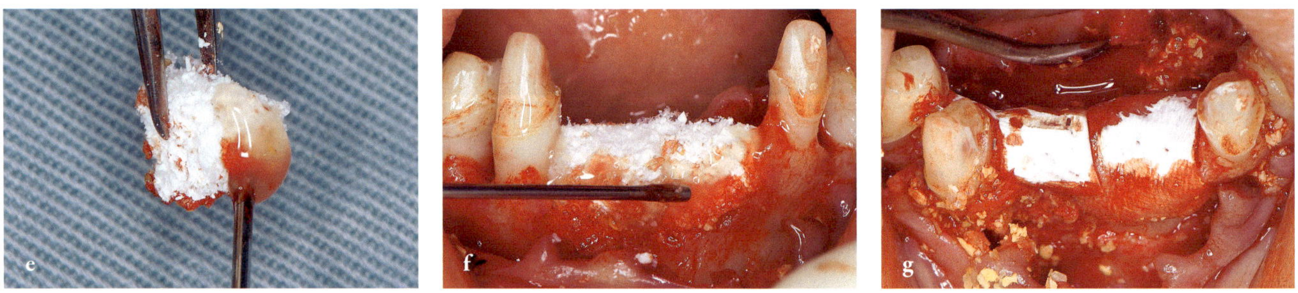

Figs 5-2e to 5-2g Bone graft material and a resorbable membrane were placed.

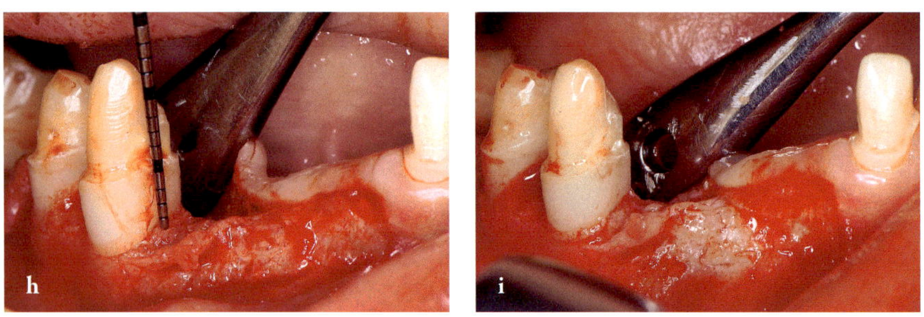

Figs 5-2h and 5-2i Reentry 1 year 3 months following GBR. The alveolar ridge was preserved and augmented.

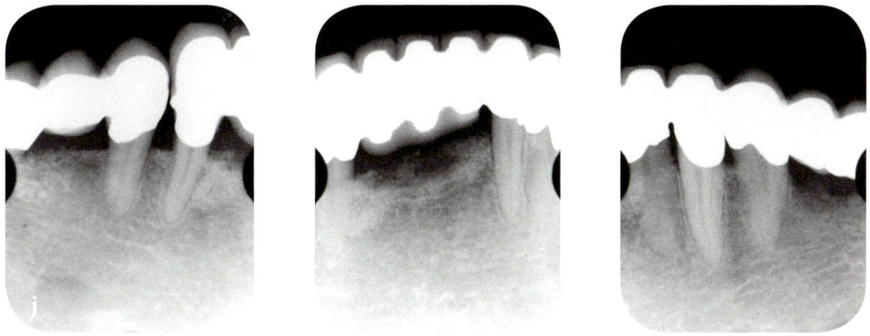

Fig 5-2j At the 5-year follow-up, the alveolar ridge was well maintained.

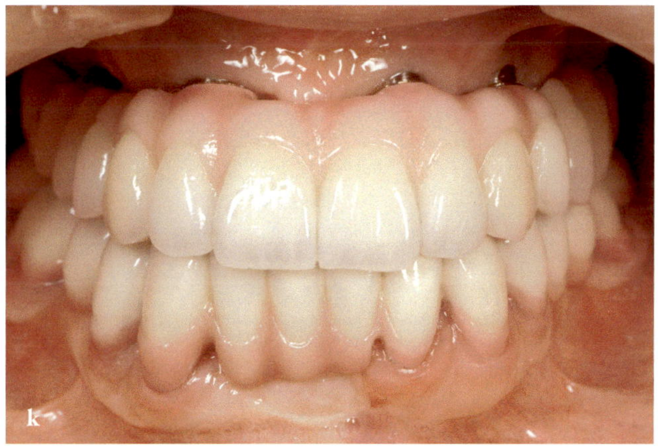

Fig 5-2k Clinical appearance 5 years after GBR, 2 years after treatment was completed, shows that the patient has performed excellent home care.

With immediate GBR, it is necessary to obtain primary closure by coronally advancing the buccal flap or by another measure, such as a soft tissue graft.

Early GBR

Early GBR is performed following soft tissue healing over the extraction socket, which is complete approximately 2 months after extraction. Woven bone occupies the majority of the extraction socket at this time. Early GBR can reduce the risk of barrier membrane exposure as well as the amount of augmentation required because of the minimal bone resorption that occurs after extraction. In full-mouth reconstructions, extraction of anterior teeth should be planned after restoring the posterior occlusion and approximately 8 weeks prior to GBR.

Delayed GBR

Delayed GBR is performed after complete healing of the extraction socket, which usually takes 6 months or longer. Soft and hard tissues have completely healed at this time. The amount of augmentation required is greatest due to the complete remodeling and resorption of the extraction socket.

Timing of implant placement and GBR

Simultaneous approach

The simultaneous approach, in which implant placement and GBR are performed at the same time, requires a 4- to 6-month healing period. This approach is possible if there is enough native alveolar bone available for primary implant stability, but it could produce complications that result in functional and esthetic problems. The 3D positioning of the implant in a compromised alveolar ridge requires a high level of skill. The vertical limit of bone augmentation is 5 mm in the mandibular molar area and 3 mm in the maxillary molar area. Anterior vertical augmentation is usually accomplished with the staged approach whereas horizontal augmentation and implant placement are often performed simultaneously.

Staged approach

The staged approach requires more treatment interventions and increases the total treatment duration: It requires a 2-month healing period for extraction, a 6-month or greater healing period for GBR, and a 4- to 6-month healing period for osseointegration. However, it also increases treatment predictability and likely results in fewer complications.

Goals of GBR in the 4D Concept

Under the four-dimensional (4D) concept of treatment, the objectives of GBR differ depending upon considerations such as location and esthetic and functional requirements (Box 5-3). Because pressure must be relieved from the GBR site during the healing period, fixed provisional restoration is preferable whenever possible. Further, posterior occlusal support is critical for the longevity of the esthetic anterior definitive restoration. Accordingly, in a given treatment plan, posterior GBR should be considered first, keeping functional and occlusal restoration as its primary goals. Anterior GBR should then be considered with the goal being an esthetic result.

GBR in the posterior region

One goal of GBR in the posterior region is to augment the alveolar ridge to adequately accommodate the diameter, length, and number of implants (Fig 5-3). Another goal is to achieve a definitive restoration that has an appropriate crown and embrasure form so that the patient may have better accessibility for oral hygiene procedures.

Box 5-3 Objectives of GBR in the 4D concept

1. Posterior region: Occlusal and functional rehabilitation
2. Anterior region: Esthetics

Vertical ridge augmentation in the molar region

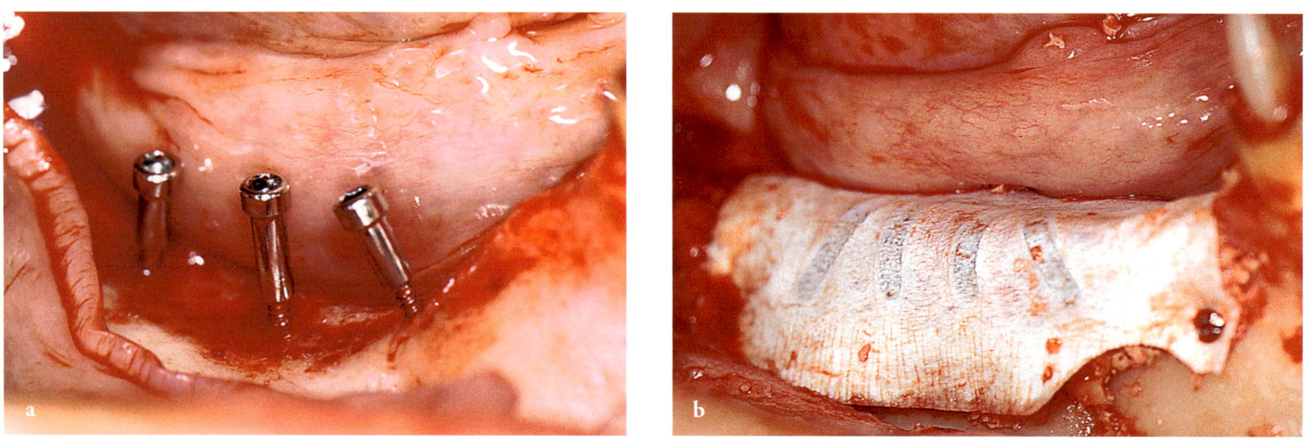

Figs 5-3a and 5-3b A 63-year-old woman required vertical ridge augmentation in the right premolar-molar area. There was not enough residual bone for primary implant stability.

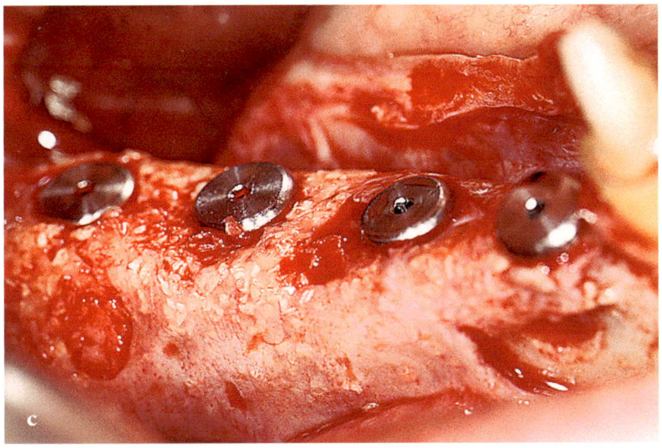

Fig 5-3c Ten months later, implants were placed in an ideal position.

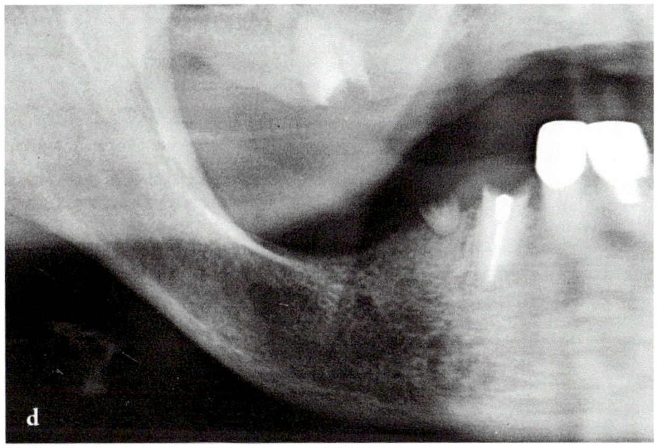

Fig 5-3d Pretreatment radiograph.

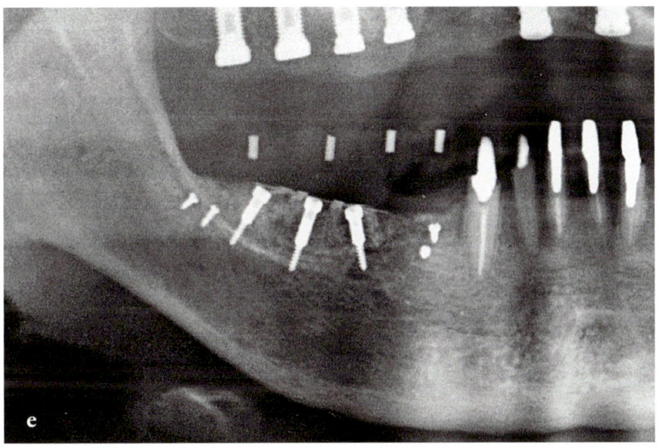

Fig 5-3e Radiograph 9 months after GBR.

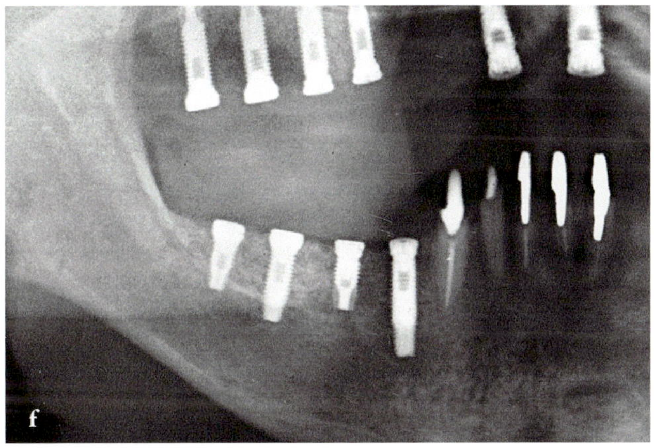

Fig 5-3f Radiograph immediately following implant placement. The implants in the first and second molar sites were placed almost entirely in regenerated bone.

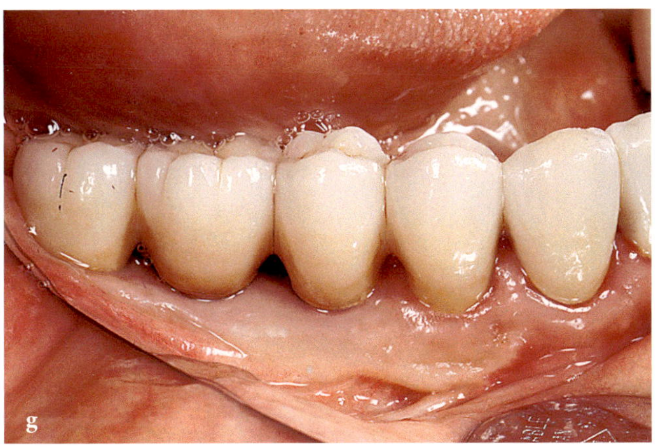

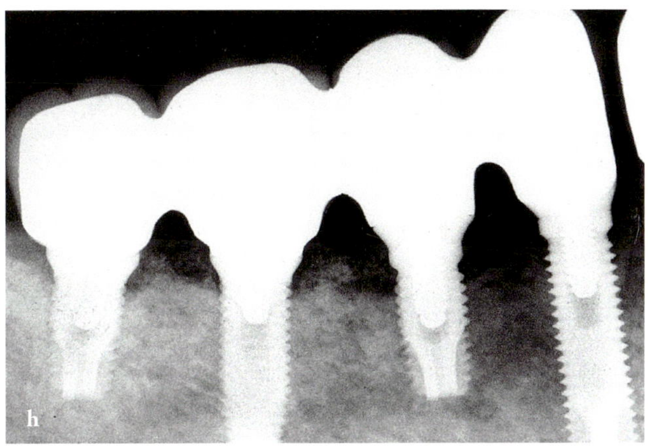

Figs 5-3g and 5-3h Clinical *(g)* and radiographic *(h)* views at the 2-year follow-up.

Horizontal and vertical augmentation goals of GBR

Horizontal width requirements

- 2 mm or greater buccal bone width at platform level.
- Buccal bone beyond the implant body should be even with or buccal to the definitive crown margin.

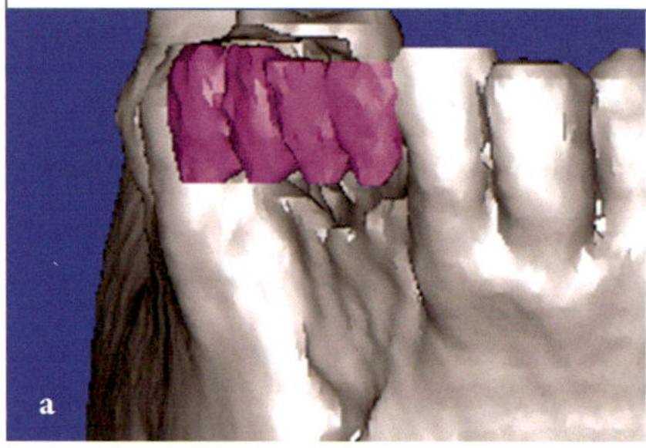

Fig 5-4a 3D image before GBR.

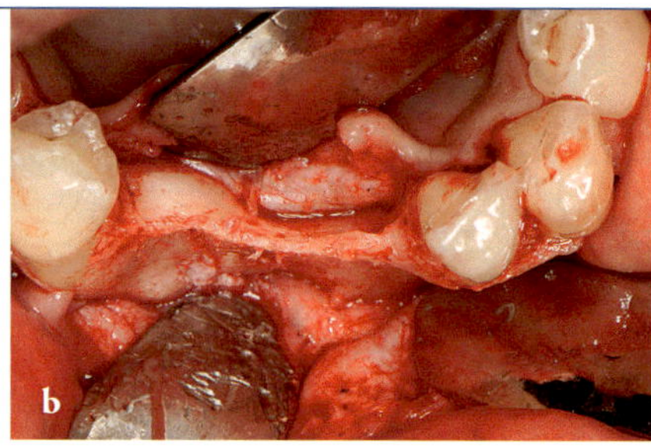

Fig 5-4b Occlusal view before GBR.

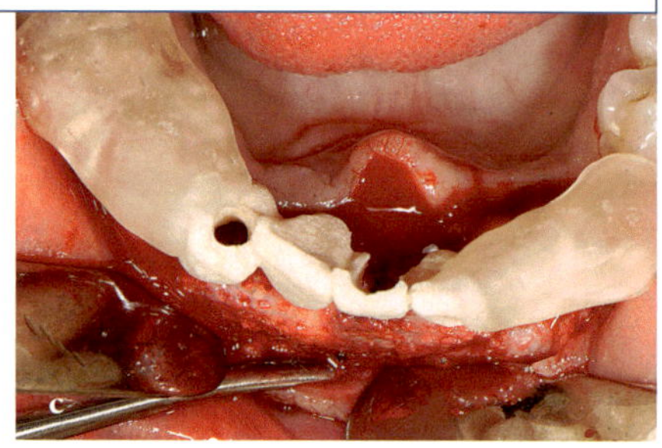

Fig 5-4c Occlusal view after GBR. The alveolar ridge augmentation created bone buccal to the definitive crown margin.

Vertical height requirements

The following reference points indicate vertical augmentation goals:

- Upper lip position
- Contact point (interproximal height of bone [IHB])
- Line connecting the adjacent intact proximal bone levels
- Ideally positioned implant platform

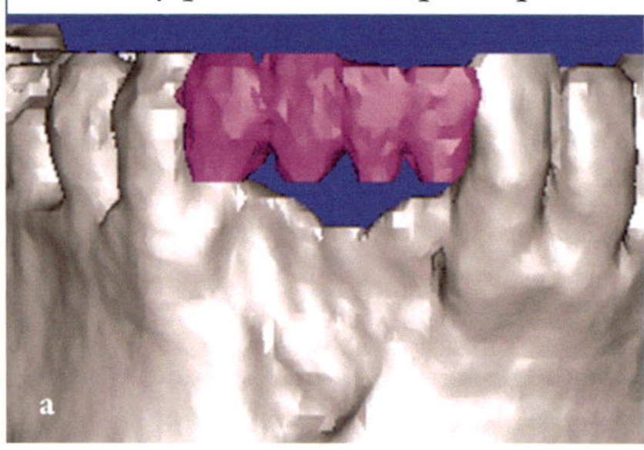

Fig 5-5a 3D image before GBR.

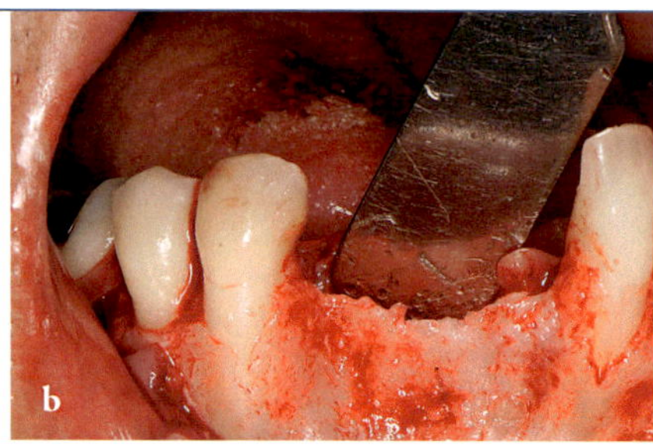

Fig 5-5b Facial view before GBR

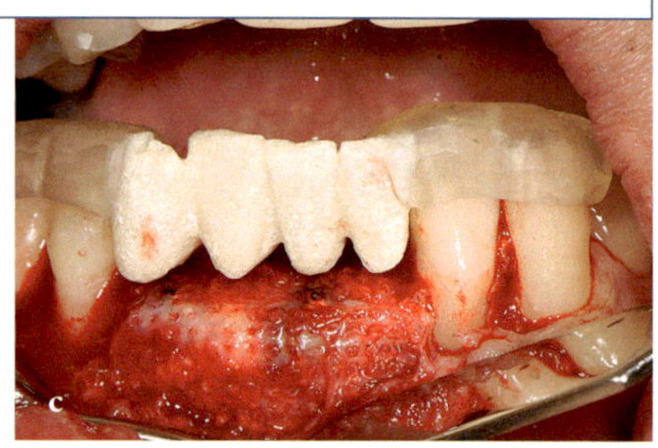

Fig 5-5c Facial view after GBR. Vertical height was augmented so that it would be level with a line connecting the adjacent intact proximal bone levels.

GBR in the anterior region

The 3D requirements of implant placement, including the width (Fig 5-4) and height (Fig 5-5) of the alveolar ridge, must be an integral part of the goals of anterior GBR. These goals, in both single-tooth (Figs 5-6 and 5-7) and multiple-tooth (Figs 5-8 and 5-9) defect cases, are to support a definitive restoration that resembles the natural dentition and has longevity.

Width of alveolar ridge

Spray et al[9] reported that buccal crestal bone height would be reduced with implant placement unless more than 1.8 to 2 mm of buccal bone was present. Grunder et al[10] stated that at least 2 mm of buccal bone must be present at platform level to compensate for the effects of bone remodeling. They also found that if the buccal bone was kept sufficiently wide, adjoining implants still could support papillae, even if the

GBR in the anterior region: Single-tooth implant cases

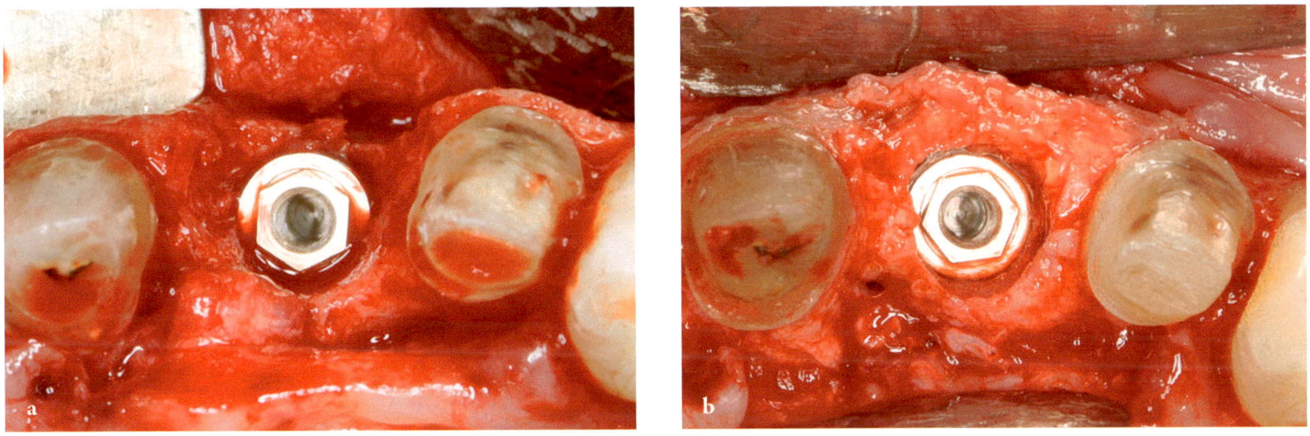

Fig 5-6 Before *(a)* and after *(b)* GBR with a titanium-reinforced nonresorbable membrane.

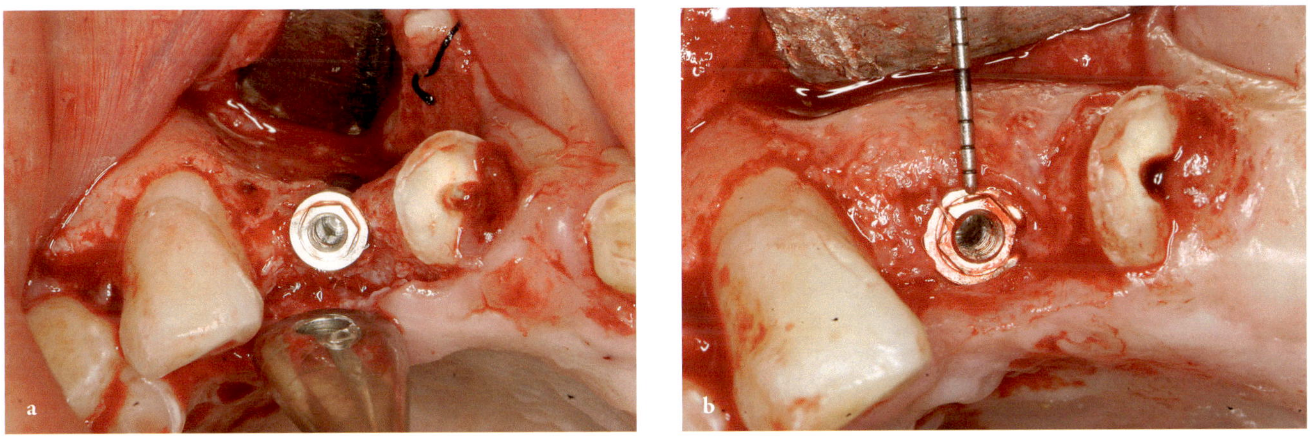

Fig 5-7 Before *(a)* and after *(b)* GBR with titanium mesh and a resorbable membrane. At least 2 mm of buccal bone was regenerated in both this case and that shown in Fig 5-6.

space between them normally would have been deemed inadequate. The ideal buccolingual implant position is about 2 mm lingual of the definitive crown margin. Buccal bone beyond the implant body should be even with or buccal to the definitive crown margin.

Height of alveolar ridge

The goal for the height achieved by GBR is affected by four reference points (see Fig 5-5).

GBR in the anterior region: Multiple-tooth implant cases

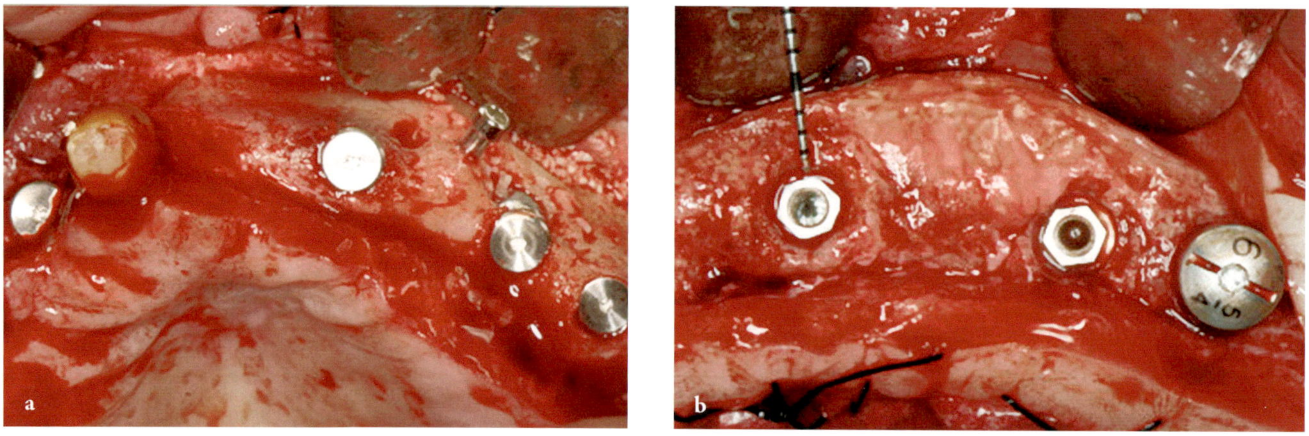

Fig 5-8 Before *(a)* and after *(b)* GBR treatment.

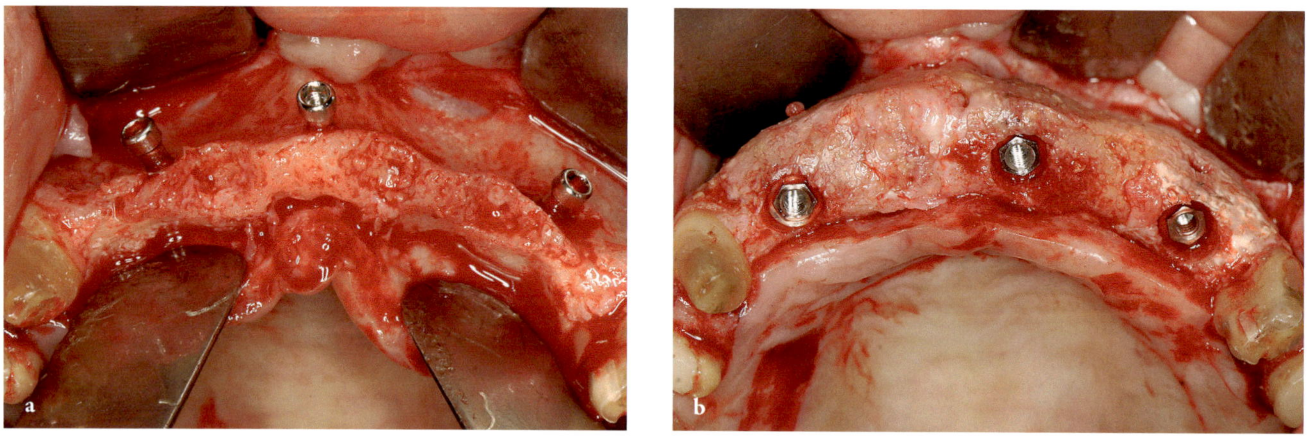

Fig 5-9 Before *(a)* and after *(b)* GBR treatment. Adequate buccal bone was regenerated in this case as well as the one shown in Fig 5-8. Bone remodeling at the platform level would not affect the buccal parameter of the alveolar ridge.

Upper lip position

The position of the central incisor and the incisal edge can be determined based upon the upper lip position (Fig 5-10). After this determination is made, the occlusal plane and the position of the other teeth may be established. Facial and lip analyses are a fundamental component of prosthetic treatment, just as they are in implant treatment.

Contact point (interproximal height of bone)

Salama et al[11] developed a classification system for the interproximal height of bone (IHB) measured from the contact point in six different prosthetic environments. As described in chapter 1, IHB and papilla height differ depending upon the particular prosthetic environment. In a clinical situation, a 4-mm IHB is a realistic goal (Fig 5-11).

Facial and lip line analysis

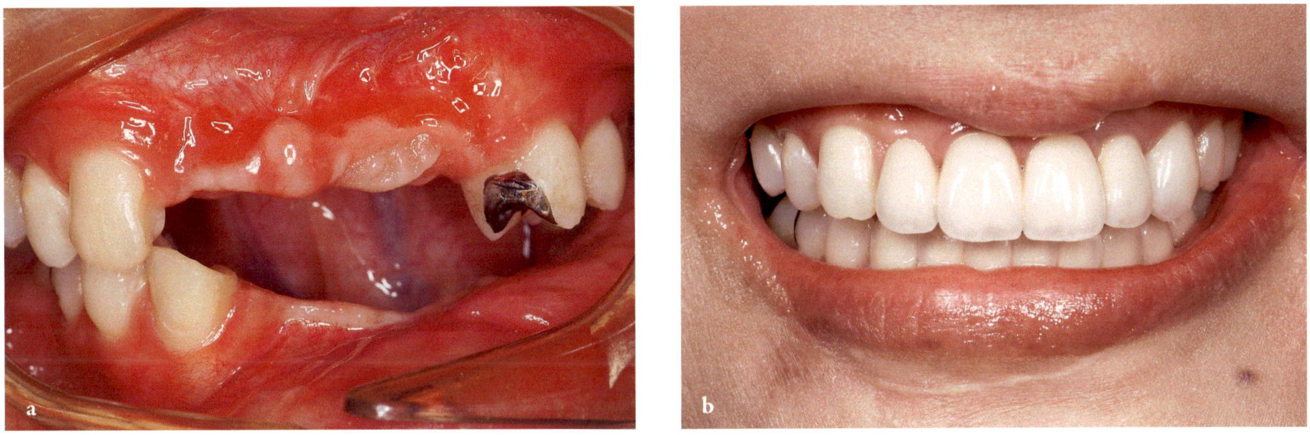

Figs 5-10a and 5-10b Harmonious relationship between upper lip and incisal edge of the definitive restorations. Adequate crown size and form were achieved. Careful facial and smile analysis helped determine the vertical goal of GBR.

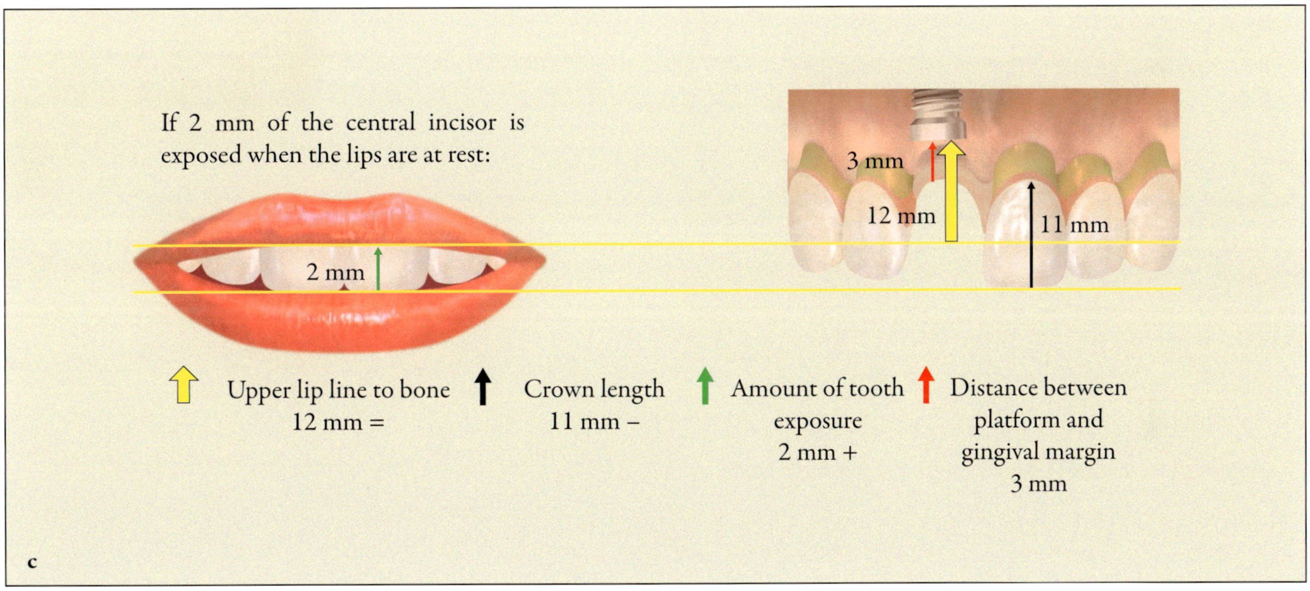

Fig 5-10c Establishing the vertical goal of GBR using the upper lip line. If 2 mm of central incisor is exposed when the lips are at rest and the crown length is 11 mm, the distance between the upper lip line and the bone level at the implant platform should be 12 mm. Interproximal bone should be 2 to 3 mm coronal to the implant platform.

Contact point (IHB)

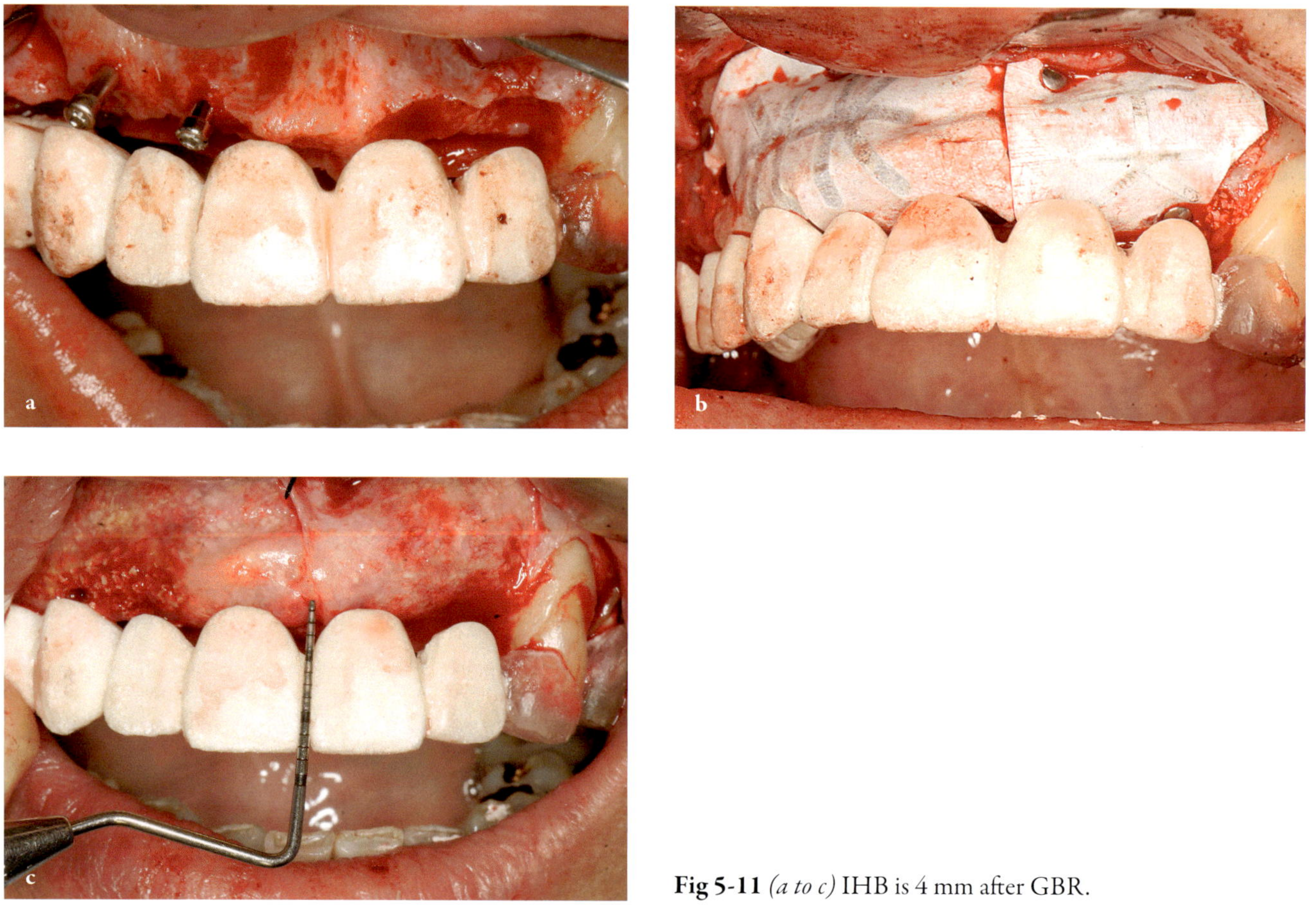

Fig 5-11 *(a to c)* IHB is 4 mm after GBR.

Line connect the adjacent intact proximal bone levels

A line across the edentulous ridge at the level of the adjacent intact proximal bone heights can serve as the vertical goal for GBR (Fig 5-12).

Implant platform position

An ideally positioned implant platform should be located approximately 2 to 3 mm apical to the most apical point of the definitive crown margin (or free gingival margin, *red arrow* in Fig 5-13) and the IHB (*yellow arrow* in Fig 5-13). Facial bone height should be at the implant platform level. Figure 5-14 shows a case in which a bone level 2 mm coronal to the implant platform was achieved.

Ideally, these reference points should converge at almost the same point. This point should correspond to the clinician's goal for the height level of GBR. When the primary concern is esthetics, GBR should provide more vertical height. However, when functional goals are more important, the vertical height does not need to be as great. Having realistic goals and understanding the objectives and limitations of GBR, as well as the 3D requirements of implant placement, are necessary for proper treatment planning and sequencing.

Adjacent intact proximal bone levels

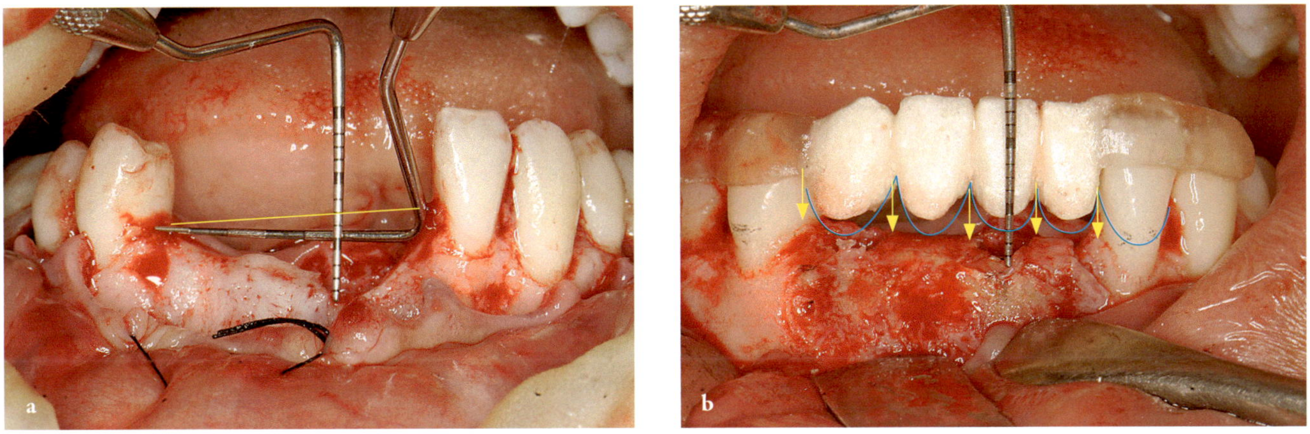

Fig 5-12 *(a)* Patient presented with tooth loss following a motor vehicle accident. The definitive restorations must resemble the adjacent dentition. The implant platform should be positioned 2 to 3 mm from the definitive crown margin. The *yellow line* connecting the adjacent intact proximal bone level indicates the vertical goal of GBR. *(b) An* IHB of 4 mm was established following GBR, and the implant platforms were positioned 2 to 3 mm apical of this level. The *blue scalloped line* indicates the definitive restoration margin.

Implant platform level

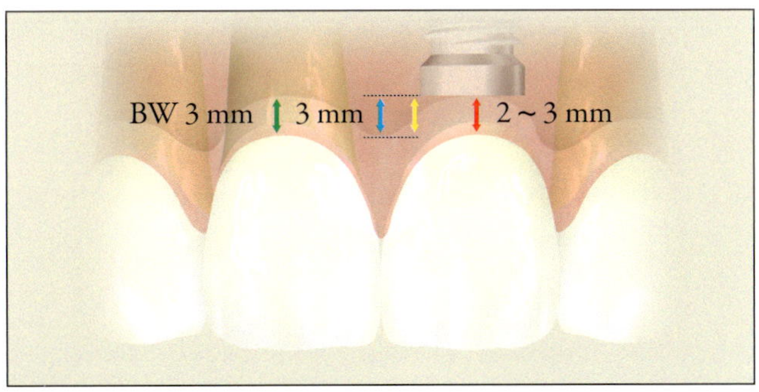

Fig 5-13 The biologic width (BW), measured from the free gingival margin to the bone crest, should be about 3 mm *(green arrow)*. The measurement from the bone crest to the IHB should also be about 3 mm *(blue arrow)*. The implant platform should be 2 to 3 mm apical to the IHB *(yellow arrow)* and the free gingival margin *(red arrow)*.

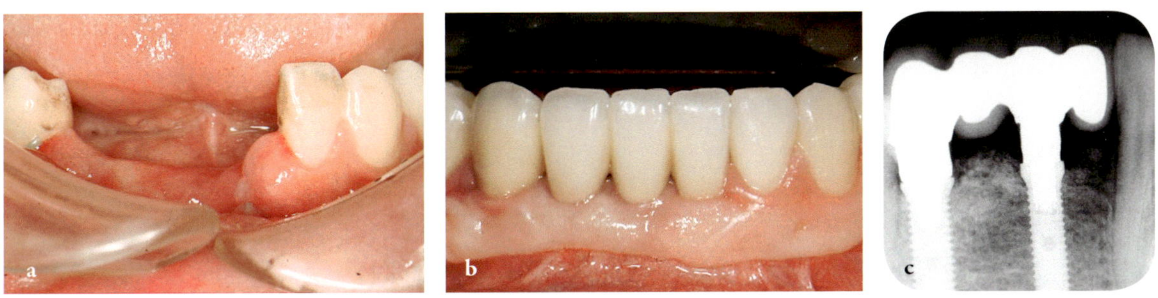

Fig 5-14 *(a)* Initial facial view. *(b)* Facial view of definitive restorations. *(c)* Periapical radiograph of the definitive restorations. In the pontic areas, the bone level is 2 mm coronal to the implant platform. Platform switching was used to minimize bone remodeling around implants.

GBR Materials

Barrier membranes

The guiding principle of GBR is to create and maintain space for bone regeneration using cell occlusive membranes, which prevent soft tissue migration. Primary closure of the GBR site and membrane is the key to successful GBR.

Nonresorbable membranes

A nonresorbable membrane maintains its function until it is removed. The resilient nature of the material allows for easy space maintenance of the GBR site. Its efficacy has been very well documented in the literature. Even an exposed nonresorbable membrane will maintain its barrier function, and bone regeneration is possible if there is no infection at the site. Simion et al[12] demonstrated that if the patient rinses with 0.2% chlorhexidine for 1 minute twice daily, exposed membranes are able to prevent bacterial invasion to the GBR site for 4 weeks. Poor management of an exposed membrane will lead to infection and possibly to a more compromised ridge than before treatment began. Primary closure of the soft tissue at the GBR site prevents membrane exposure, which is why it is critical to a successful result.[13]

Resorbable membranes

The resorbable membranes available today have either a collagen base or a polylactic acid–polyglycolic acid base. The authors do not use the latter type for two reasons. First, it has lower biocompatibility. Second, the byproducts that it produces during the resorption process may negatively affect regeneration. Collagen-based membranes are generally soft and are unable to maintain the necessary space on their own. However, they adapt well to the regeneration site and often require no additional fixation. They also have a higher biocompatibility and less membrane exposure.

Non–cross-linked or weak–cross-linked collagen membranes maintain their function for about 2 months, which is not a sufficient length of time if a large amount of regeneration is required.[14,15] These membranes will resorb quickly and lose their barrier function when they are exposed. They do, however, have a high biocompatibility that is ideal for guided tissue regeneration around the natural dentition.

A cross-linked collagen membrane maintains its barrier function for more than 6 months, even if it is exposed.[16] Its histologic properties are comparable to those of nonresorbable membranes.[17] It has been reported that cross-linked collagen membranes with early exposure allow for more bone regeneration than nonresorbable or non-cross-linked collagen membranes.[18,19] Cross-linked collagen membranes have lower biocompatibility than non–cross-linked membranes and have been reported to have a higher incidence of membrane exposure.[20] Table 5-1 summarizes the authors' clinical impressions and comparisons of these materials.

Compared with titanium-reinforced nonresorbable membranes, resorbable membranes are less able to maintain space for GBR. Therefore, they are not suitable for GBR when an esthetic result is the primary goal.

Bone graft materials

The authors prefer a mixture of autogenous and xenogeneic bone graft materials for GBR. Autogenous bone contains osteogenic cells and growth factor, and xenograft acts as a scaffold for bone formation and as a space maintainer because of its slow resorption process (Fig 5-15).

Table 5-1 Comparison of nonresorbable and collagen membranes

Parameter	Nonresorbable membrane	Cross-linked collagen membrane	Non–cross-linked collagen membrane
Membrane function	Until removed	> 6 months	2 months
Handling	Difficult	Easy	Easy
Biocompatibility	Low	Moderate	High
Cost	High	Low	Low
Complications	High	Moderate	Low
3D GBR	Easy	Difficult	Difficult

GBR case using xenograft

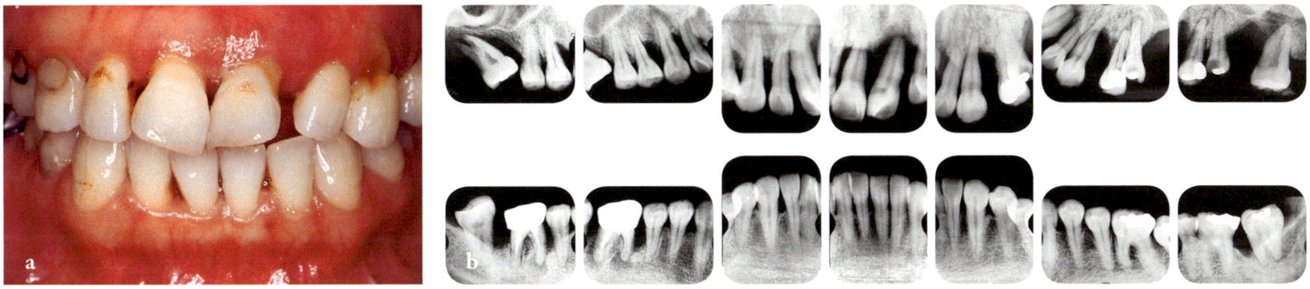

Figs 5-15a and 5-15b At the initial examination, severe bone loss was observed in most of the dentition.

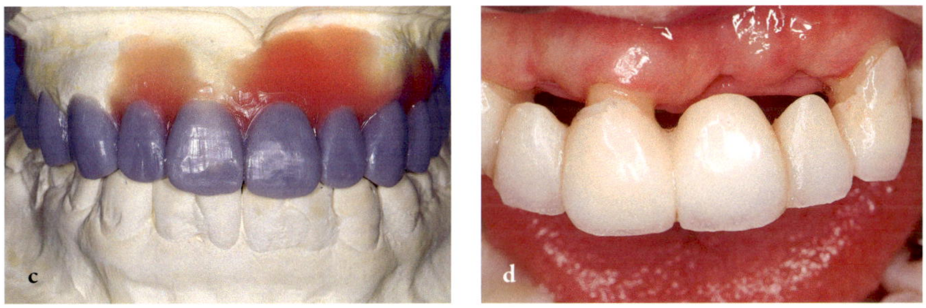

Fig 5-15c and 5-15d *(c)* Diagnostic wax-up. *(d)* The second premolars, right first premolar, canines, and right central incisor were used to support the provisional restoration.

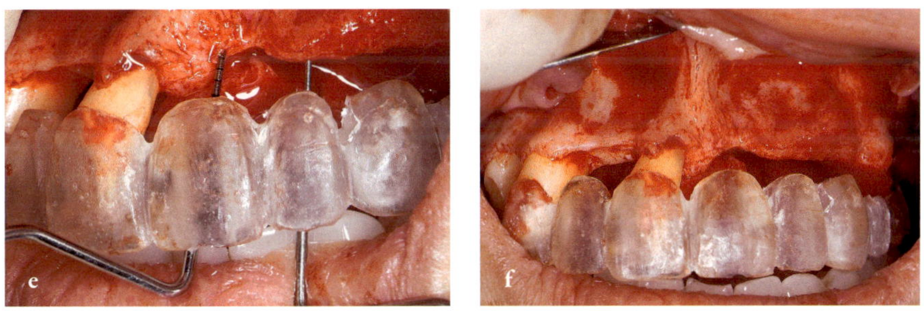

Figs 5-15e and 5-15f Before GBR. Horizontal and vertical bone loss was observed.

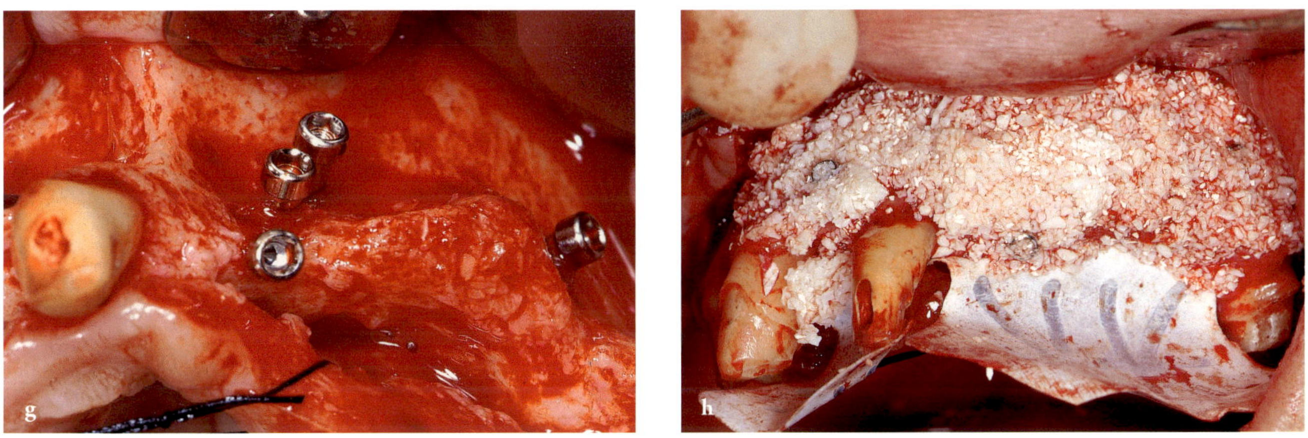

Figs 5-15g and 5-15h GBR with a titanium reinforced membrane and 90% xenograft mixture was performed 2 months following extractions and socket preservation.

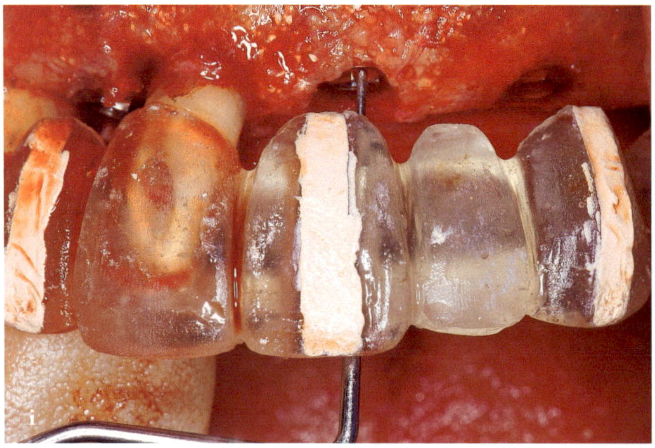

Fig 5-15i Seven months after GBR, following implant placement. Adequate buccal bone volume was achieved. The IHB is 2 to 3 mm coronal to the ideally positioned implant. Papillae will be supported by this interproximal bone.

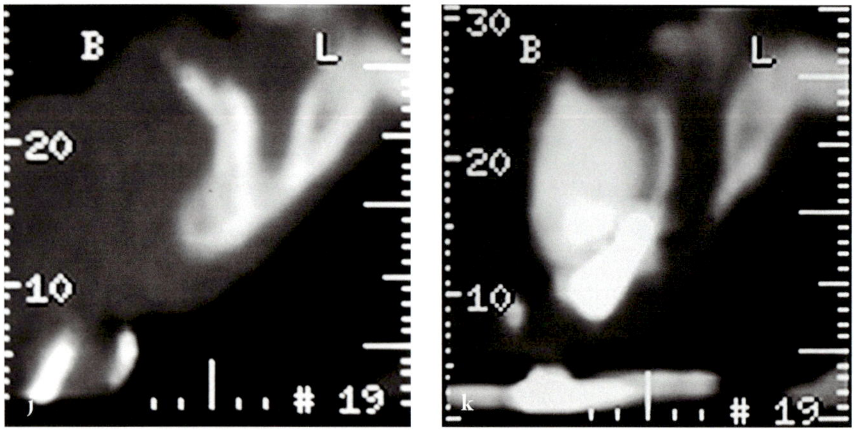

Figs 5-15j and 5-15k Computed tomographic evaluation before *(j)* and after *(k)* GBR. The alveolar ridge has been 3D augmented.

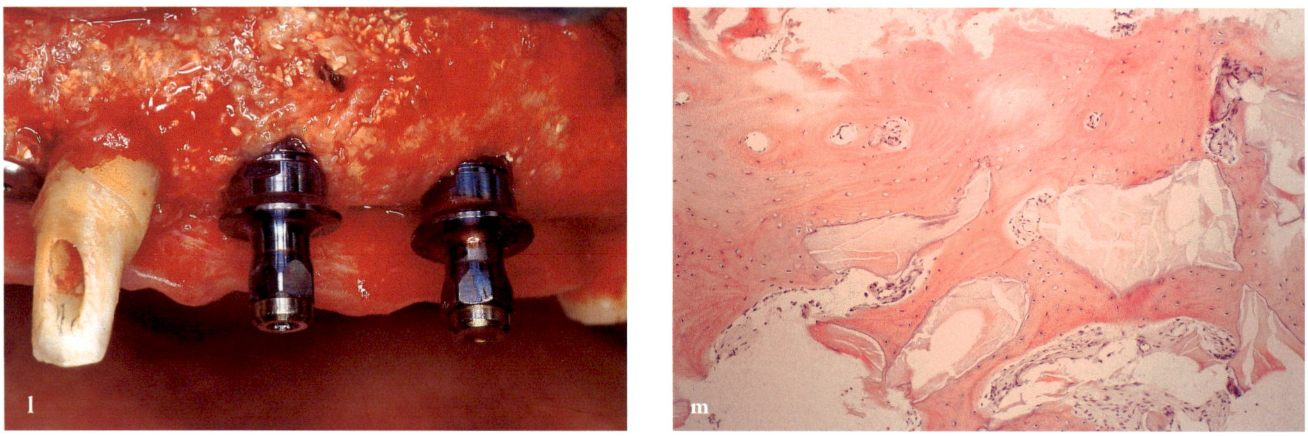

Figs 5-15l and 5-15m A sample from the implant osteotomy site *(l)* shows new bone formation *(m)*. (Courtesy of Dr Takeshi Ishida.)

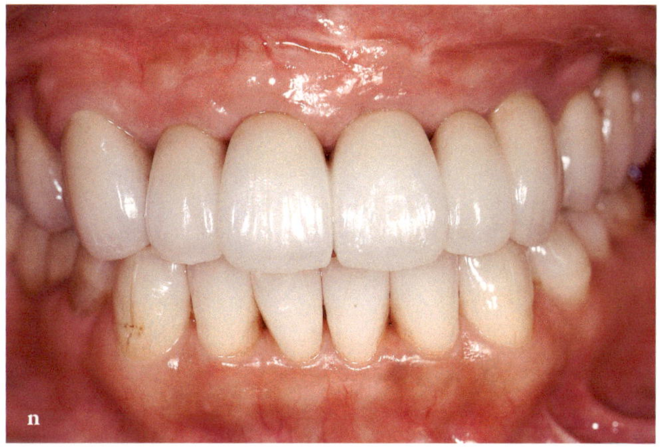

Fig 5-15n Facial view of definitive restorations, which resemble the diagnostic wax-up.

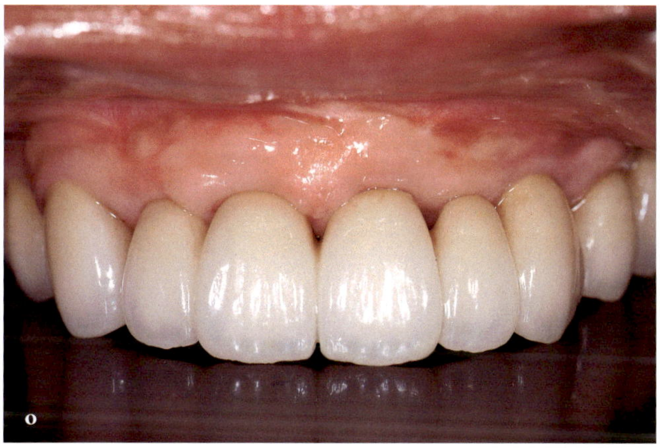

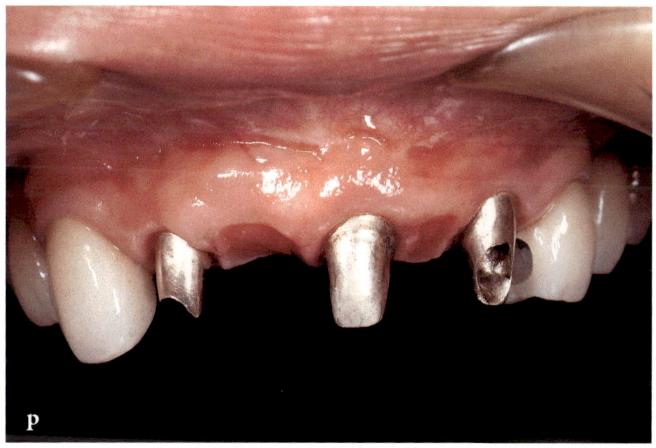

Figs 5-15o and 5-15p The esthetic final result was maintained 7 years after GBR and 5 years after the definitive restoration.

Autogenous bone

Harvested with a bone scraper

Autogenous bone can be harvested with a bone scraper (Fig 5-16), which is less invasive than using autogenous bone block harvesting. Harvested bone is mainly cortical in nature, but cancellous bone can be harvested. Usually the mandibular ramus area serves as a donor site. It is preferable to wait at least 6 months after extraction of the third molar before harvesting bone from this area.

Harvested at the implant osteotomy site

When GBR is performed simultaneously with implant placement, autogenous bone can be harvested from the implant osteotomy site (Fig 5-17). When used at 50 rpm with no irrigation, an implant drill will retain autogenous bone from the osteotomy site. This protocol reduces the risk of contaminating the harvested bone, which is cancellous in nature and contains osteogenic cells and growth factors.[21]

Xenogeneic bone

Xenogeneic bone graft materials with slow resorption properties allow the shape and form created by GBR to be maintained for a longer period of time. The authors have been using xenograft in sinus lift procedures for about 10 years. Their radiographic observations of the dimensional stability of the sinus lift area concur with the findings generally published in the literature.[22–24] Simion et al[25] demonstrated a comparable vertical ridge augmentation result using a titanium-reinforced expanded polytetrafluoroethylene (e-PTFE) membrane with autogenous bone graft alone or with a mixture of autogenous bone and xenograft in a 1:1 ratio.

Autogenous bone harvest using a bone scraper

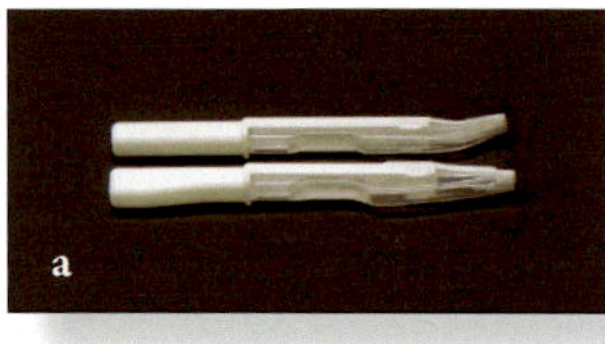

Advantages
- Low surgical morbidity
- Low risk

Disadvantage
- Harvested bone consists mainly of cortical bone

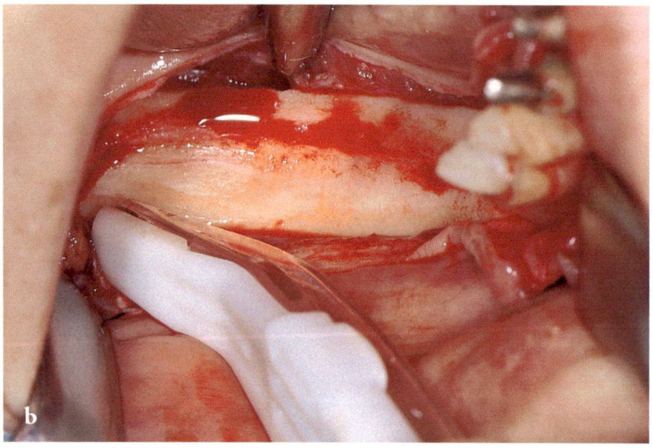

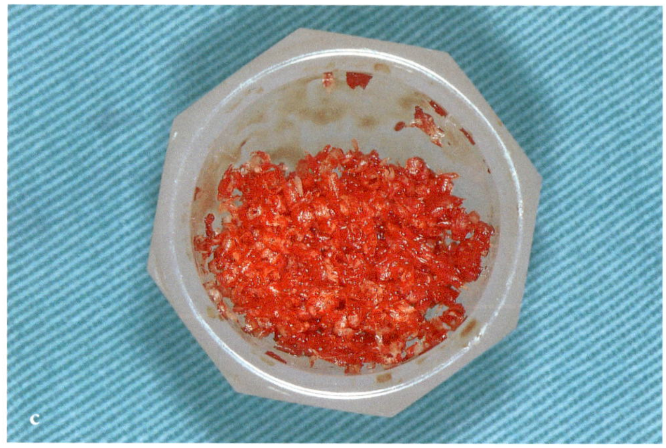

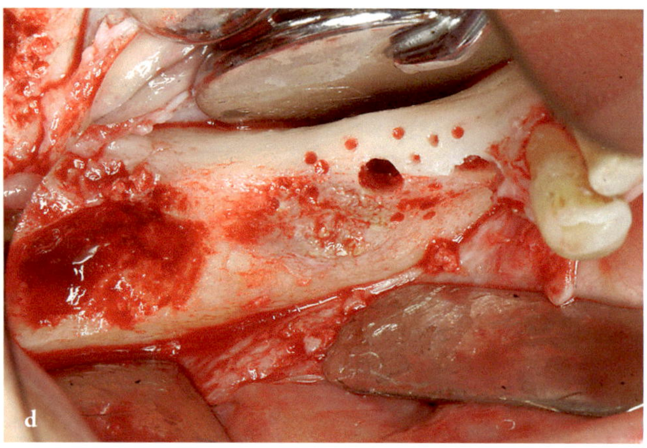

Fig 5-16 *(a)* Bone scrapers. *(b)* Autogenous bone harvesting with a bone scraper. *(c)* Autogenous bone and xenograft mixture. *(d)* After bone scraping.

New GBR Protocol

As summarized in Table 5-1, a resorbable membrane has superior biocompatibility but is not suitable to maintain 3D shape for GBR. So, the authors have created a new surgical protocol for GBR in the esthetic region, consisting of a combination of titanium mesh with a resorbable cross-linked collagen membrane and bone graft (autogenous bone and xenograft) placed at the same time for a predictable 3D GBR result.

Titanium mesh

In implant treatment, an atrophic alveolar ridge must be augmented to meet 3D requirements and support an esthetic final restoration. In 1985, after 10 years of observation, Boyne et al[26] published an effective technique for reconstructing a deficient maxillary edentulous ridge using titanium mesh and autogenous particulate cancellous bone grafts from the iliac. Since then, predictable 3D ridge augmentation, using titanium mesh with extraoral or intraoral autogenous bone and xenograft, has been well demonstrated in the literature.[27–39]

Bone graft materials were completely covered with titanium mesh and stabilized to the ridge in most

Autogenous bone harvest from implant osteotomy sites

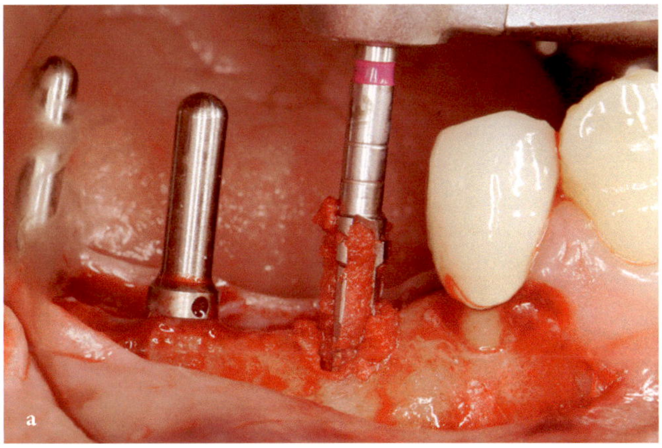

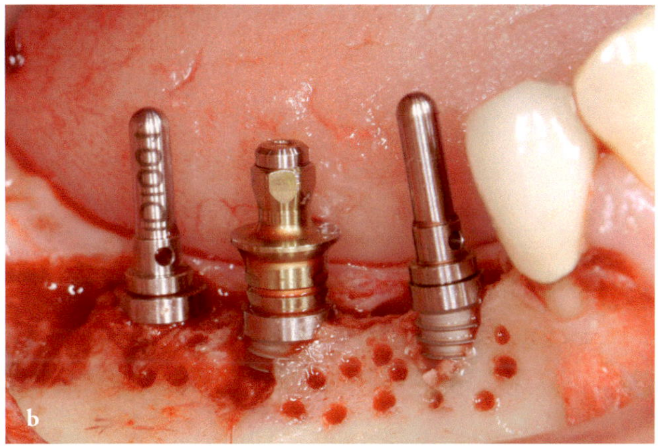

Figs 5-17a and 5-17b Following use of 2710 and 2-mm twist drills, implant site osteotomy is completed with a shaping drill at 50 rpm and no irrigation. This drilling protocol enables autogenous bone harvesting.

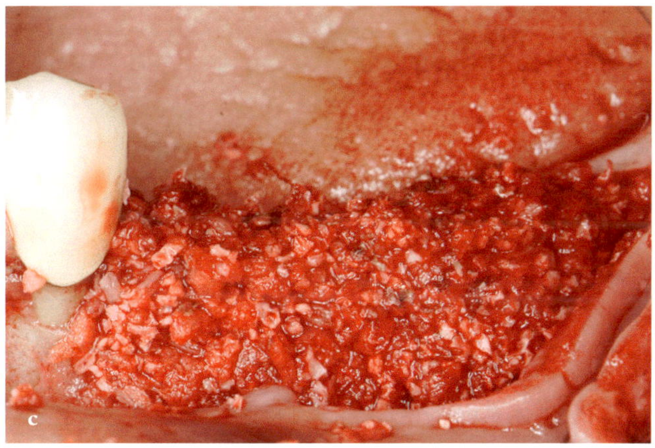

Fig 5-17c After implant placement, a mixture of autogenous bone from the osteotomy site and xenograft is placed at the implant sites to be covered with a resorbable membrane.

publications. That requires higher clinical skills than using a barrier membrane, especially in the anterior region, which generally has a more curved arch form. Alternatively, titanium mesh can be used to provide a framework for a resorbable membrane. It is not necessary to cover the entire GBR site or to stabilize the mesh. However, it is important to use titanium mesh to provide sufficient support for the resorbable membrane, especially at the facial line angle of the ridge. The mesh can be applied in multiple independent frames (Figs 5-18 and 5-19) or in one piece with a long slit for 3D shaping (Fig 5-20).

The following measures reduce complications with titanium mesh:

- Adapting and adjusting the mesh on the cast (Fig 5-21)
- Staged augmentation
- Using thin (0.1-mm) titanium mesh while assuring space maintenance by placing an implant with a healing abutment and/or tenting screws (Fig 5-22).

A combination of collagen membrane and titanium mesh in GBR has the advantages of both materials and provides a superior result with fewer complications (Fig 5-23).

Application of titanium mesh

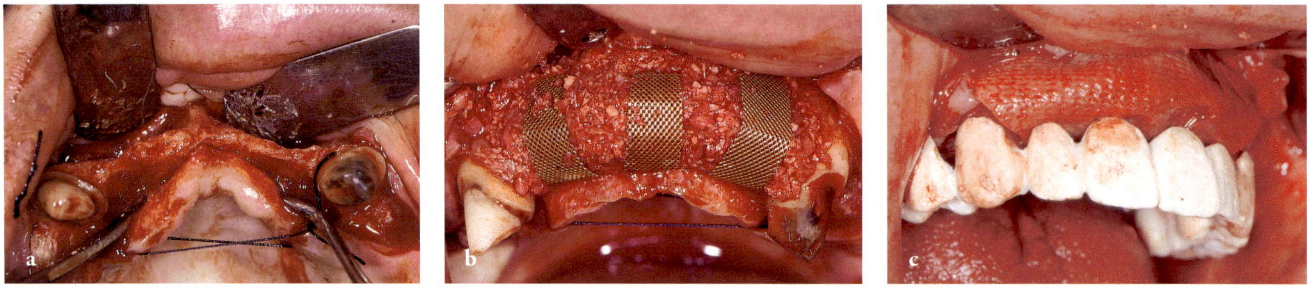

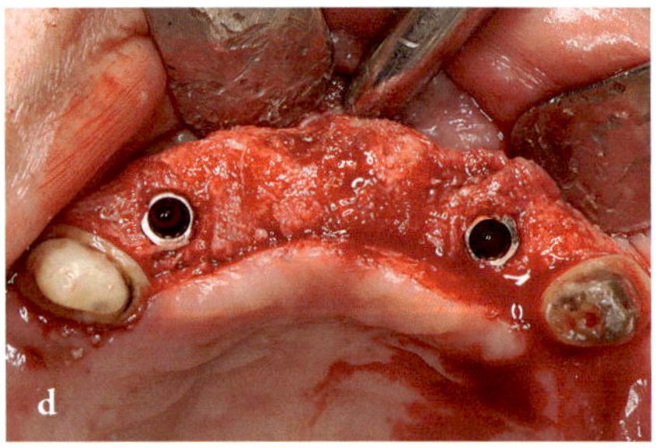

Fig 5-18a to 5-18d *(a)* The alveolar ridge was too narrow to place implants. *(b)* The autogenous bone and xenograft mixture was grafted, and titanium mesh was positioned. *(c)* The bone graft and mesh were completely covered with collagen membranes. *(d)* Seven months later, implants were placed in the augmented ridge. Less bone volume was observed where mesh was not placed.

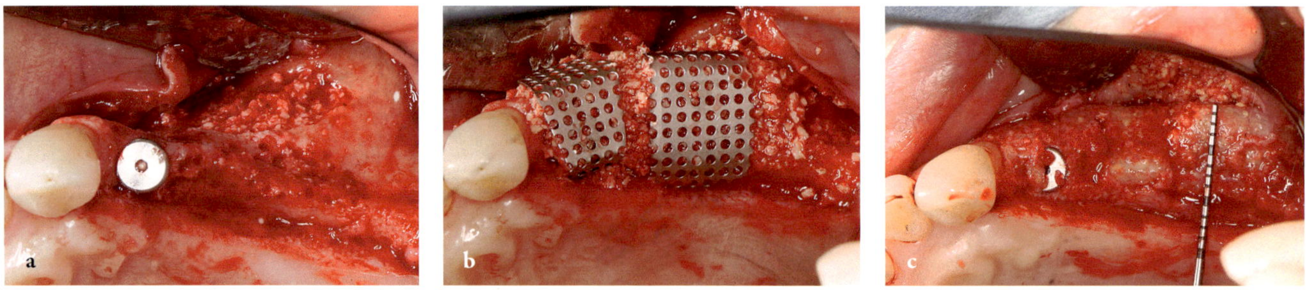

Fig 5-19 *(a to c)* GBR with multiple independent titanium mesh frames.

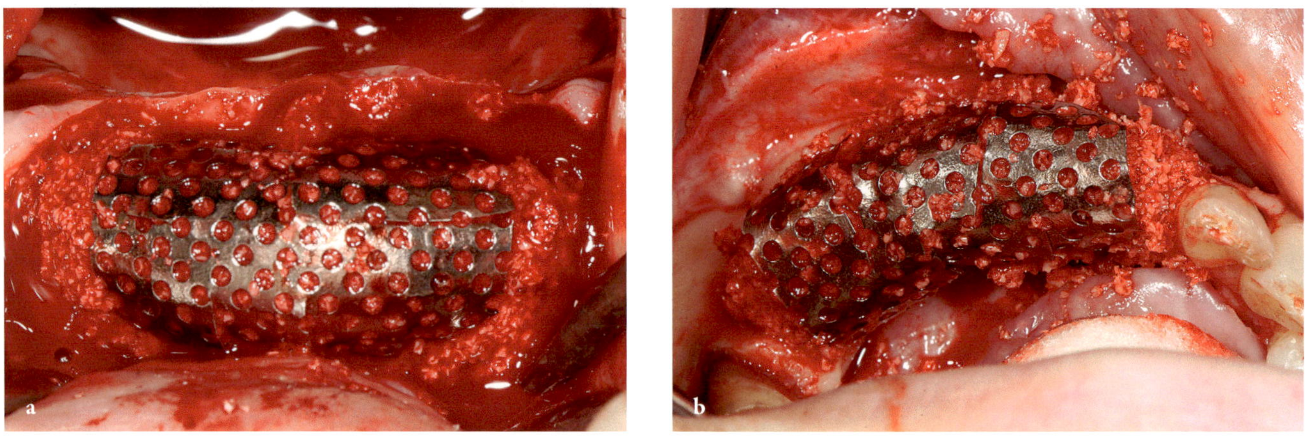

Fig 5-20 *(a and b)* Two examples of GBR with a single titanium mesh frame fitted to the proper 3D form using slits.

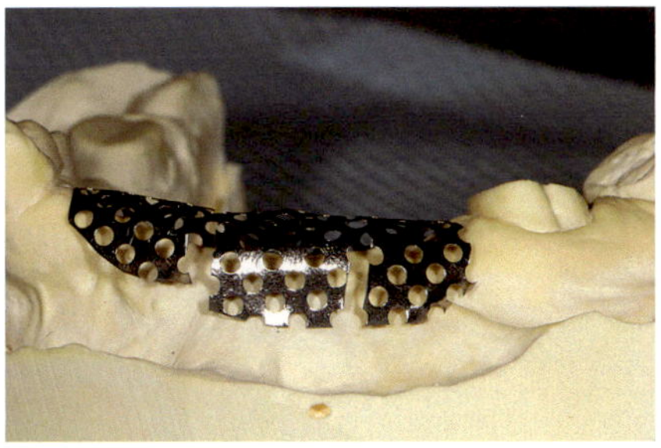

Fig 5-21 Mesh preparation on cast before surgery.

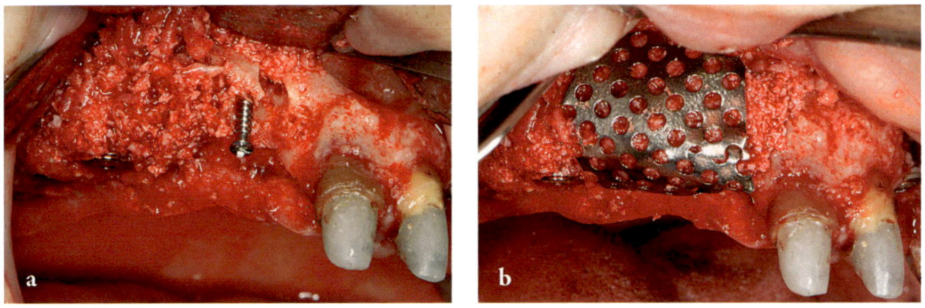

Fig 5-22 *(a and b)* Implants with healing abutments and tenting screws help assure space maintenance with the use of thin mesh.

Use of new GBR protocol to achieve significant horizontal and vertical bone augmentation

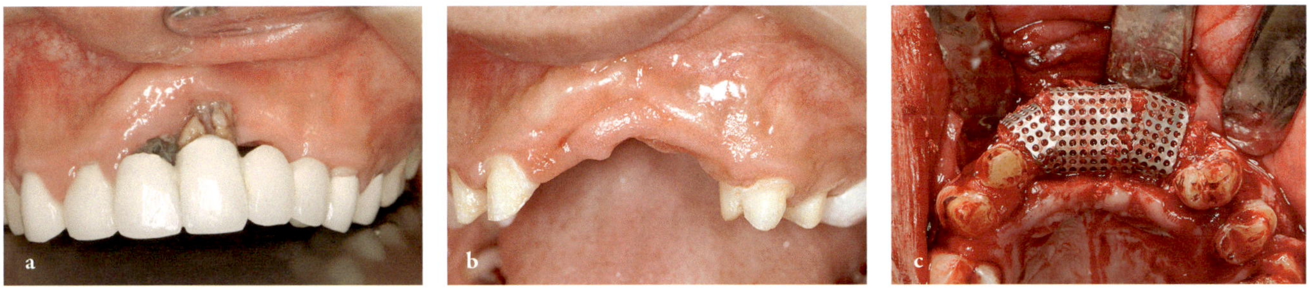

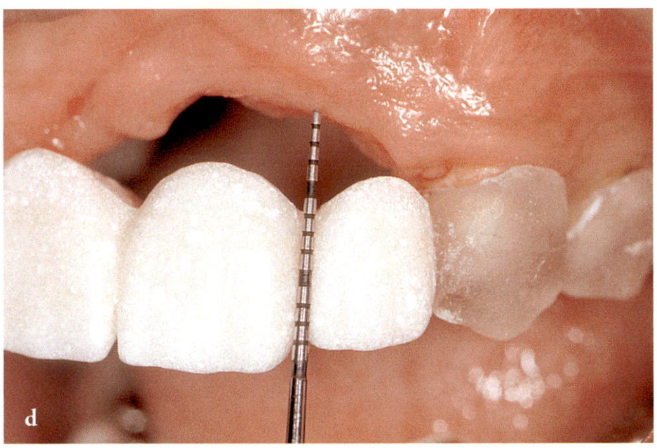

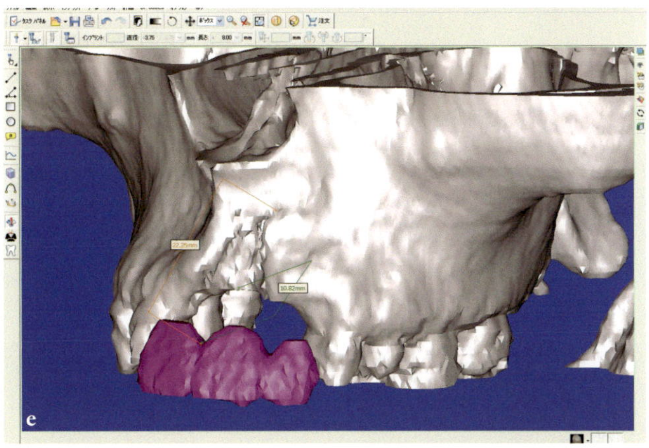

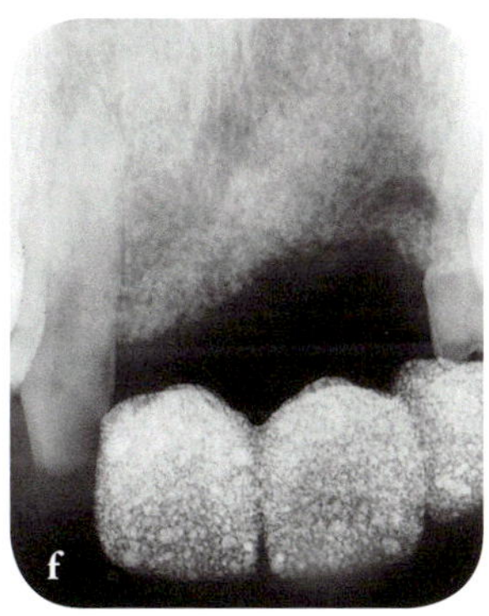

Figs 5-23a to 5-23f A 23-year-old man presented with a severe bone defect in the incisor area. Clinical *(a to d)*, 3D imaging *(e)*, and radiographic *(f)* views revealed the extent of the defect.

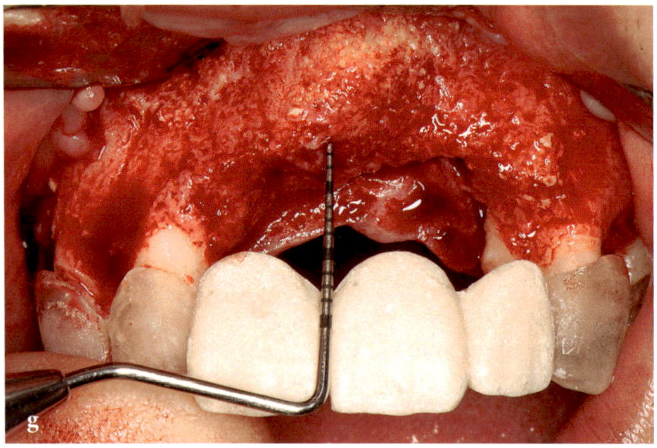

Fig 5-23g It was determined that 9 to 10 mm of vertical GBR was necessary to achieve an esthetic final result.

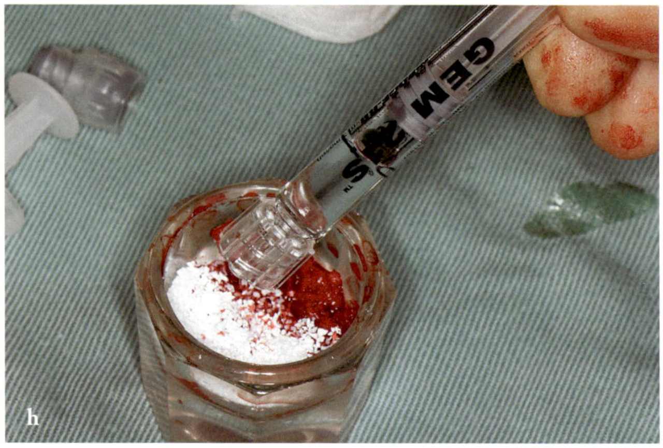

Fig 5-23h Autogenous bone and xenograft were mixed with recombinant human platelet-derived growth factor (rhPDGF).

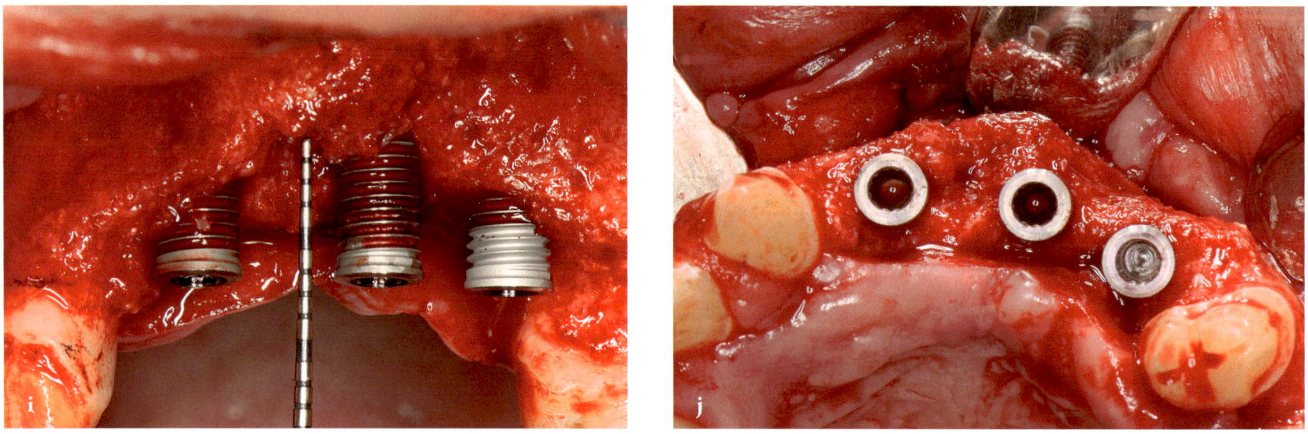

Figs 5-23i and 5-23j Implants were placed in the ideal prosthetic position. A significant volume of vertical and horizontal bone defect was observed.

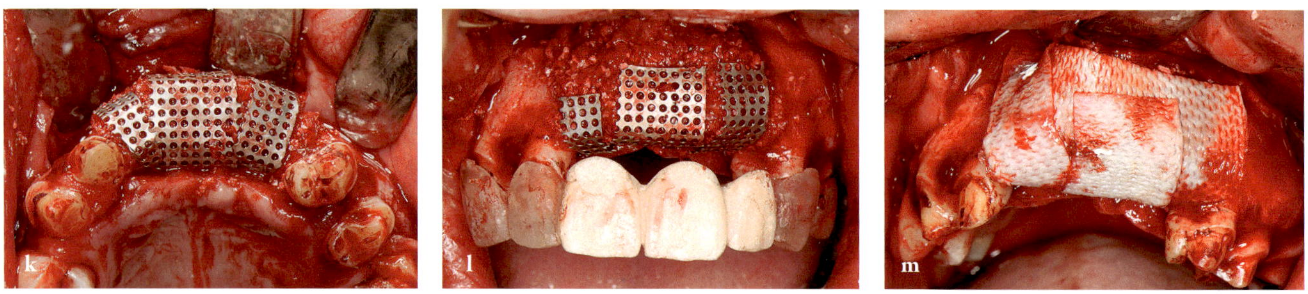

Figs 5-23k to 5-23m Three independent titanium mesh frames were placed over the bone graft material *(k and l)*, then completely covered with collagen membranes *(m)*.

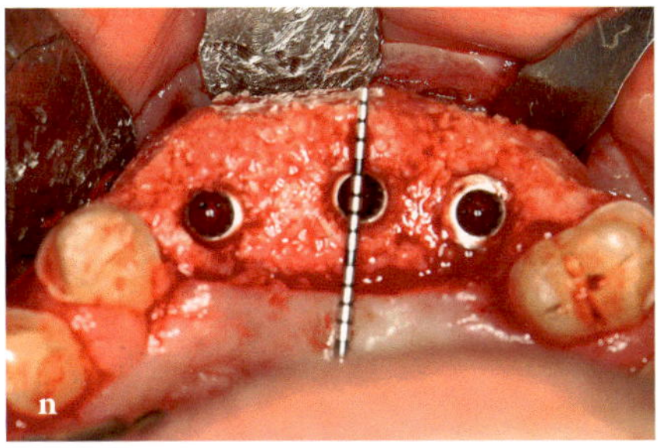

Fig 5-23n Nine months later, sufficient width of buccal bone had been regenerated.

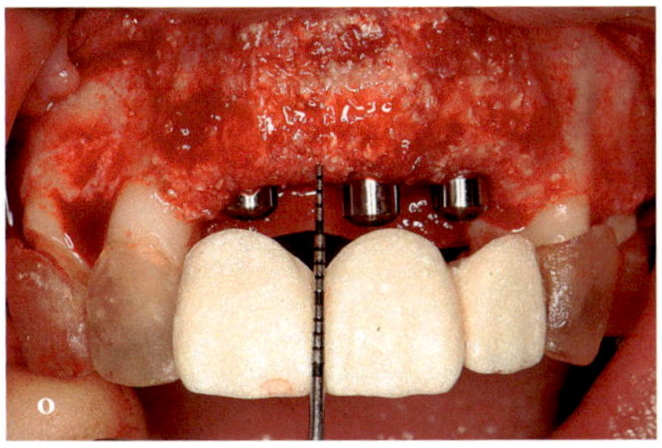

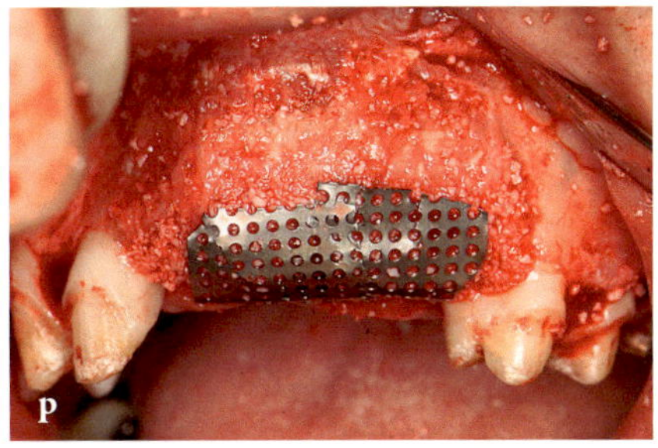

Figs 5-23o and 5-23p In order to achieve an esthetic definitive restoration with a natural soft tissue profile, an additional 3 mm of vertical bone augmentation was necessary.

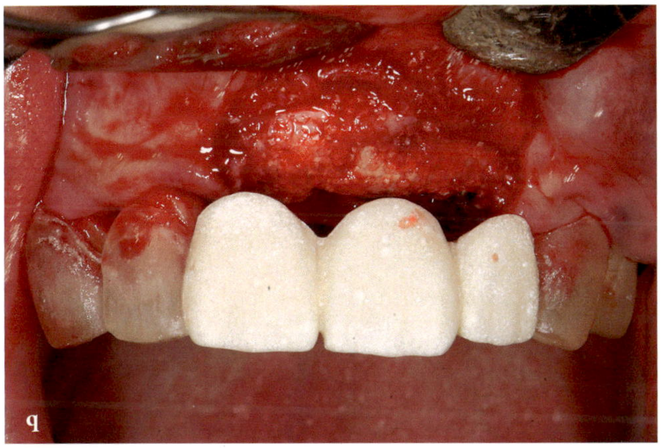

Fig 5-23q Six months later, sufficient vertical height of bone had been regenerated around the implants and healing abutments. An impressive 9 to 10 mm of vertical GBR was successfully achieved with a staged approach using titanium mesh and the cross-linked collagen membrane.

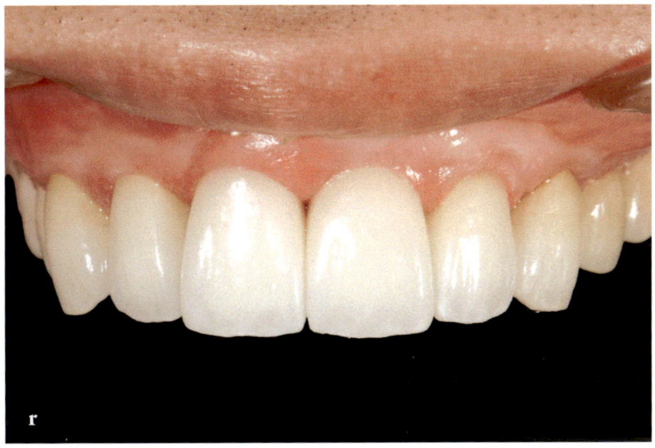

Fig 5-23r Facial view. An esthetic definitive restoration and soft tissue profile was achieved.

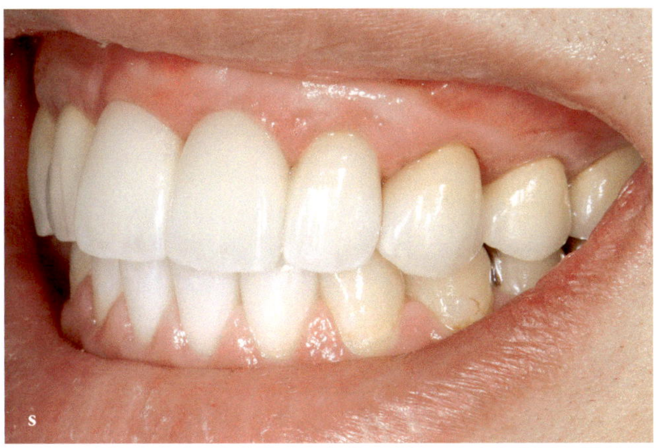

Fig 5-23s Lateral view of definitive restoration.

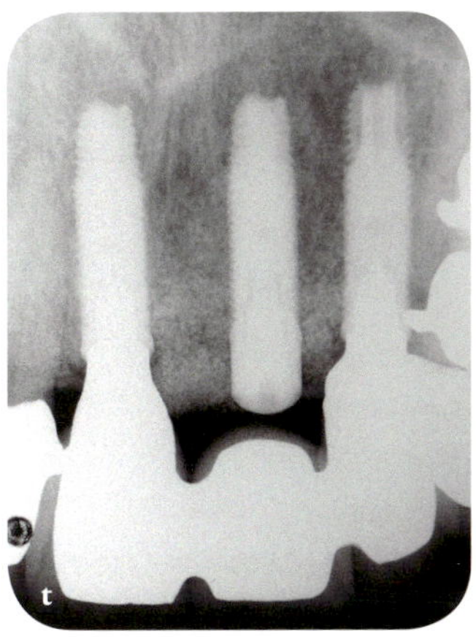

Fig 5-23t Periapical radiograph with definitive restoration. Significant vertical bone augmentation was achieved. Surrounding bone at the implant-abutment junction was maintained with platform switching.

FT Wing

Funato and Tonotsuka developed a titanium frame, called the FT wing, that features a 0.15-mm-thick titanium plate. By easily bending the frame and stabilizing it with an implant cover screw, they created a facial space that measured 2 mm from the implant body. This is a very effective approach when implant placement and GBR are performed simultaneously in the esthetic region (Figs 5-24 and 5-25).

GBR with FT wing: Multiple-tooth implant case

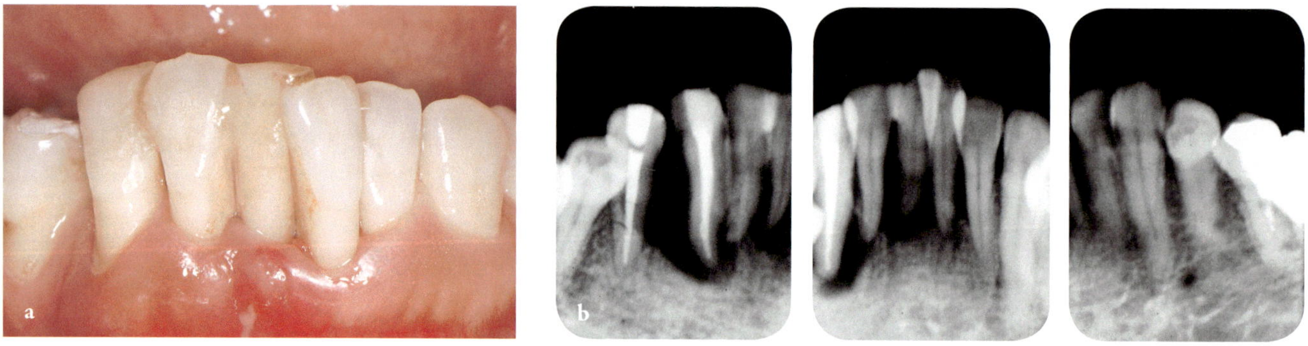

Figs 5-24a and 5-24b All teeth from the right first premolar to the left lateral incisor were diagnosed as hopeless because of severe periodontal disease.

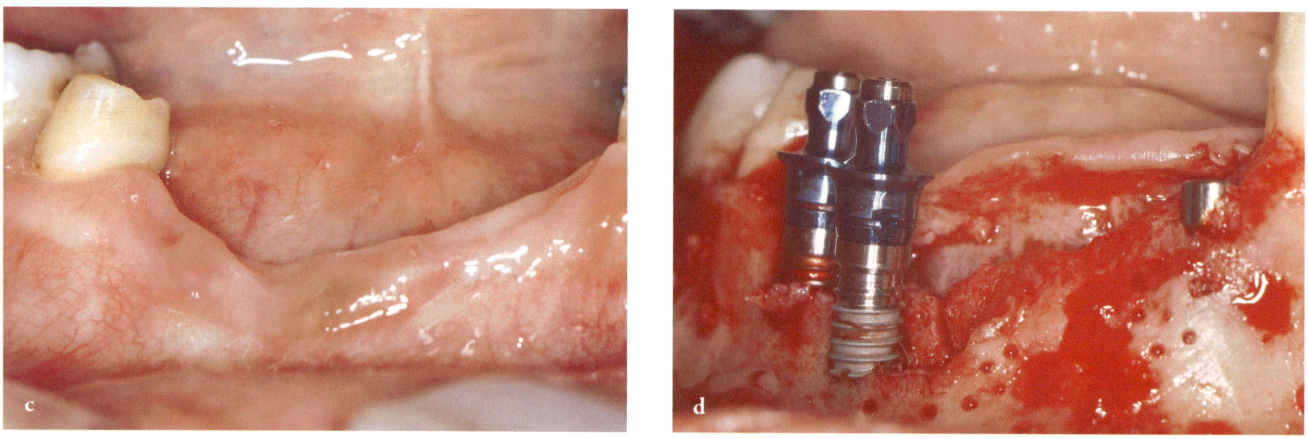

Figs 5-24c and 5-24d Implants were placed in the right first premolar and canine and left lateral incisor positions.

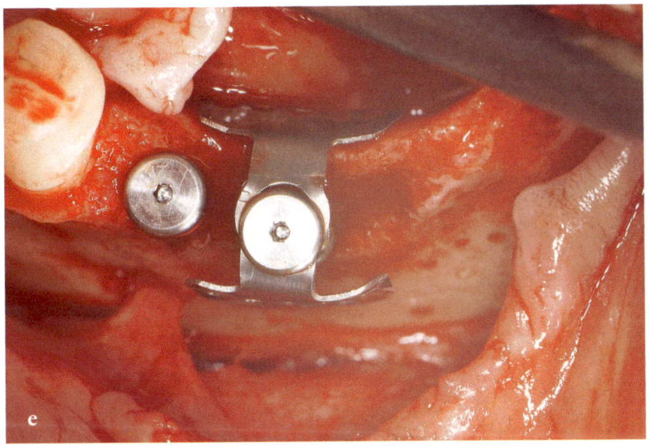

Fig 5-24e The FT wing was placed on the right canine implant.

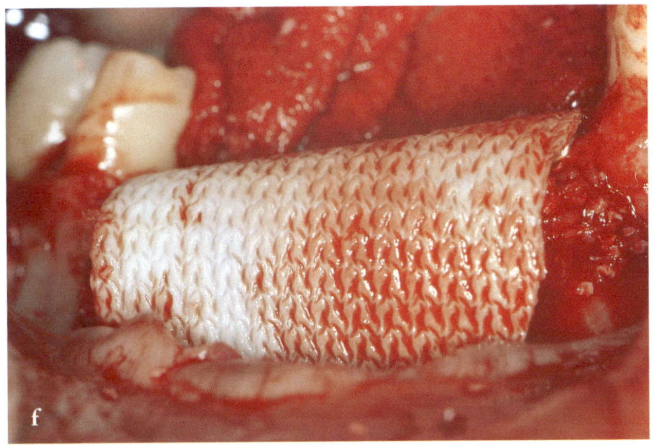

Fig 5-24f Autogenous bone and xenograft were placed and covered with a collagen membrane.

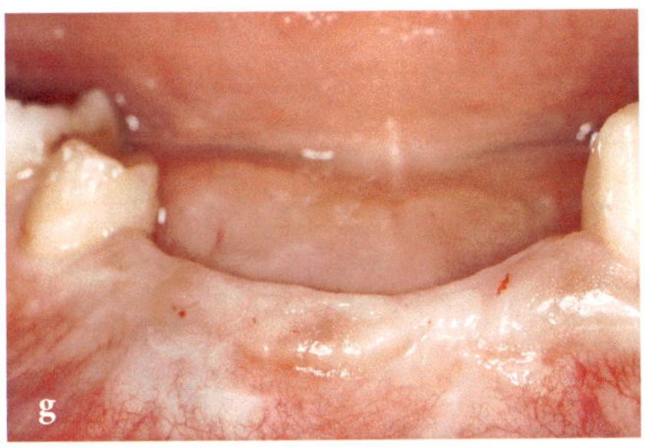

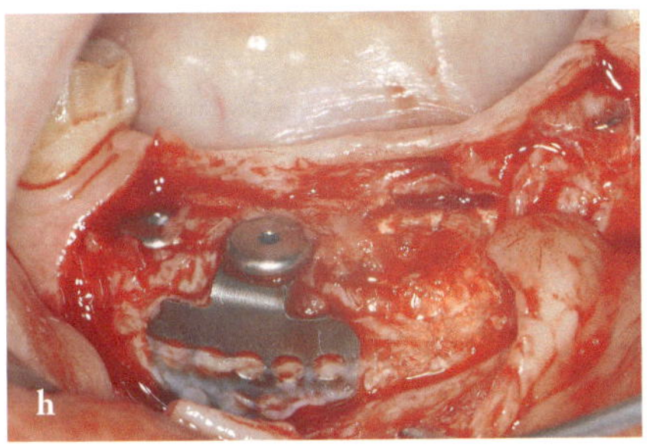

Figs 5-24g and 5-24h Six months later, sufficient bone regeneration was confirmed at stage-two surgery.

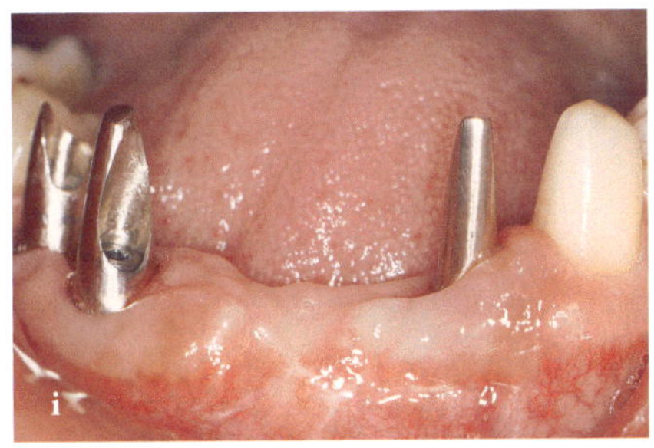

Fig 5-24i Facial view with definitive abutments.

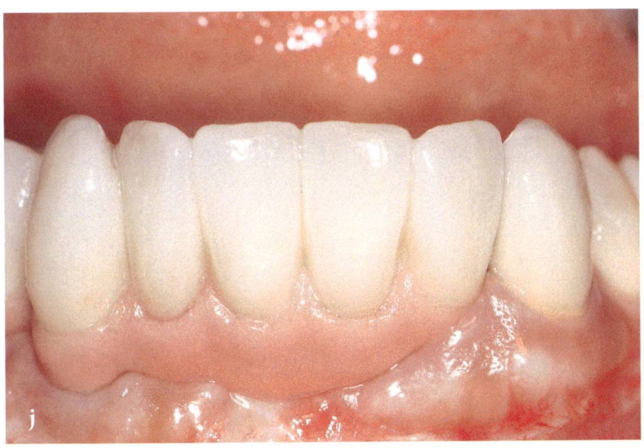

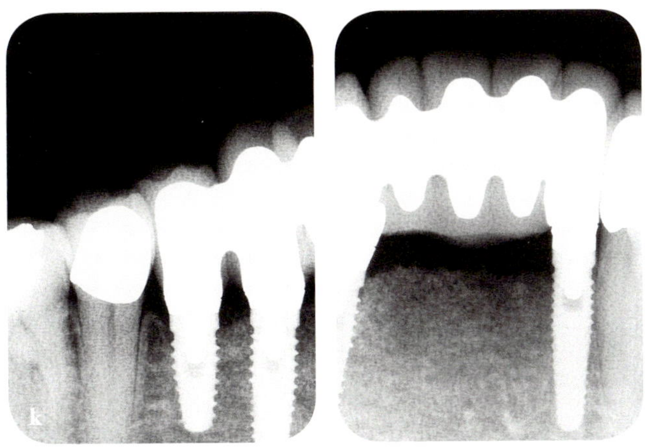

Figs 5-24j and 5-24k Facial view *(j)* and periapical radiographs *(k)* with the definitive restoration.

GBR with FT wing: Single-tooth implant case

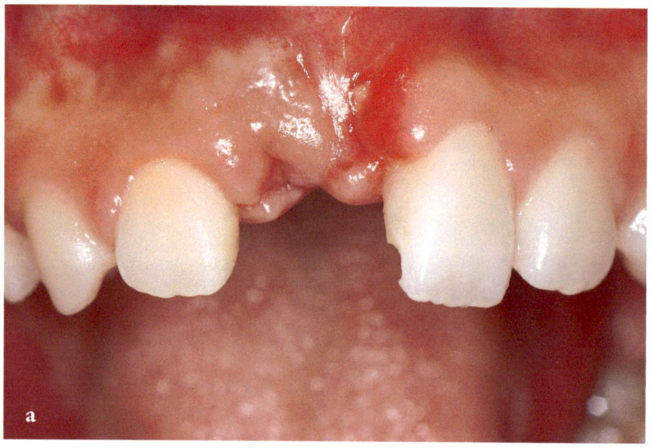

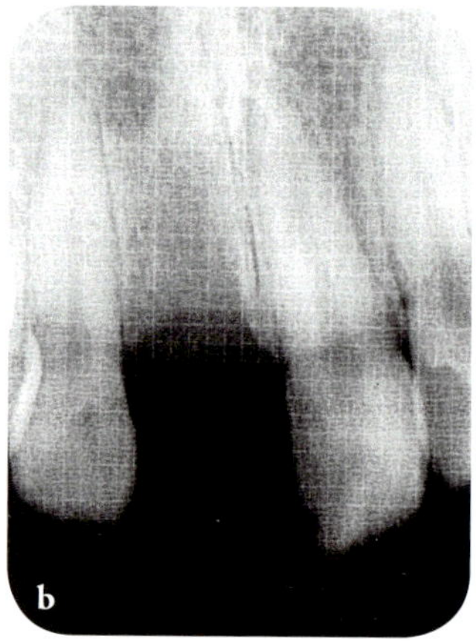

Figs 5-25a and 5-25b Initial examination. The right central incisor had been lost in a motor vehicle accident.

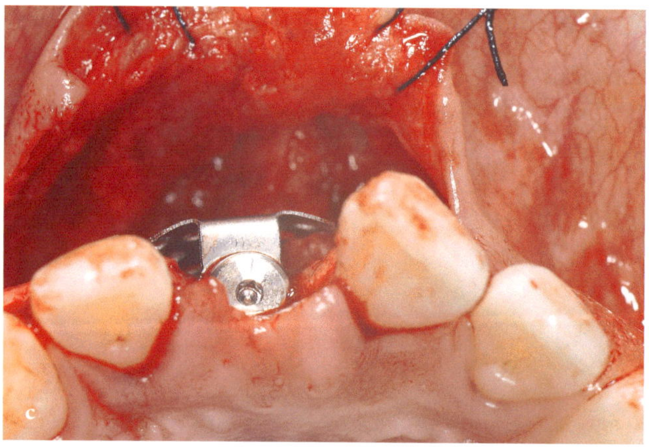

Fig 5-25c Occlusal view of implant and FT wing positioning. Autogenous bone graft was harvested from the ramus and grafted.

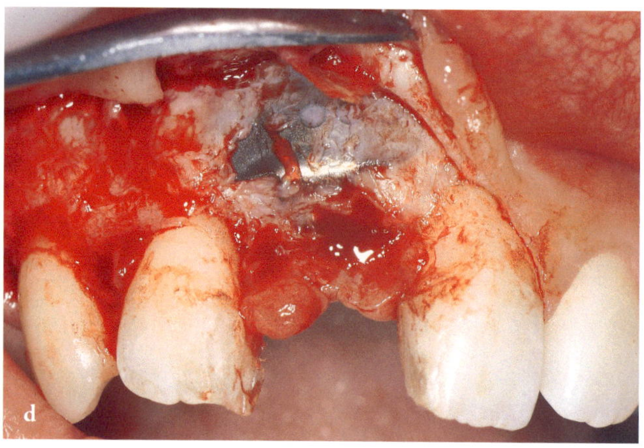

Fig 5-25d Six months later, the FT wing was removed.

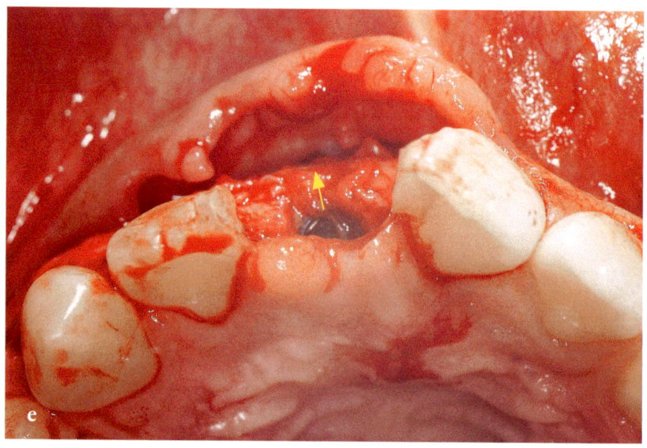

Fig 5-25e A sufficient buccal "balcony" *(yellow arrow)* was regenerated.

Summary

GBR has enabled 3D ridge augmentation with less surgical trauma. It is important to reduce risks, such as membrane exposure, through the following measures:

- Proper soft tissue management with mucogingival surgery or periodontal plastic surgery
- Clear objectives and goals of GBR
- Correct material selection
- Understanding of basic surgical principles

In a multiple-tooth implant case, ridge augmentation must be planned and sequenced with the 4D concept in mind. A multiple-tooth implant case with a severe atrophic alveolar ridge requires a staged approach to GBR, often using titanium mesh and resorbable membrane (Fig 5-26). Although complications may sometimes occur (Fig 5-27), on the whole, ridge augmentation is safe, effective, and fundamental to supporting an esthetic final restoration.

GBR with titanium mesh and resorbable membrane

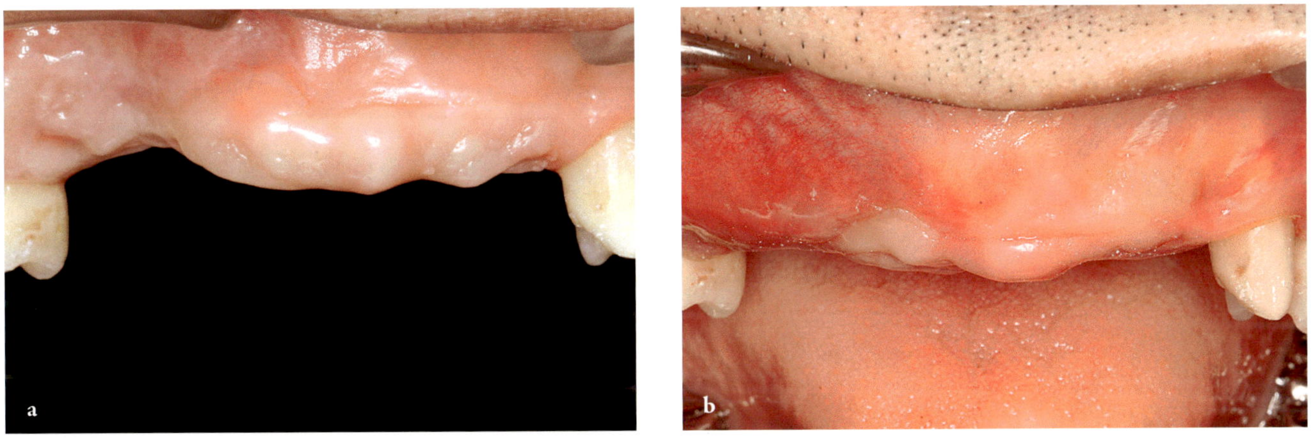

Figs 5-26a and 5-26b Before and after GBR. Due to a severe bone defect, staged GBR and implant placement were selected.

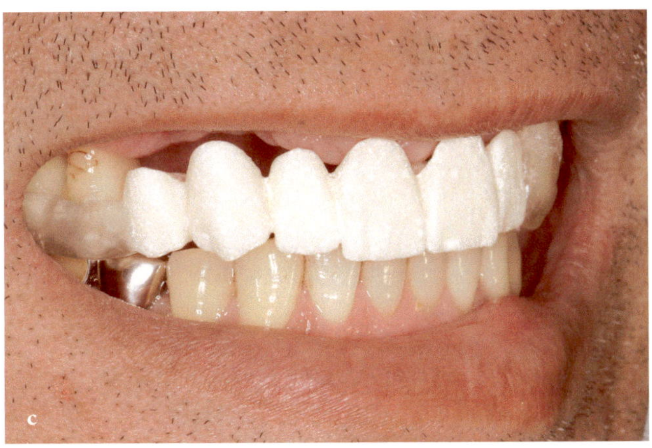

Fig 5-26c The smile line evaluation reveals a deficient alveolar ridge that will not support an esthetic definitive restoration.

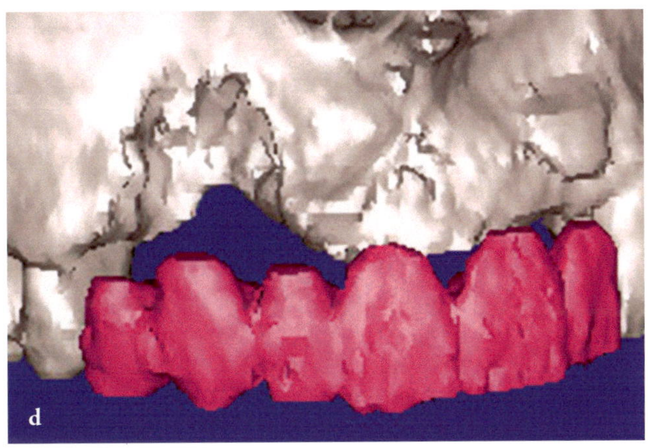

Fig 5-26d A significant horizontal and vertical bone defect was confirmed with 3D simulation software.

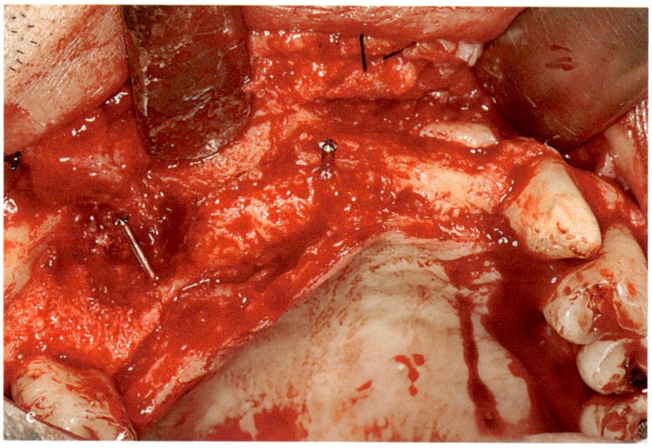

Fig 5-26e Screws were placed for space maintenance and 3D ridge augmentation.

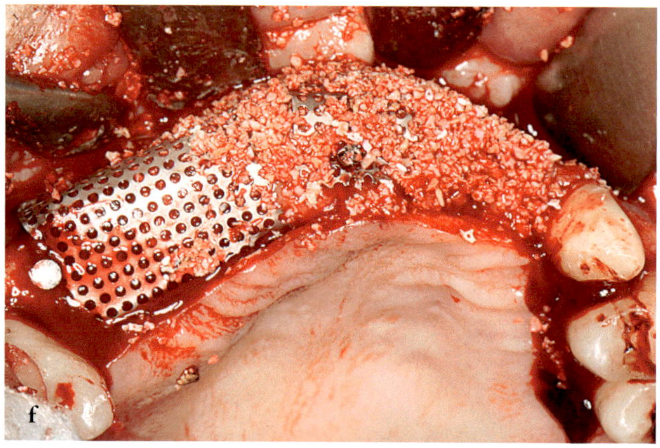

Fig 5-26f Bone graft and titanium mesh were placed.

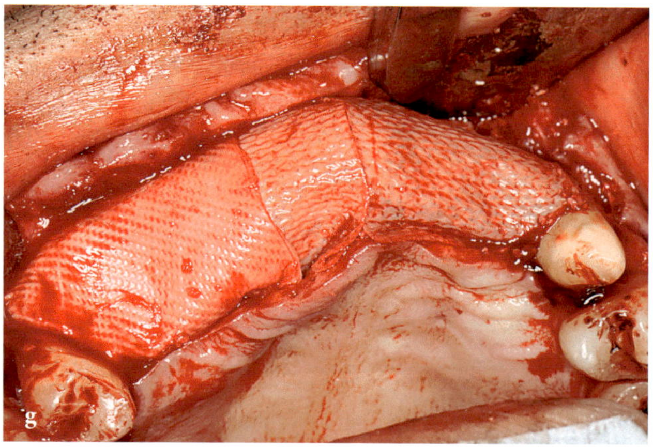

Fig 5-26g Bone graft and titanium mesh were completely covered with a cross-linked collagen membrane.

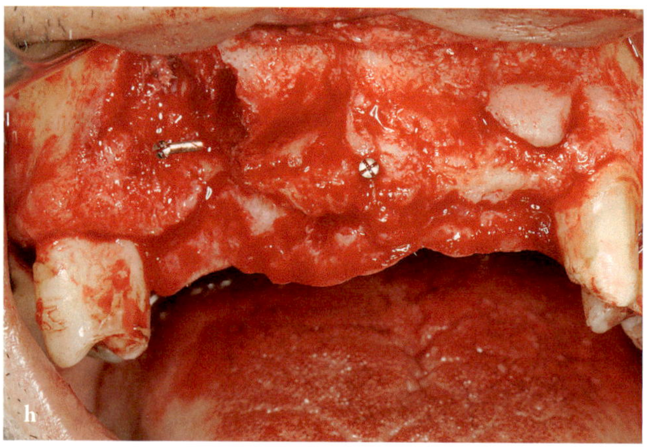

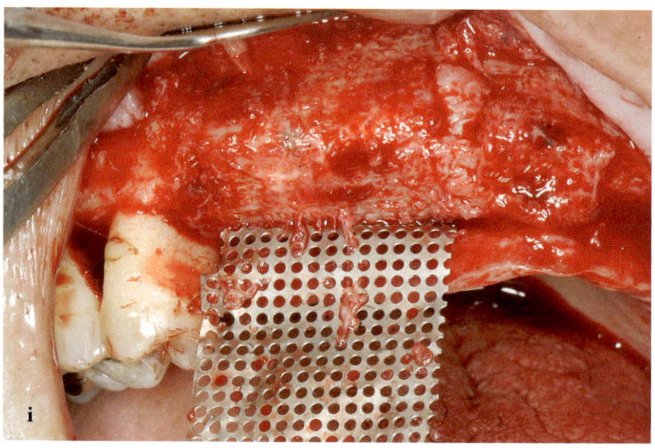

Figs 5-26h and 5-26i Before *(h)* and after *(i)* GBR.

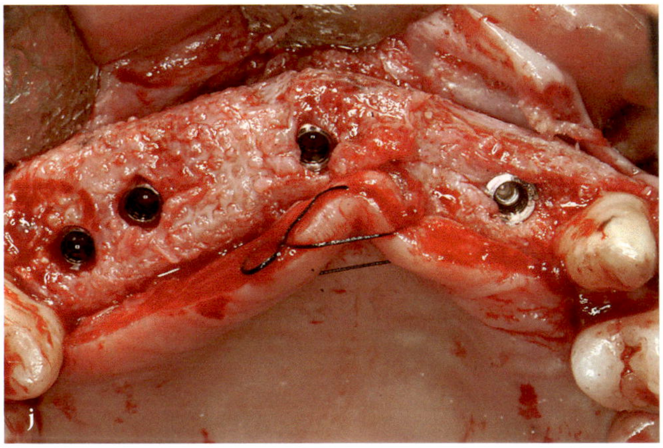

Fig 5-26j Sufficient buccal bone width was confirmed around the ideally positioned implants.

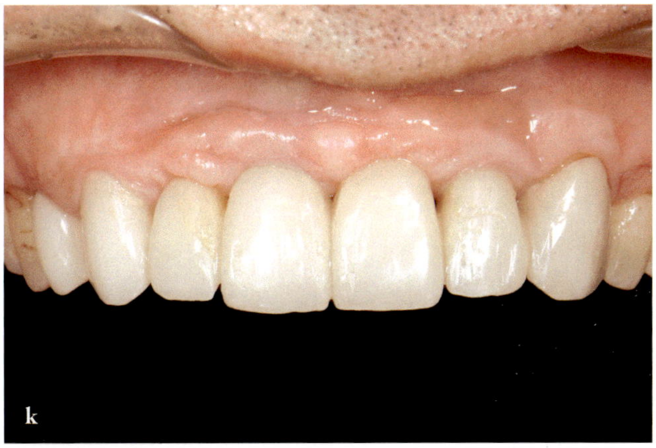

Fig 5-26k 27 months after GBR with a provisional restoration. 3D ridge augmentation was achieved.

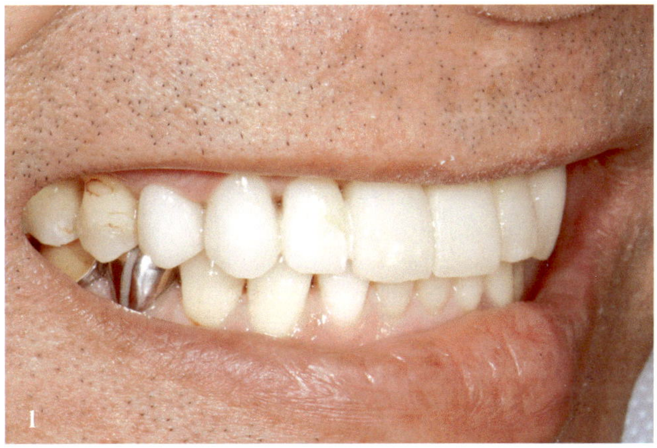

Fig 5-26l Esthetic problems were improved.

Learning from failure: GBR complications

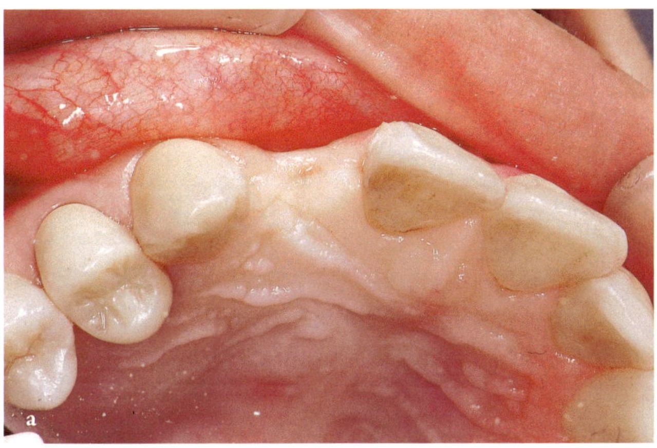

Fig 5-27a A significant ridge deformity was observed.

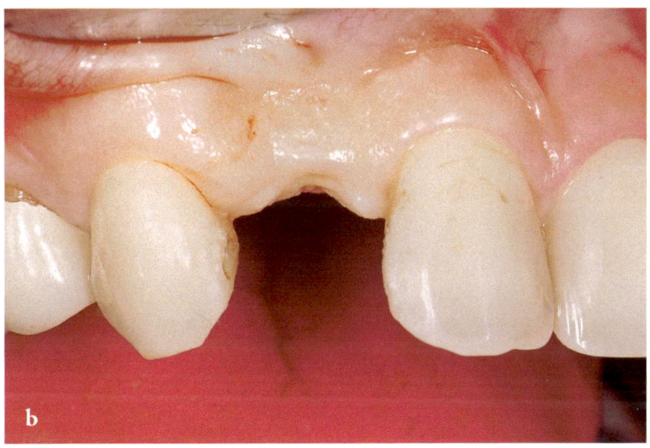

Fig 5-27b The alveolar ridge was resorbed despite socket preservation.

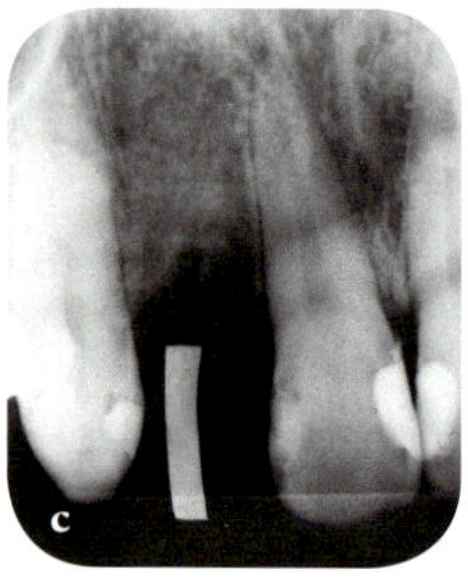

Fig 5-27c Significant horizontal and vertical bone loss were confirmed. Bone loss distal to the right central incisor was also confirmed.

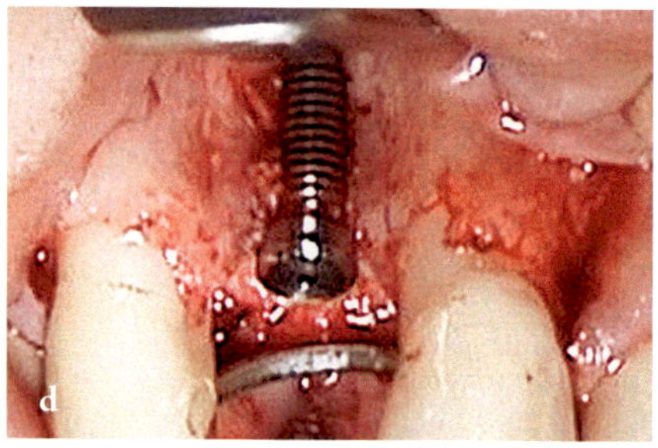

Fig 5-27d Implant placement in an ideal position.

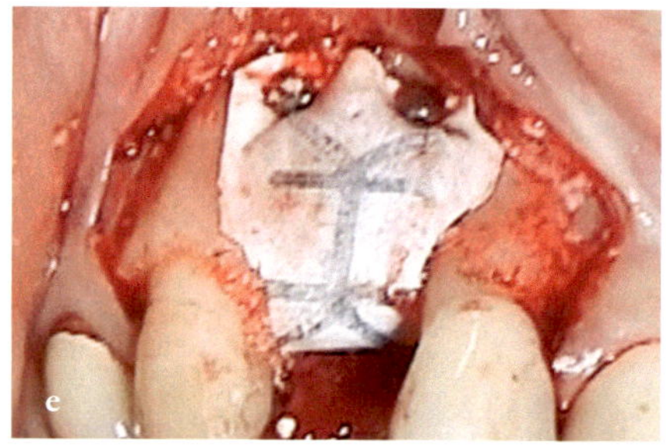

Fig 5-27e The membrane was stabilized. Note that the membrane was too close to the adjacent teeth.

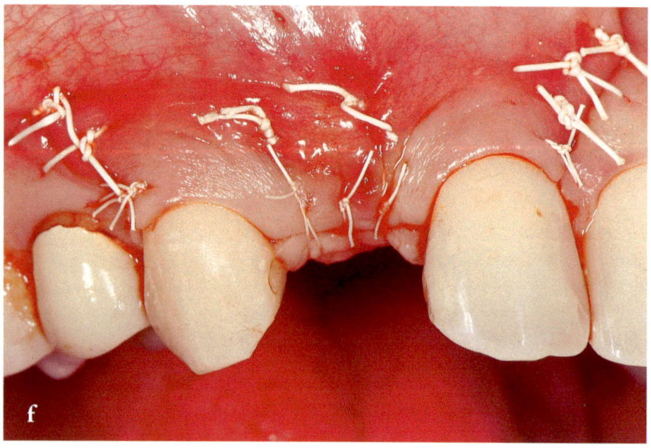

Fig 5-27f Primary closure was obtained. Note the slight tension along the incision line. The amount of distal vertical incision seems insufficient.

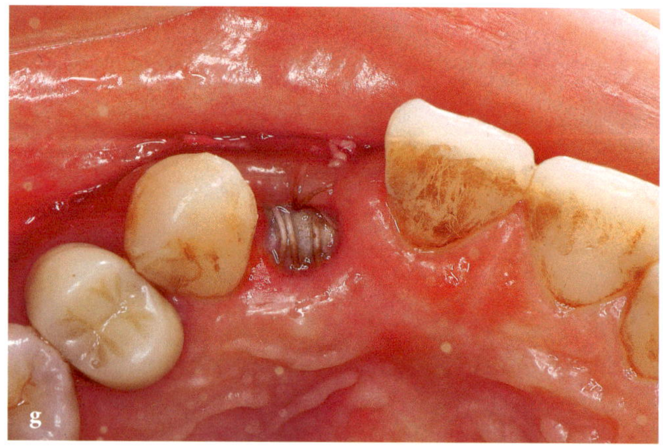

Fig 5-27g Occlusal view 6 weeks after surgery. The membrane was exposed 2 weeks after surgery but was maintained for 4 weeks with twice weekly professional cleanings and oral rinsing five times per day.

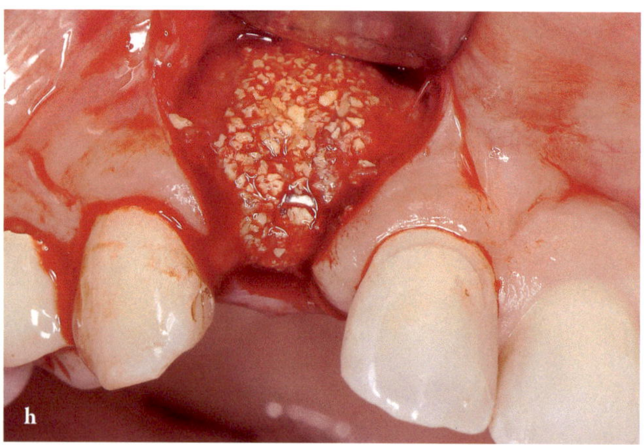

Fig 5-27h The membrane was removed, and the area was irrigated. Some of the bone graft material was removed.

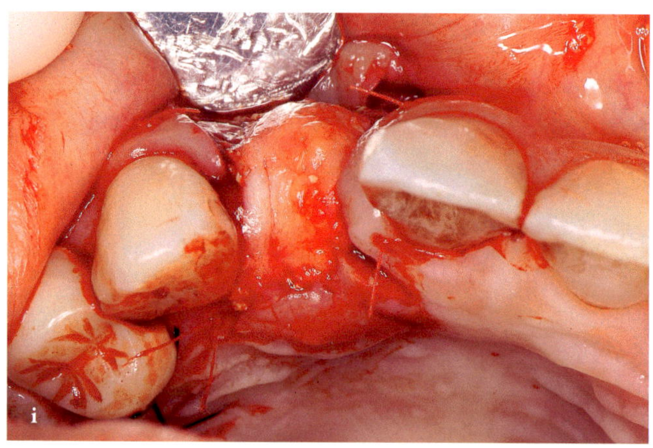

Fig 5-27i Connective tissue was harvested from the palate and placed over the implant site.

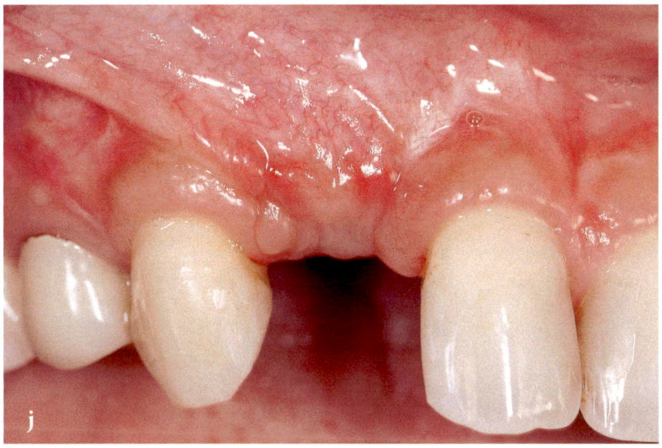

Fig 5-27j One year after connective tissue grafting. A lack of keratinized tissue was observed.

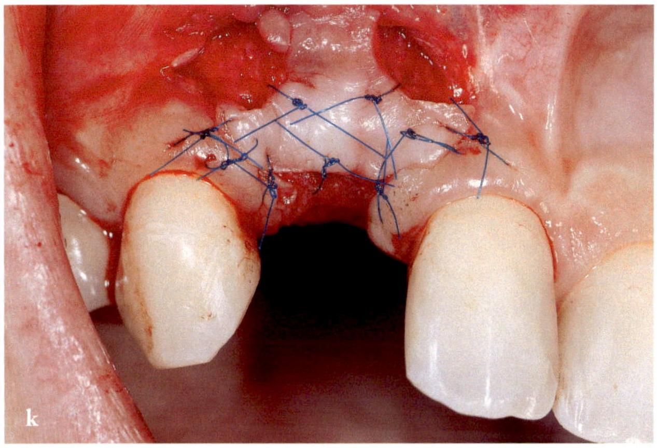

Fig 5-27k An apically positioned flap was performed to augment the keratinized tissue.

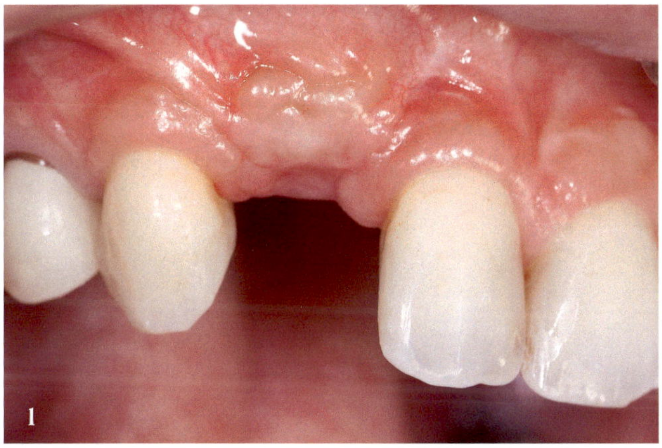

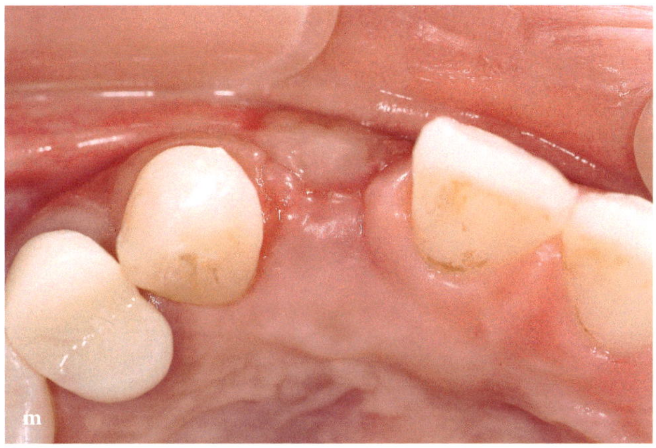

Figs 5-27l and 5-27m Three months after augmentation with apically positioned flap. Keratinized tissue was augmented, but buccal soft tissue volume was insufficient.

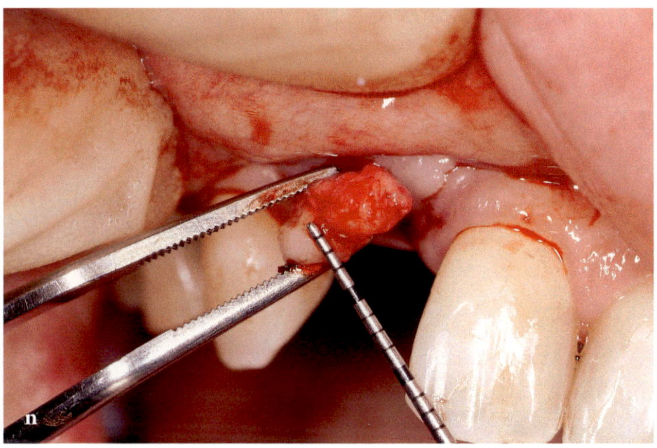

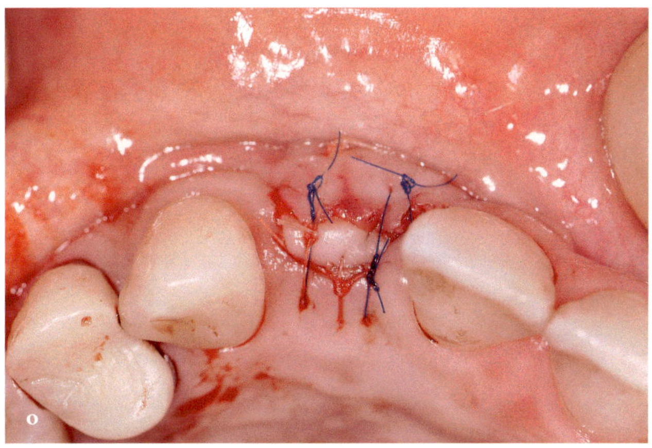

Figs 5-27n and 5-27o An interpositional graft was harvested from the tuberosity and grafted to augment the buccal soft tissue volume.

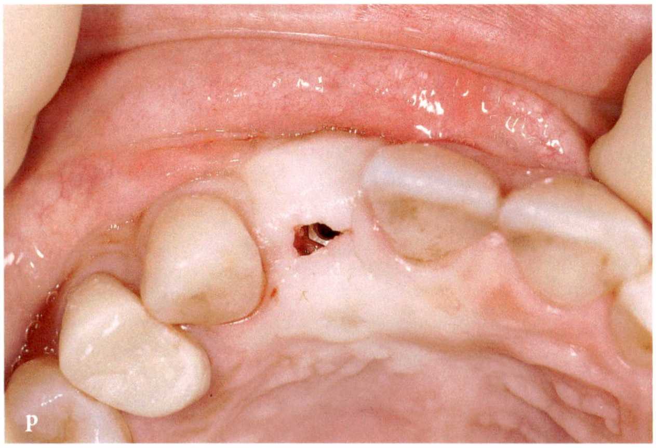

Fig 5-27p Occlusal view 8 weeks after interpositional graft placement. A provisional restoration was placed using a tissue punch technique.

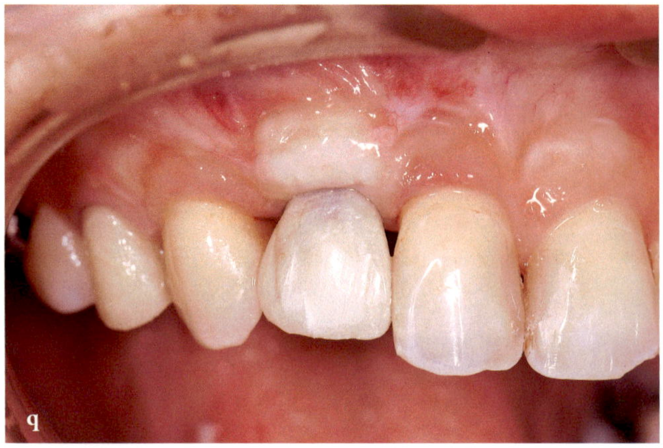

Fig 5-27q Due to the buccally inclined Class 2 implant placement (see Fig 3-10), the provisional restoration was given a concave subgingival profile.

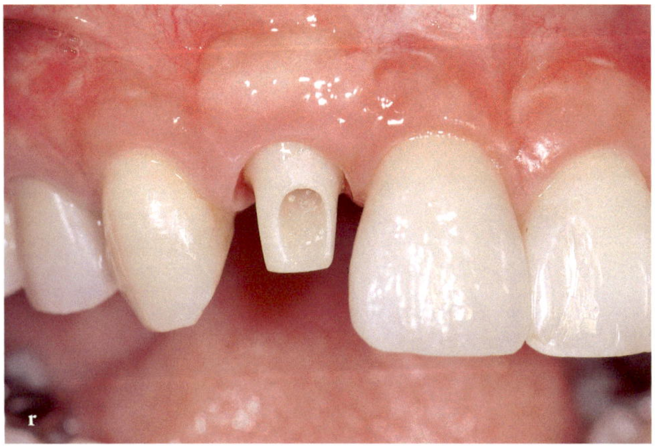

Fig 5-27r Facial view with a definitive abutment.

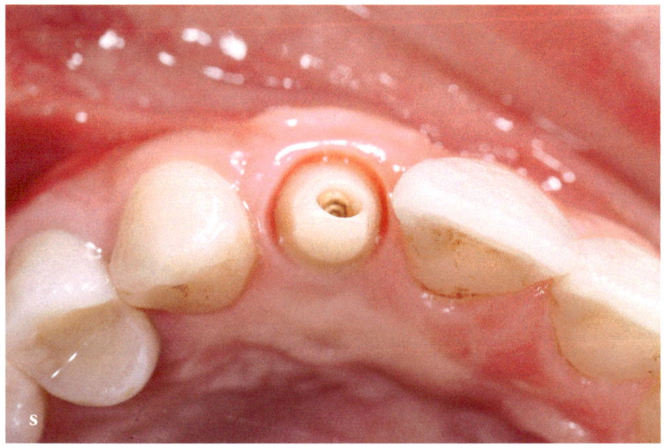

Fig 5-27s Occlusal view confirmed sufficient buccal soft tissue volume.

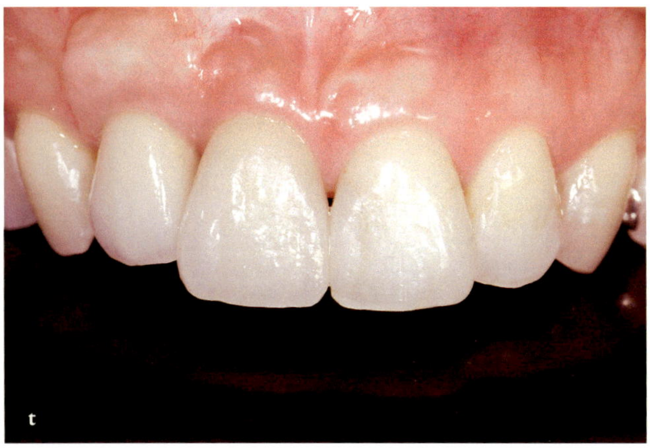

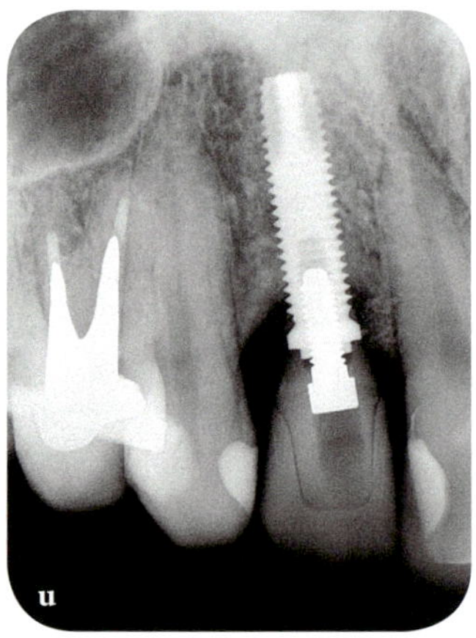

Figs 5-27t and 5-27u After 4 years of function. An acceptable esthetic result was maintained. The papilla height between the right lateral and central incisors was reduced because of attachment loss on the distal of the right central incisor. Careful follow-up was required because of the complication during GBR and the Class 2 implant positioning.

☞ Clinical tips

A series of complications occurred following challenging implant placement with simultaneous vertical GBR using a titanium membrane. These types of treatment situations have a higher risk for complications and should be avoided, especially when they involve a severe alveolar ridge defect in the esthetic region. A staged approach using a titanium frame and a resorbable membrane would reduce the risk of such complications and would also allow easier recovery should these types of complications develop.

References

1. Ishikawa T. GBR technique. In: Miyamoto Y, Yoshie H (eds). Technique and Science of Regenerative Dentistry, Periodontology, Esthetic Dentistry, and Implantology [in Japanese]. Tokyo: Quintessence, 2005:160–175.
2. Buser D, Brägger U, Lang NP, Nyman S. Regeneration and enlargement of jaw bone using guided tissue regeneration. Clin Oral Implants Res 1990;1:22–32.
3. Buser D, Dula K, Hirt HP, Schenk RK. Lateral ridge augmentation using autografts and barrier membranes: A clinical study with 40 partially edentulous patients. J Oral Maxillofac Surg 1996;54:420–432.
4. Simion M, Trisi P, Piattelli A. Vertical ridge augmentation using a membrane technique associated with osseointegrated implants. Int J Periodontics Restorative Dent 1994;14:496–511.
5. Tinti C, Parma-Benfenati S, Polizzi G. Vertical ridge augmentation: What is the limit? Int J Periodontics Restorative Dent 1996;16:220–229.
6. Simion M, Jovanovic SA, Trisi P, Scarano A, Piattelli A. Vertical ridge augmentation around dental implants using a membrane technique and autogenous bone or allografts in humans. Int J Periodontics Restorative Dent 1998;18:8–23.
7. Nevins M, Mellonig JT, Clem DS 3rd, Reiser GM, Buser DA. Implants in regenerated bone: Long-term survival. Int J Periodontics Restorative Dent 1998;18:34–45.
8. Simion M, Jovanovic SA, Tinti C, Benfenati SP. Long-term evaluation of osseointegrated implants inserted at the time or after vertical ridge augmentation. A retrospective study on 123 implants with 1–5 year follow-up. Clin Oral Implants Res 2001;12:35–45.
9. Spray JR, Black CG, Morris HF, Ochi S. The influence of bone thickness on facial marginal bone response: Stage 1 placement through stage 2 uncovering. Ann Periodontol 2000;5:119–128.
10. Grunder U, Gracis S, Capelli M. Influence of the 3-D bone-to-implant relationship on esthetics. Int J Periodontics Restorative Dent 2005;25:113–119.
11. Salama H, Salama MA, Garber D, Adar P. The interproximal height of bone: A guidepost to predictable aesthetic strategies and soft tissue contours in anterior tooth replacement. Pract Periodontics Aesthet Dent 1998;10:1131–1141.
12. Simion M, Trisi P, Maglione M, Piattelli A. Bacterial penetration in vitro through GTAM membrane with and without topical chlorhexidine application. A light and scanning electron microscopic study. J Clin Periodontol 1995;22:321–331.
13. Verardi S, Simion M. Management of the exposure of e-PTFE membranes in guided bone regeneration. Pract Proced Aesthet Dent 2007;19:111–117.
14. Owens KW, Yukna RA. Collagen membrane resorption in dogs: A comparative study. Implant Dent 2001;10:49–58.
15. Oh TJ, Meraw SJ, Lee EJ, Giannobile WV, Wang HL. Comparative analysis of collagen membranes for the treatment of implant dehiscence defects. Clin Oral Implants Res 2003;14:80–90.
16. Rothamel D, Schwarz F, Sager M, Herten M, Sculean A, Becker J. Biodegradation of differently cross-linked collagen membranes: An experimental study in the rat. Clin Oral Implants Res 2005;16:369–378.
17. Friedmann A, Strietzel FP, Maretzki B, Pitaru S, Bernimoulin JP. Histological assessment of augmented jaw bone utilizing a new collagen barrier membrane compared to a standard barrier membrane to protect a granular bone substitute material. Clin Oral Implants Res 2002;13:587–594.
18. Moses O, Pitaru S, Artzi Z, Nemcovsky CE. Healing of dehiscence-type defects in implants placed together with different barrier membranes: A comparative clinical study. Clin Oral Implants Res 2005;16:210–219.
19. Friedmann A, Strietzel FP, Maretzki B, Piratu S, Bernimoulin JP. Observations on a new collagen barrier membrane in 16 consecutively treated patients. Clinical and histological findings. J Periodontol 2001;72:1616–1623.
20. Bornstein MM, Bosshardt D, Buser D. Effect of two different bioabsorbable collagen membranes on guided bone regeneration: A comparative histomorphometric study in the dog mandible. J Periodontol 2007;78:1943–1953.

21. Anitua E, Carda C, Andia I. A novel drilling procedure and subsequent bone autograft preparation: A technical note. Int J Oral Maxilliofac Implants 2007;22:138–145 [erratum 2007;22:309].
22. Sartori S, Silvestri M, Forni F, Icaro Cornaglia A, Tesei P, Cattaneo V. Ten-year follow-up in a maxillary sinus augmentation using anorganic bovine bone (Bio-Oss). A case report with histomorphometric evaluation. Clin Oral Implants Res 2003;14:369–372.
23. Maiorana C, Beretta M, Salina S, Santoro F. Reduction of autogenous bone graft resorption by means of bio-oss coverage: A prospective study. Int J Periodontics Restorative Dent 2005;25:19–25.
24. Artzi Z, Weinreb M, Givol N, et al. Biomaterial resorption rate and healing site morphology of inorganic bovine bone and beta-tricalcium phosphate in the canine: A 24-month longitudinal histologic study and morphometric analysis. Int J Oral Maxilliofac Implants 2004;19:357–368.
25. Simion M, Fontana F, Rasperini G, Maiorana C. Vertical ridge augmentation by expanded-polytetrafluoroethylene membrane and a combination of intraoral autogenous bone graft and deproteinized anorganic bovine bone (Bio Oss). Clin Oral Implants Res 2007;18:620–629.
26. Boyne PJ, Cole MD, Stringer D, Shafqat JP. A technique for osseous restoration of deficient edentulous maxillary ridges. J Oral Maxillofac Surg 1985;43(2):87–91.
27. Gongloff RK, Cole M, Whitlow W, Boyne PJ. Titanium mesh and particulate cancellous bone and marrow grafts to augment the maxillary alveolar ridge. Int J Oral Maxillofac Surg 1986;15:263–268.
28. von Arx T, Hardt N, Wallkamm B. The TIME technique: A new method for localized alveolar ridge augmentation prior to placement of dental implants. Int J Oral Maxillofac Implants 1996;11:387–394.
29. von Arx T, Kurt B. Implant placement and simultaneous peri-implant bone grafting using a micro titanium mesh for graft stabilization. Int J Periodontics Restorative Dent 1998;18:117–127.
30. von Arx T, Wallkamm B, Hardt N. Localized ridge augmentation using a micro titanium mesh: A report on 27 implants followed from 1 to 3 years after functional loading. Clin Oral Implants Res 1998;9:123–130.
31. von Arx T, Kurt B. Implant placement and simultaneous ridge augmentation using autogenous bone and a micro titanium mesh: A prospective clinical study with 20 implants. Clin Oral Implants Res 1999;10:24–33.
32. Maiorana C, Santoro F, Rabagliati M, Salina S. Evaluation of the use of iliac cancellous bone and anorganic bovine bone in the reconstruction of the atrophic maxilla with titanium mesh: A clinical and histologic investigation. Int J Oral Maxillofac Implants 2001;16:427–432.
33. Lozada J, Proussaefs P. Clinical radiographic, and histologic evaluation of maxillary bone reconstruction by using a titanium mesh and autogenous iliac graft: A case report. J Oral Implantol 2002;28:9–14.
34. Artzi Z, Dayan D, Alpern Y, Nemcovsky CE. Vertical ridge augmentation using xenogenic material supported by a configured titanium mesh: Clinicohistopathologic and histochemical study. Int J Oral Maxillofac Implants 2003;18:440–446.
35. Proussaefs P, Lozada J, Kleinman A, Rohrer MD, McMillan PJ. The use of titanium mesh in conjunction with autogenous bone graft and inorganic bovine bone mineral (bio-oss) for localized alveolar ridge augmentation: A human study. Int J Periodontics Restorative Dent 2003;23:185–195.
36. Degidi M, Scarano A, Piattelli A. Regeneration of the alveolar crest using titanium micromesh with autologous bone and a resorbable membrane. J Oral Implantol 2003;29:86–90.
37. Roccuzzo M, Ramieri G, Spada MC, Bianchi SD, Berrone S. Vertical alveolar ridge augmentation by means of a titanium mesh and autogenous bone grafts. Clin Oral Implants Res 2004;15:73–81.
38. Proussaefs P, Lozada J. Use of titanium mesh for staged localized alveolar ridge augmentation: Clinical and histologic-histomorphometric evaluation. J Oral Implantol 2006;32:237–247.
39. Roccuzzo M, Ramieri G, Bunino M, Berrone S. Autogenous bone graft alone or associated with titanium mesh for vertical alveolar ridge augmentation: A controlled clinical trial. Clin Oral Implants Res 2007;18:286–294.

Chapter 6

Peri-implant Soft Tissue Management

in the Esthetic Region

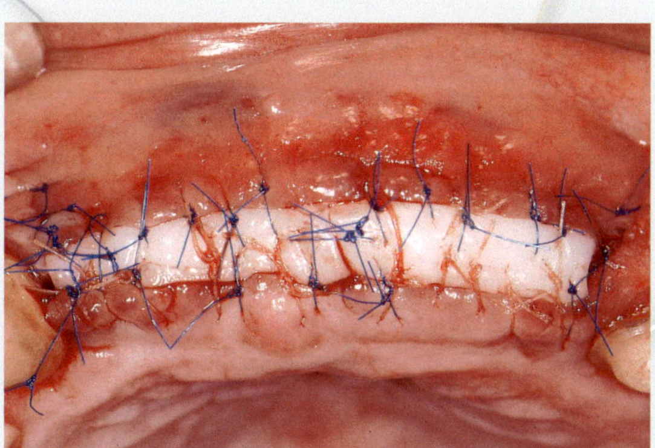

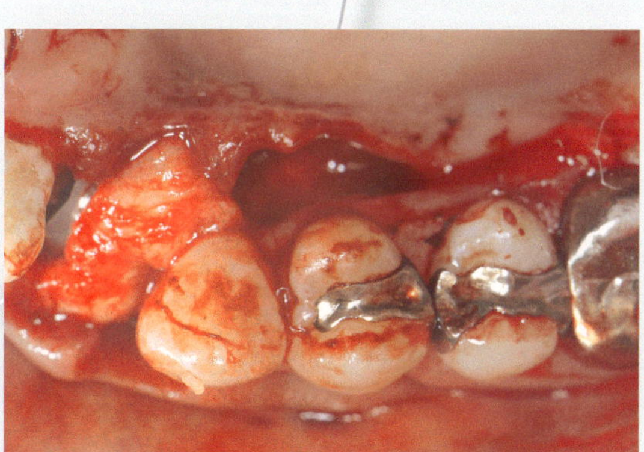

The esthetic soft tissue profile around an implant restoration is supported by the alveolar bone. Alveolar ridge preservation and augmentation, which were discussed in chapters 4 and 5, often result in a deficiency of the soft tissue, such as a thin mucosa or a lack of keratinized tissue. Because it does not share the same attachment apparatus or anatomy as the soft tissue around the natural dentition, it is important to understand how to manage the soft tissue around an implant to produce an esthetic definitive restoration.

Characteristics of Peri-implant Soft Tissue

The soft tissue barrier around an implant is generally described as having a biologic width similar to that around the natural dentition.[1–3] However, they have some important differences. The soft tissue around an implant, unlike the one around the natural dentition, is not supplied with blood from the periodontal ligament space (Fig 6-1). Further, connective tissue fiber inside the peri-implant soft tissue runs parallel to the implant but perpendicular to the natural tooth root[4] (Fig 6-2).

Biologic width around the natural dentition is located coronal to the alveolar crest. The biologic width around a two-piece implant, however, is located apical to the implant-abutment junction and alveolar crest (see Fig 6-2). As a result, bone remodeling at the implant-abutment junction and alveolar bone resorption occur.[5] In addition, the soft tissue around an implant and the soft tissue around the natural dentition do not share the same attachment apparatus. Therefore, soft tissue management for an esthetic definitive implant restoration requires special attention.

Goals of Peri-implant Soft Tissue Management

The goals of soft tissue management around an implant are determined by the location of the implant and the extent to which esthetics are a concern for the definitive restoration. In the mandibular molar region, the priority is to restore function and to maintain accessibility for oral hygiene by augmenting the keratinized tissue[6] (Fig 6-3).

In the esthetic region, the soft tissue around an implant requires natural three-dimensional (3D) form, color, and texture. A coronal shift of the mucogingival junction (Fig 6-4) and a deficiency of the keratinized tissue occur as a result of alveolar bone augmentation. Moreover, the guided bone regeneration (GBR) barrier membrane suppresses the blood supply to the soft tissue above the membrane, which tends to decrease the thickness of this tissue. Berglundh and Lindhe[7] observed consistent bone resorption at sites where the ridge mucosa was surgically thinned prior to abutment connection. This implies that a certain minimum width and thickness of the peri-implant mucosa may be required and that bone resorption may take place to allow a stable soft tissue attachment to form. It is therefore important to maintain adequately wide and thick soft tissue around the implant to maintain underlying osseous support.

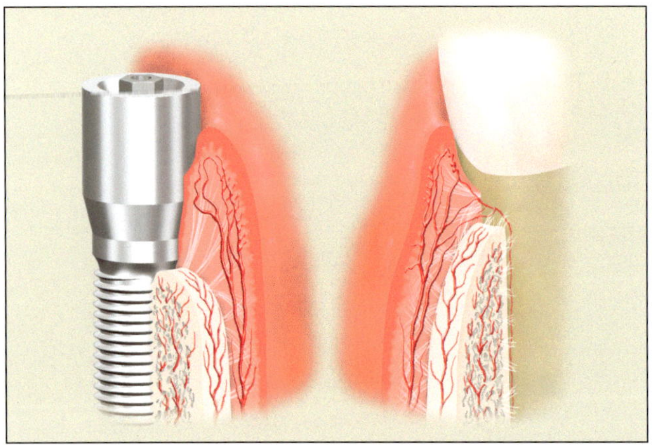

Fig 6-1 The blood supply to the soft tissue around the natural tooth comes from the periosteum, connective tissue, and periodontal ligament space. The soft tissue around the implant does not have a blood supply from the periodontal ligament space.

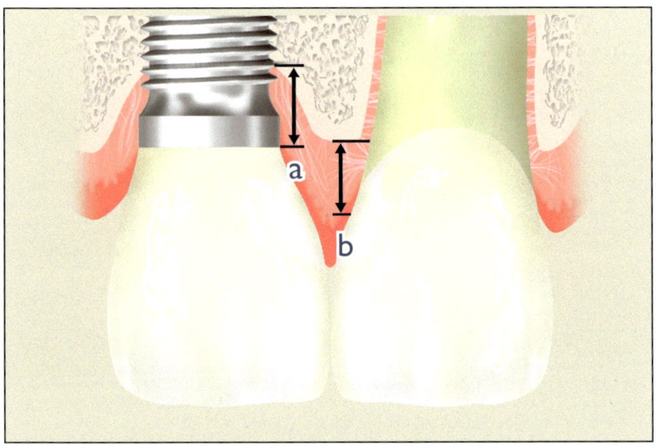

Fig 6-2 Connective tissue fiber runs perpendicular to natural teeth and parallel to implants. For implants, biologic width is located apical to the implant-abutment junction (a), and for natural teeth it is located coronal to the alveolar crest (b).

Augmenting keratinized tissue around implants

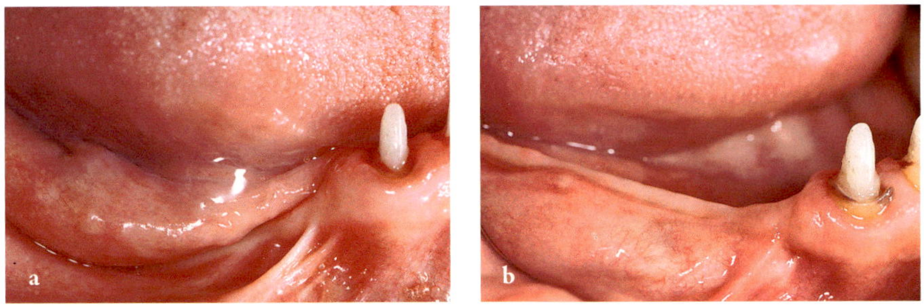

Figs 6-3a and 6-3b Same case as presented in Fig 5-3. Before *(a)* and after *(b)* guided bone regeneration. There is a limited amount of keratinized tissue present at the alveolar crest.

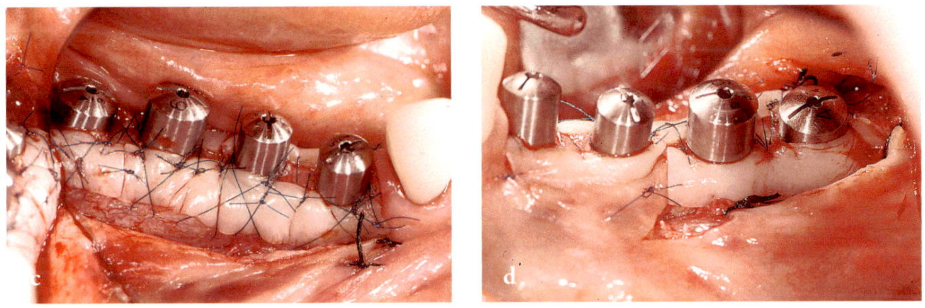

Figs 6-3c and 6-3d Keratinized tissue was augmented with a free gingival graft and an apically positioned flap.

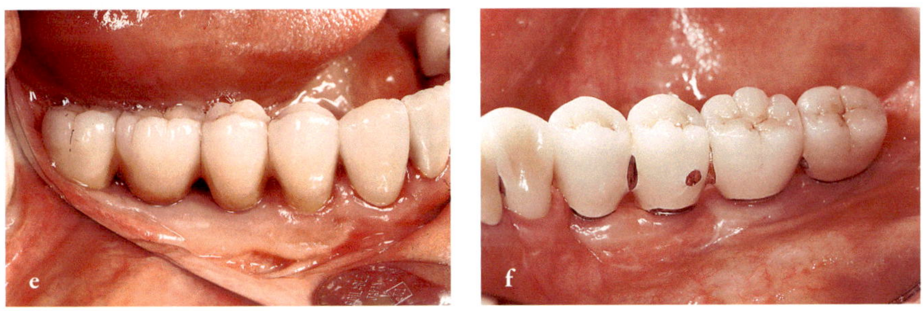

Figs 6-3e and 6-3f Buccal *(e)* and lingual *(f)* views show an adequate zone of keratinized tissue around the definitive restorations.

Coronal shift of mucogingival junction with guided bone regeneration (GBR)

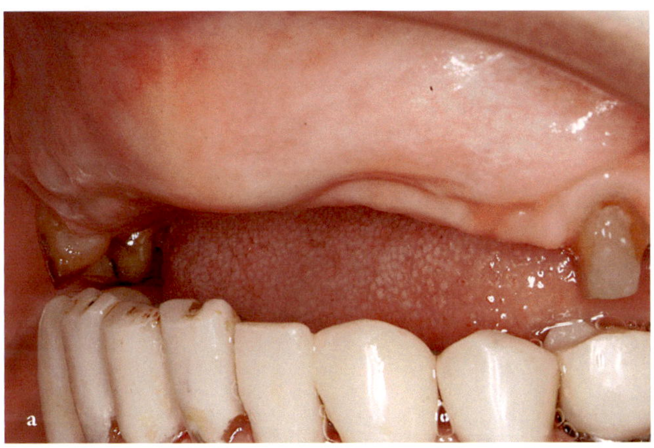

Fig 6-4a The mucogingival junction has shifted coronally toward the palatal side as a complication of GBR.

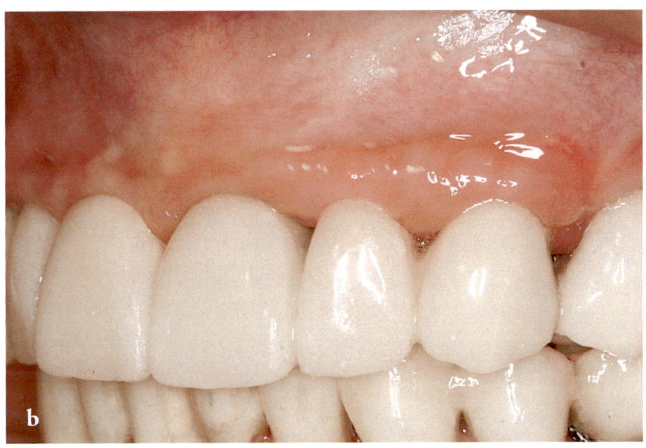

Fig 6-4b The soft tissue problems were corrected by a laterally positioned flap and an interpositional graft.

Determinants of Peri-implant Soft Tissue Profile

The soft tissue profile around the implant restoration is determined by the quality and quantity of the soft tissue, the anatomy and morphology of the abutment, and the subgingival morphology of the implant suprastructure. A patient's biotype also significantly affects the treatment result.[8–10] Kan et al[10] suggested that greater soft tissue dimension around the implant was noted in patients with a thick biotype as opposed to those with a thin biotype.

Predicted papilla height is in part determined by whether the papilla is between teeth, pontics, implants, or some combination thereof[11] (see Table 2-1). Tarnow et al[5] measured from the highest point of the soft tissue to the crest of bone between two adjacent implants and found that 72.8% of the sites demonstrated 3- or 4-mm soft tissue height. In a single-tooth implant case, the natural tooth's periodontium adjacent to the implant supports the papilla. In cases with multiple adjacent implants and pontics, the soft tissue profile is only supported by the restorations (Fig 6-5).

Esthetic soft tissue profile around definitive implant restorations

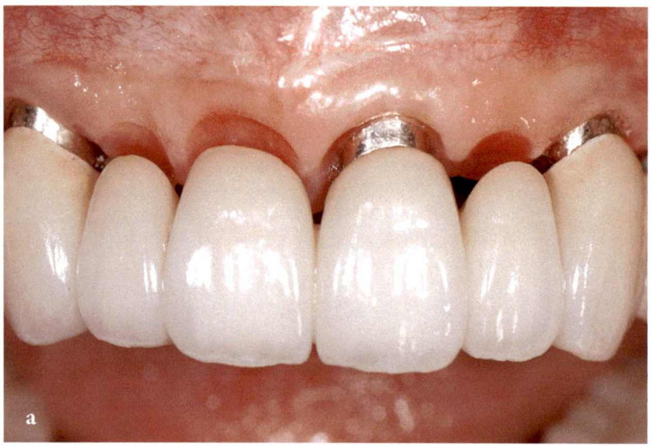

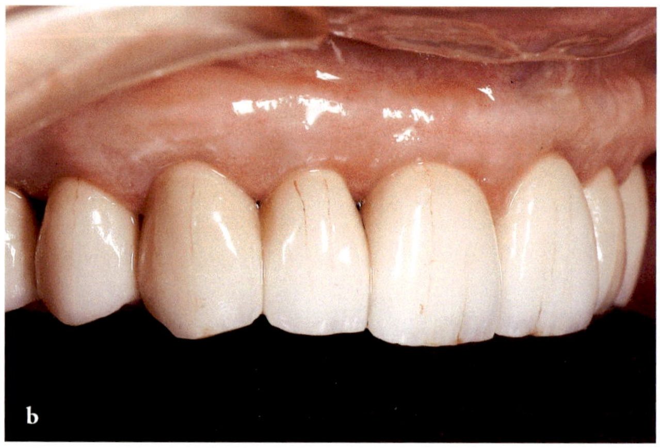

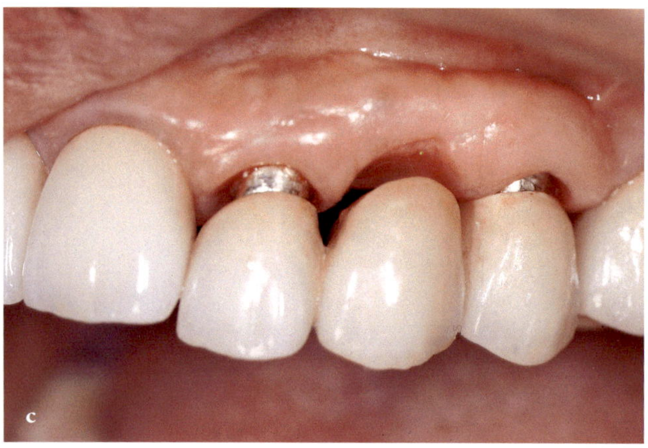

Figs 6-5a to 6-5c Clinical views of three patients for whom esthetic papilla form was created between implant and pontic, between pontics, and between implants.

Timing of Soft Tissue Augmentation Under the 4D Concept

The timing and sequence of soft tissue augmentation is important.[12] Under the four-dimensional (4D) concept, soft tissue augmentation could occur at any one of seven points[13] (Box 6-1).

Point 1: Extraction

To seal the extraction socket and to augment facial tissue, the practitioner may perform a connective tissue graft, a socket seal procedure, or a pedicle connective tissue graft. The decision whether to reflect the gingival flap depends upon the goals of augmentation and preservation as well as the surrounding tissue condition.

Point 2: Bone augmentation

Soft tissue augmentation immediately prior to bone augmentation is not advisable because it may cause soft tissue trauma to the area. Soft tissue augmentation at the same time as bone augmentation may also seem ill advised because areas with a GBR membrane have a reduced blood supply. However, if a pedicle connective tissue graft, which maintains blood supply from the donor site, is used, soft tissue augmentation can be performed simultaneously with a bone augmentation procedure.

Point 3: Implant placement

With immediate implant placement, the extraction socket can be closed with a soft tissue graft. After bone augmentation with a nonresorbable membrane or titanium mesh, the clinician often needs to perform the implant placement and a connective tissue graft simultaneously to augment the soft tissue thickness. Slight facial concavity could be corrected with a soft tissue graft at implant placement. The advantage of following this approach is that it reduces surgical interventions.

Box 6-1 Seven points at which soft tissue augmentation can occur under the 4D concept

1. Extraction
2. Bone augmentation
3. Implant placement
4. Implant integration
5. Stage-two surgery
6. Provisional restoration
7. Definitive restoration

Point 4: Implant integration

When implant placement and bone augmentation are done at the same time, a soft tissue graft can be performed while removing the membrane and/or mesh. Placing healing abutments with a 2- to 3-mm height helps to augment the soft tissue height as well.

Point 5: Stage-two surgery

A soft tissue graft and the gingival flap can be anchored to the healing abutment with sutures. This approach is effective for facial tissue augmentation.

Point 6: Provisional restoration

After stage-two surgery with abutment connection, bone remodeling commences, and the soft tissue profile changes. Tissue sculpting will promote soft tissue changes. Major soft tissue changes occur within 3 months; however, 6 months or more of soft tissue observation is preferable with provisional restorations. Soft tissue changes beyond the anticipated amount should be corrected with a soft tissue graft when necessary, often employing an envelope technique (as described in the next section) so as not to damage the surrounding soft tissue profile. When soft tissue height needs to be increased at this stage, the abutment has to be replaced with a cover screw to allow soft tissue coverage over the implant. Then, the soft tissue height should be augmented with an envelope technique. Soft tissue sculpting is necessary again upon the healing of the soft tissue graft.

Point 7: Definitive restoration

Unexpected soft tissue changes that occur after a patient is in the maintenance period should be corrected with a connective tissue graft using a minimally invasive protocol.

Soft Tissue Augmentation Protocols Under the 4D Concept

Soft tissue management procedures and their optimal timing are listed in Box 6-2.

Roll technique

The roll technique was introduced by Abrams in 1972. Thick palatal tissue can be rolled inside the buccal flap to augment buccal soft tissue thickness (Fig 6-6). To achieve an esthetic result, care must be taken not to extend the incisions too far buccally.

Envelope technique

Buccal soft tissue volume can be augmented with an envelope technique with connective tissue grafting (Figs 6-7 and 6-8). This technique is less invasive than some of the other options; interproximal tissues are not affected.[14,15]

Flap technique

A connective tissue graft needs to be positioned at the alveolar crest in order to augment vertical height. Using a low-profile healing abutment helps vertical soft tissue augmentation in some cases. The implant should be submerged after soft tissue augmentation, then stage-two surgery with a tissue punch technique should be performed. Treatment period and number of surgical interventions increase. With a large amount of augmentation, the mucogingival junction shifts, and buccal keratinized tissue decreases (Figs 6-9 and 6-10). An additional procedure such as an apically positioned flap may be necessary in order to augment keratinized tissue.

Interpositional graft

Keratinized tissue as well as the width and height of the alveolar ridge can be augmented using a connective tissue graft with a wide band of keratinized tissue. A buccal flap, including the keratinized tissue, should be elevated from the alveolar crest. The keratinized tissue portion of the graft should be positioned at the alveolar crest, then a buccal flap sutured over the connective tissue portion of the graft (Fig 6-11). Today, the authors mainly select this technique as a soft tissue management option because it allows augmentation of the soft tissue thickness as well as the amount of keratinized tissue. It does so without esthetic complications such as failure of soft tissue color to match.

Pedicle connective tissue graft

Vertical height and buccal soft tissue thickness can be augmented at the same time with a pedicle connective tissue graft (Fig 6-12). The pedicle connective tissue graft maintains blood supply from the palatal donor site. This technique is effective with immediate implant placement, which has a reduced blood supply to the gingival flap because of the extraction socket.[16–21]

Laterally positioned flap

In multiple-tooth implant cases, maxillary buccal tissue can be augmented with a laterally positioned flap (Fig 6-13). The flap should include palatal tissue, which usually consists of thick, dense connective tissue. Palatal tissue can be securely sutured in the buccal position using temporary healing abutments as an anchor, as described by Tinti and Benfenati.[22] However, the mesiodistal dimension of the flap often becomes insufficient. Note that a palatal open wound has no significant effect on the buccal soft tissue profile.[23]

Laterally positioned flap + interpositional graft

In addition to the laterally positioned flap, a connective tissue graft with a wide bank of keratinized tissue can be used to augment soft tissue thickness (Fig 6-14). Soft tissue augmentation of the pontic site can be performed with this protocol.

Tissue punch technique

The tissue punch technique can preserve soft tissue during stage-two surgery when soft tissue quality and quantity are sufficient (Fig 6-15). Performing the tissue punch slightly palatally allows for preservation of buccal tissue. Soft tissue sculpting is necessary after the tissue punch. An esthetic soft tissue profile can be created with an ovate pontic prior to the tissue punch.

Box 6-2 Soft tissue management techniques and timing under the 4D concept

1. Roll technique (point 5)
2. Envelope technique (point 5, 6, or 7)
3. Flap technique (point 3 or 4)
4. Interpositional graft (multiple-tooth implant cases in the esthetic region) (point 3 or 4)
5. Pedicle connective tissue graft (point 1, 2, 3, or 4)
6. Laterally positioned flap (multiple-tooth implant cases in the esthetic region) (point 5)
7. Laterally positioned flap + interpositional graft (multiple-tooth implant cases in the esthetic region) (point 5)
8. Tissue punch technique (multiple-tooth implant cases in the esthetic region) (point 5)

Roll technique performed at point 5 (stage-two surgery)

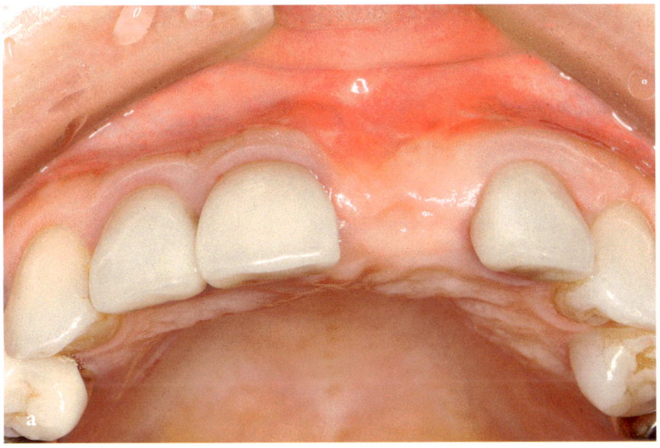

Fig 6-6a Occlusal view 6 months after socket preservation and implant placement. The buccal soft tissue volume was insufficient.

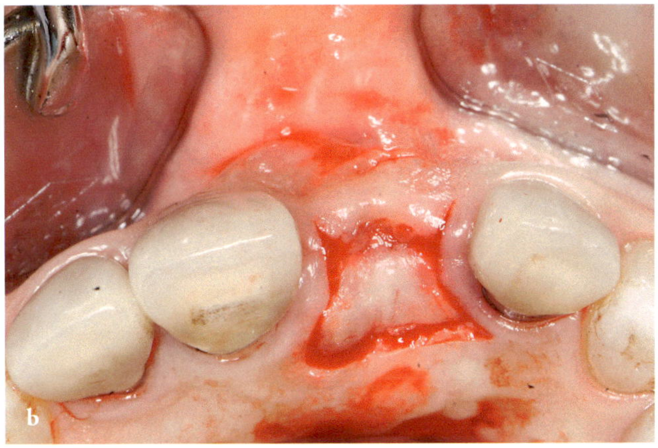

Fig 6-6b The palatal donor area was deepithelialized.

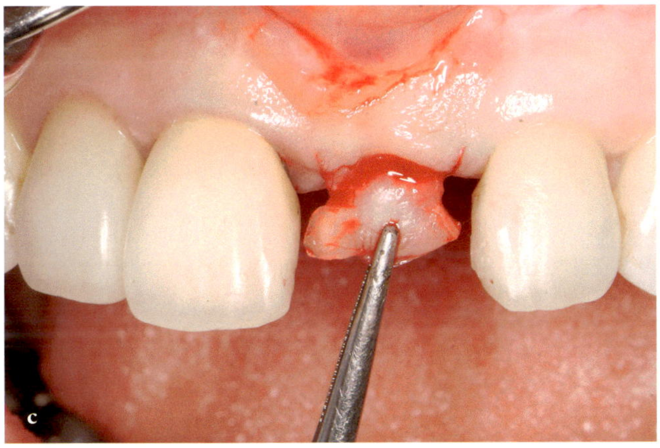

Fig 6-6c The donor tissue was reflected, and a pouch was created buccally.

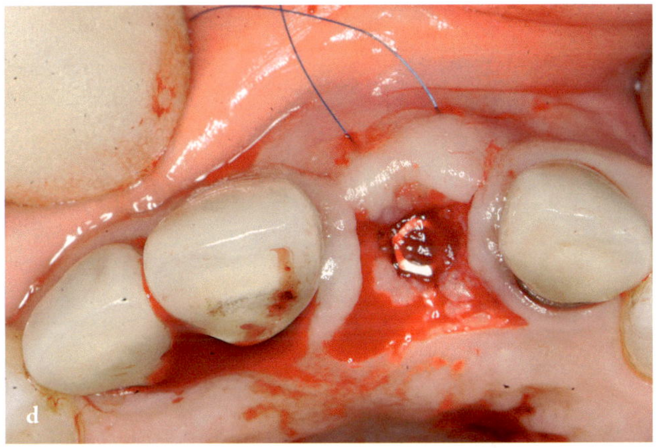

Fig 6-6d The donor tissue was rolled into the inside of the buccal pouch and stabilized with a suture. Note that the incisions were not extended too far buccally.

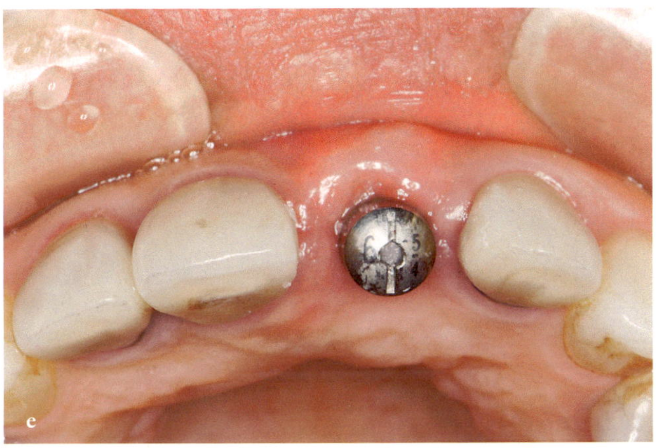

Fig 6-6e Adequate soft tissue volume was observed 3 months after surgery.

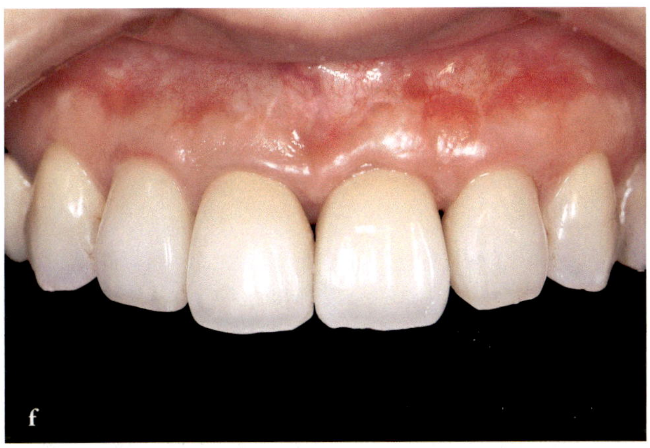

Fig 6-6f At the 2-year follow-up, an esthetic soft tissue profile was maintained.

Envelope technique performed at point 7 (definitive restoration)

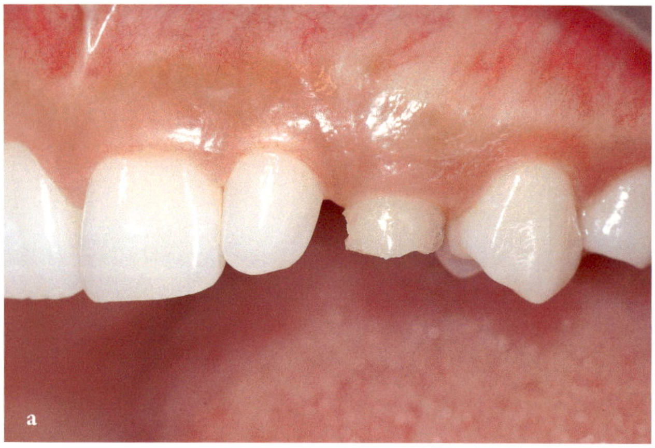

Fig 6-7a The patient presented with a retained primary tooth, which created an esthetic problem.

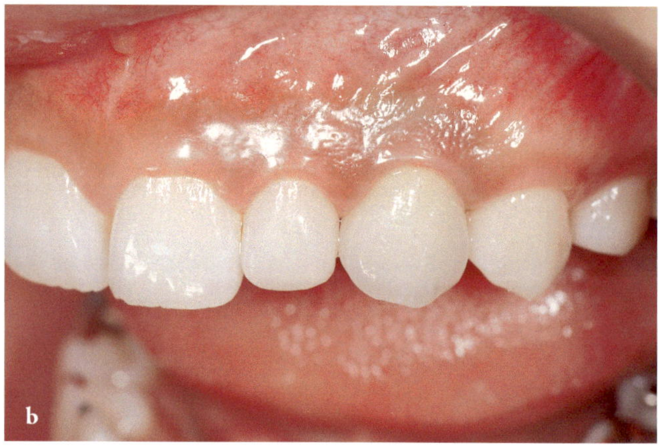

Fig 6-7b Facial view of definitive restoration. Prior to placement of the definitive restoration, immediate implant placement was performed, and a provisional restoration was placed immediately.

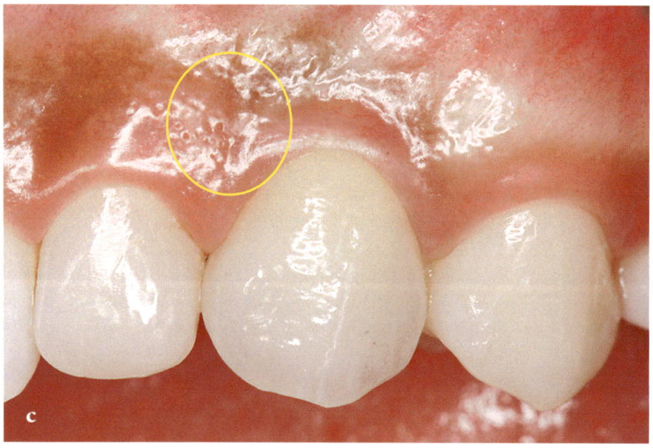

Fig 6-7c Two years later, a small perforation of the soft tissue *(circled area)* was observed at the implant-abutment connection level.

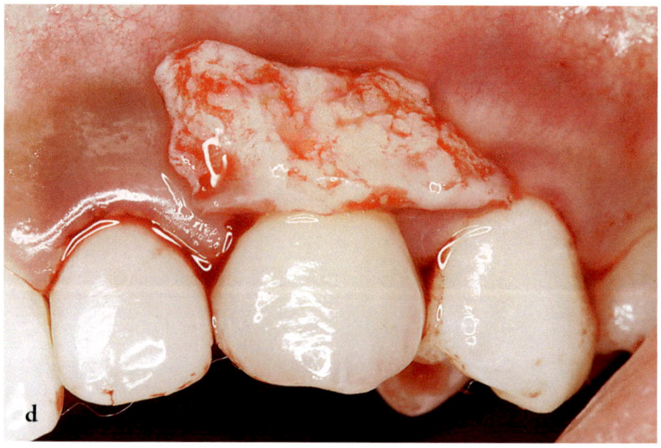

Fig 6-7d Envelope technique and connective tissue grafting were performed.

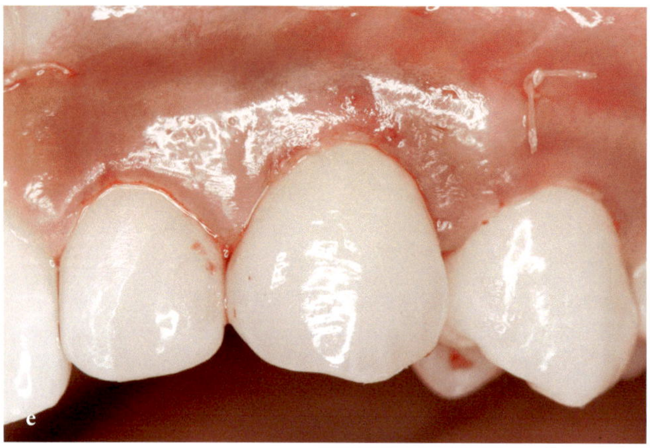

Fig 6-7e Clinical appearance immediately after suturing.

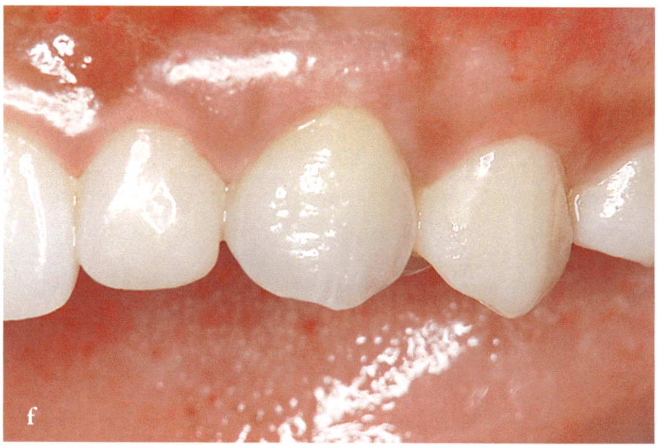

Fig 6-7f Good results were maintained 3 years after implant placement and 1 year after soft tissue augmentation.

Envelope technique performed at point 6 (provisional restoration)

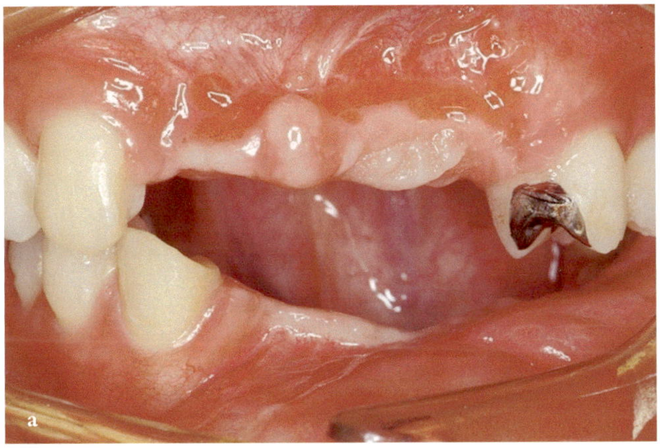

Fig 6-8a Patient presented with multiple missing teeth following a motor vehicle accident.

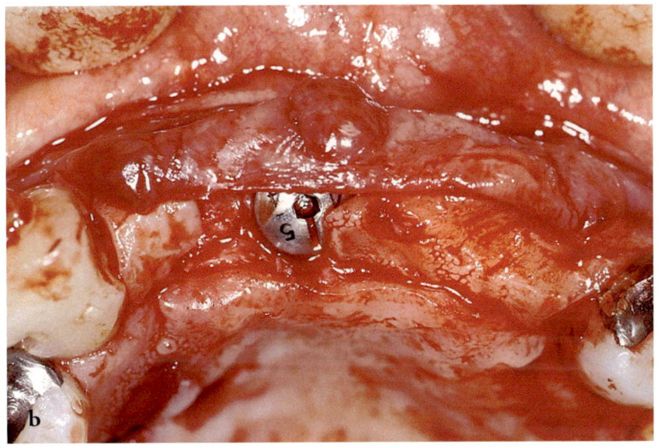

Fig 6-8b Implants were placed after bone augmentation. A laterally positioned flap and interpositional graft were performed at stage-two surgery. Note the thin buccal flap.

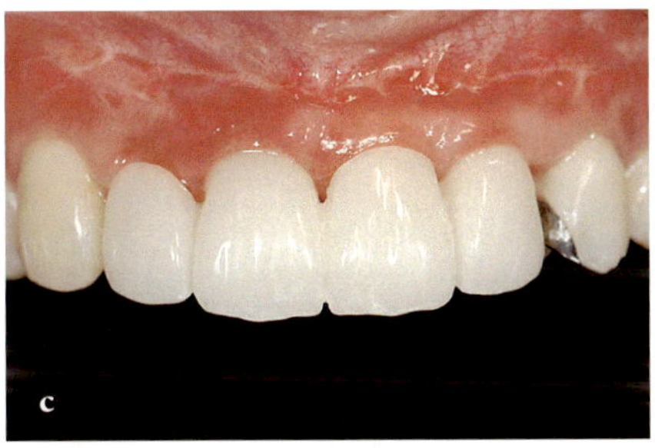

Fig 6-8c Eight weeks after the provisional restoration was placed, a soft tissue perforation was observed distal to the right central incisor.

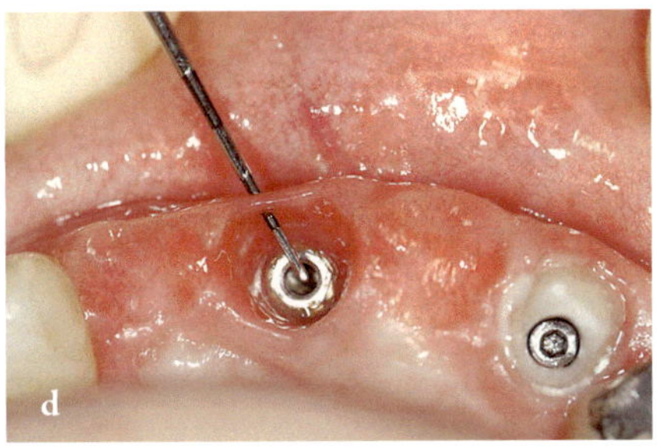

Fig 6-8d The soft tissue thickness was less than 1 mm.

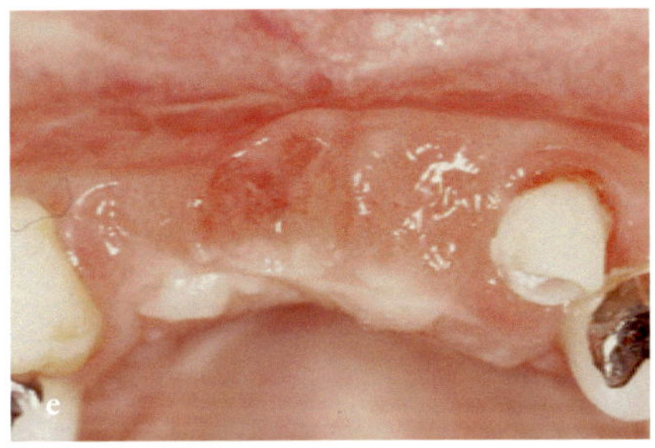

Fig 6-8e The implant was completely covered with soft tissue 3 weeks after the provisional restoration was removed.

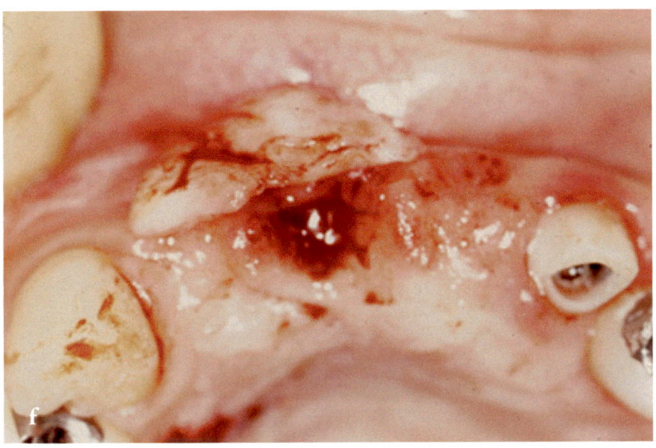

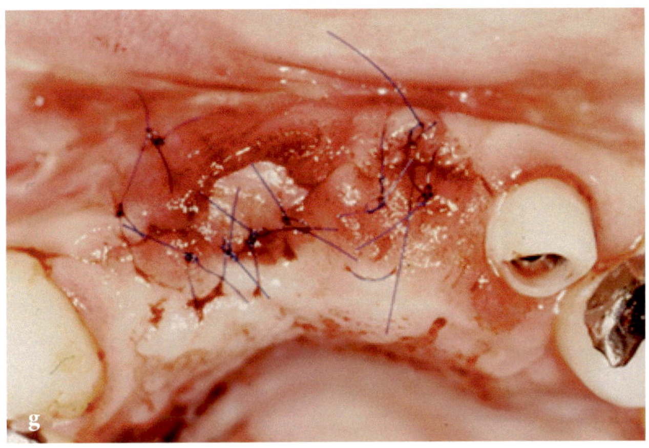

Figs 6-8f and 6-8g Connective tissue grafting with an envelope technique was performed.

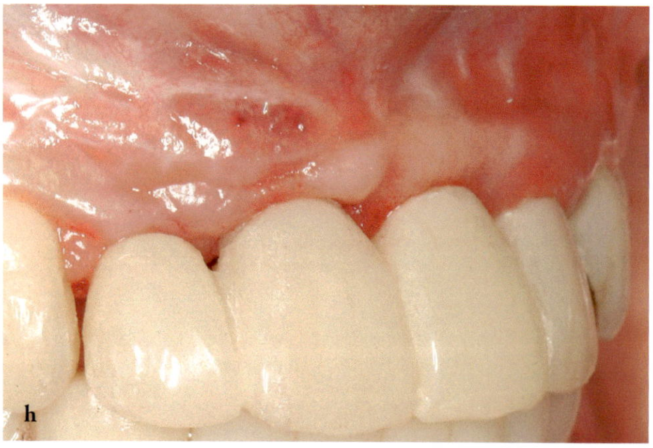

Fig 6-8h Two months after connective tissue grafting, the same provisional custom abutment and provisional restoration were placed. The facial subgingival contour of the provisional custom abutment was reduced. Papilla form was flat. A provisional restoration margin was exposed at this stage. Adequate pressure was applied to the tissue.

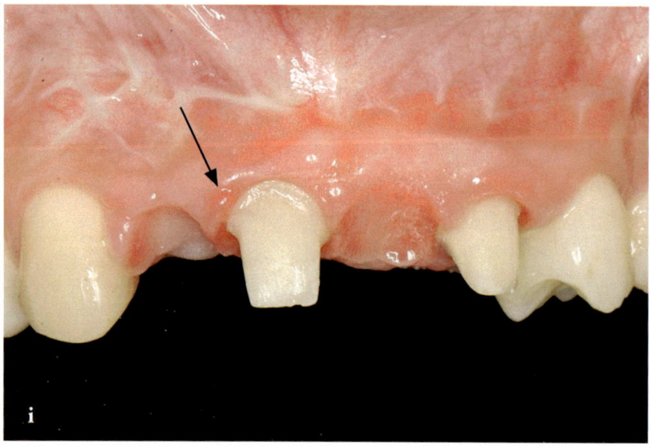

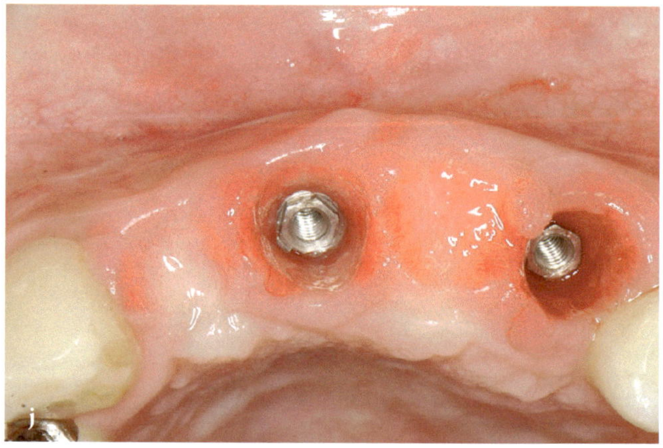

Figs 6-8i and 6-8j Two weeks later, an appropriate soft tissue profile was reestablished. The provisional restoration margin was subgingival, and adequate soft tissue thickness was obtained.

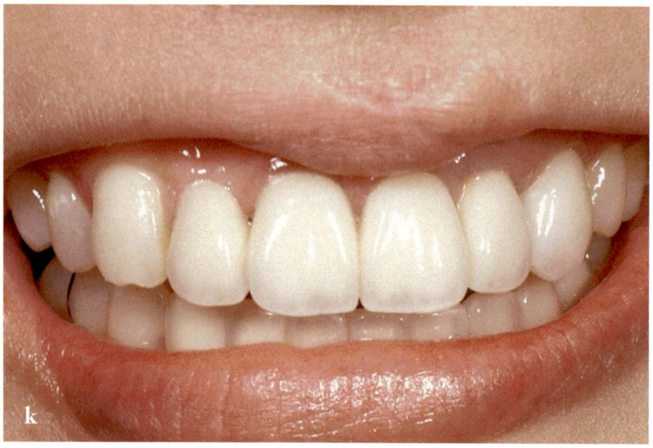

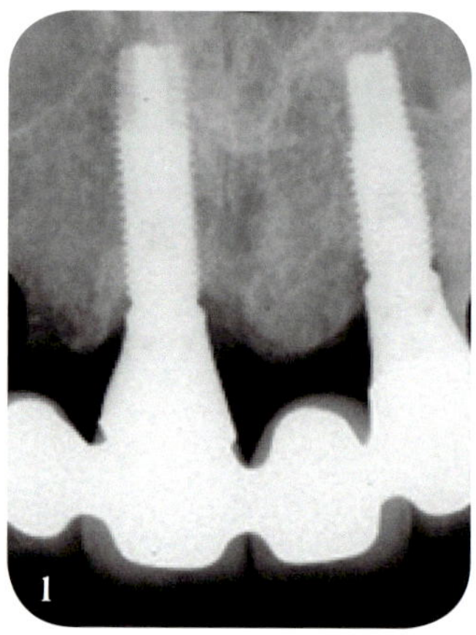

Figs 6-8k and 6-8l Definitive restoration.

Flap technique: No mucogingival junction shift

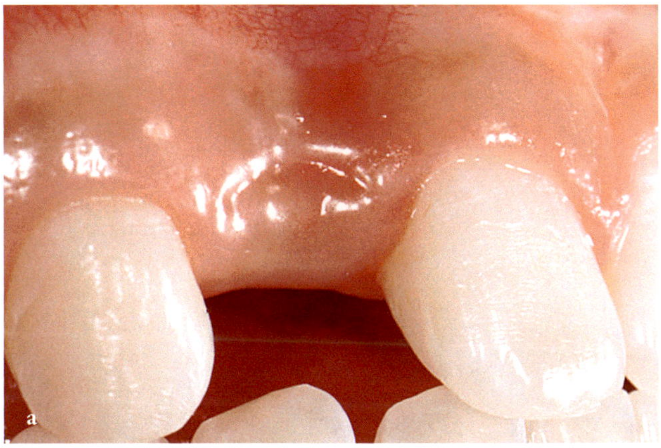

Fig 6-9a Initial examination. The right lateral incisor was congenitally missing, and a buccal concavity was observed.

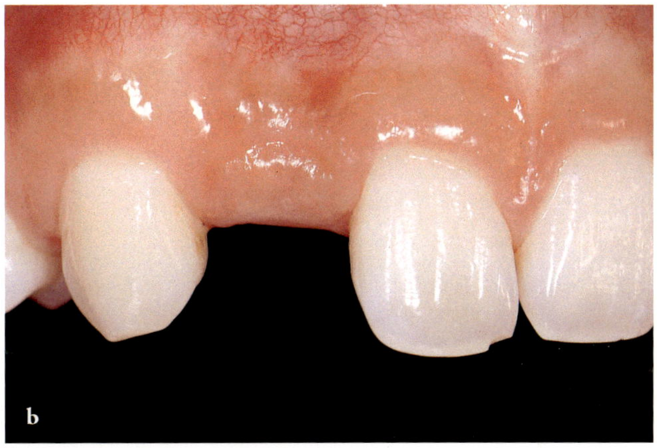

Fig 6-9b After implant placement and GBR, the mucogingival junction did not shift.

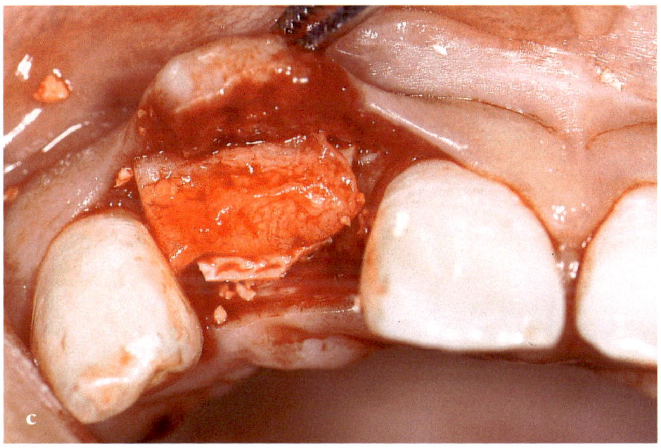

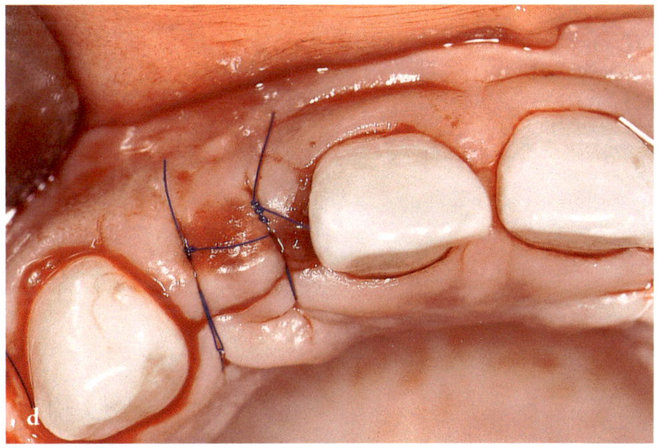

Figs 6-9c and 6-9d After flap elevation, the connective tissue graft was positioned buccally beginning at the alveolar crest. The flap was sutured, and the implant was submerged.

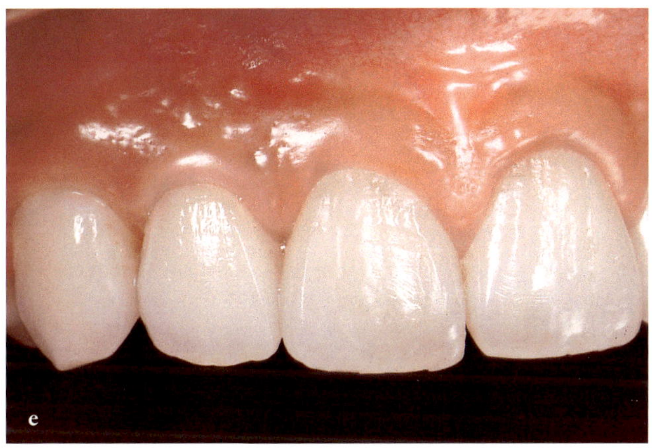

Fig 6-9e Facial view of definitive restoration. An esthetic soft tissue profile was established.

Flap technique: Large mucogingival junction shift

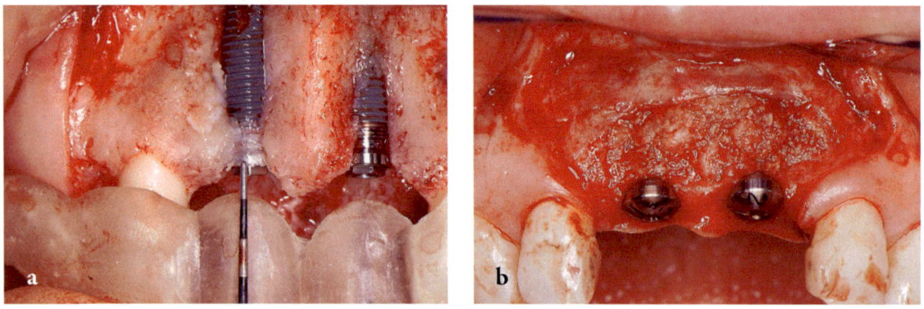

Figs 6-10a and 6-10b Adequate buccal bone was augmented.

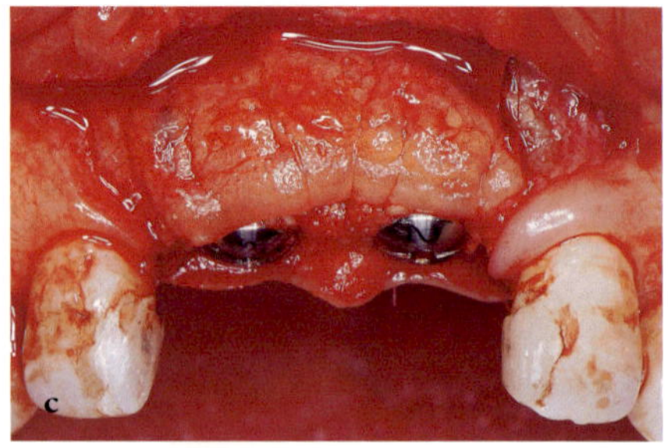

Fig 6-10c Healing abutments (2 mm in height) were placed, and the connective tissue graft was stabilized.

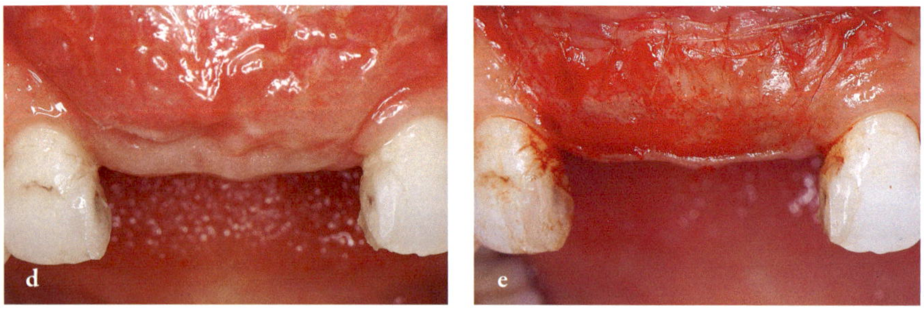

Figs 6-10d and 6-10e *(d)* The mucogingival junction was shifted coronally, and the amount of buccal keratinized tissue was decreased. *(e)* A partial thickness flap was elevated from the alveolar crest, and keratinized tissue was apically positioned and sutured.

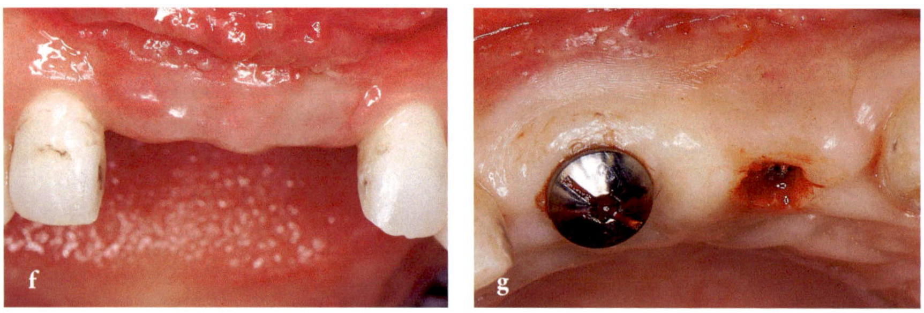

Figs 6-11f and 6-11g *(f)* Two months later, an adequate amount of keratinized tissue was gained. *(g)* Healing abutments were connected following a tissue punch technique.

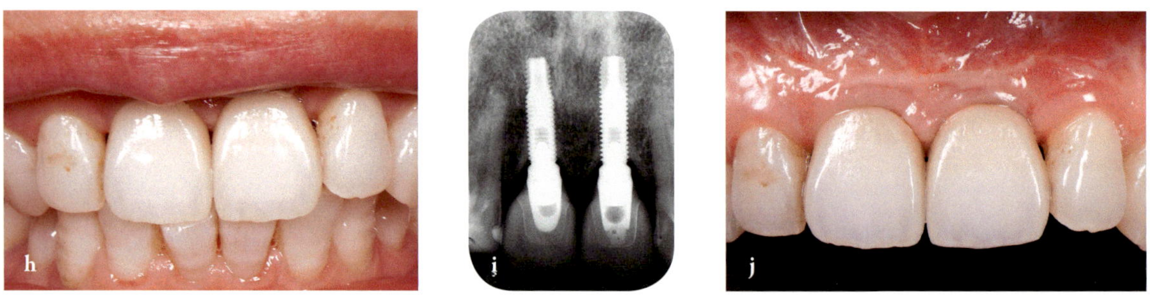

Figs 6-10h to 6-10j An esthetic soft tissue profile was maintained at the 6-year follow-up.

Interpositional graft

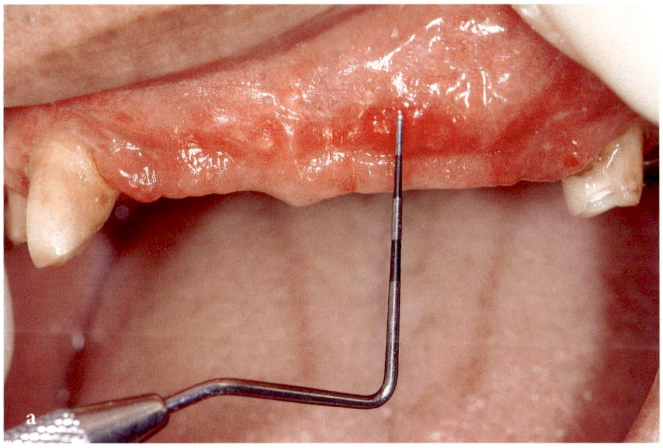

Fig 6-11a After ridge augmentation, keratinized tissue was deficient by 4 to 5 mm.

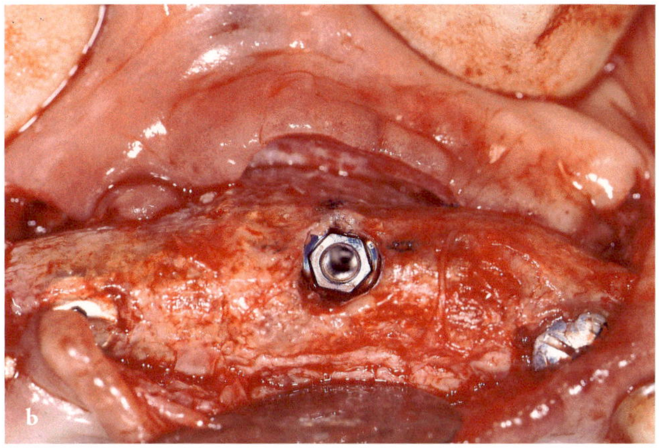

Fig 6-11b Buccal soft tissue augmentation was necessary.

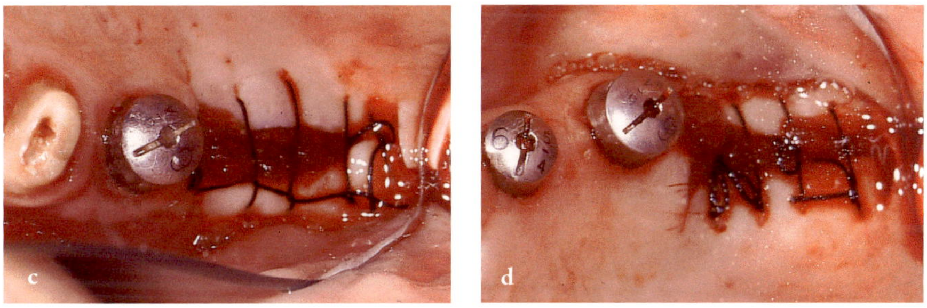

Figs 6-11c and 6-11d A connective tissue graft with 5 mm of keratinized tissue was harvested from both sides of the palate.

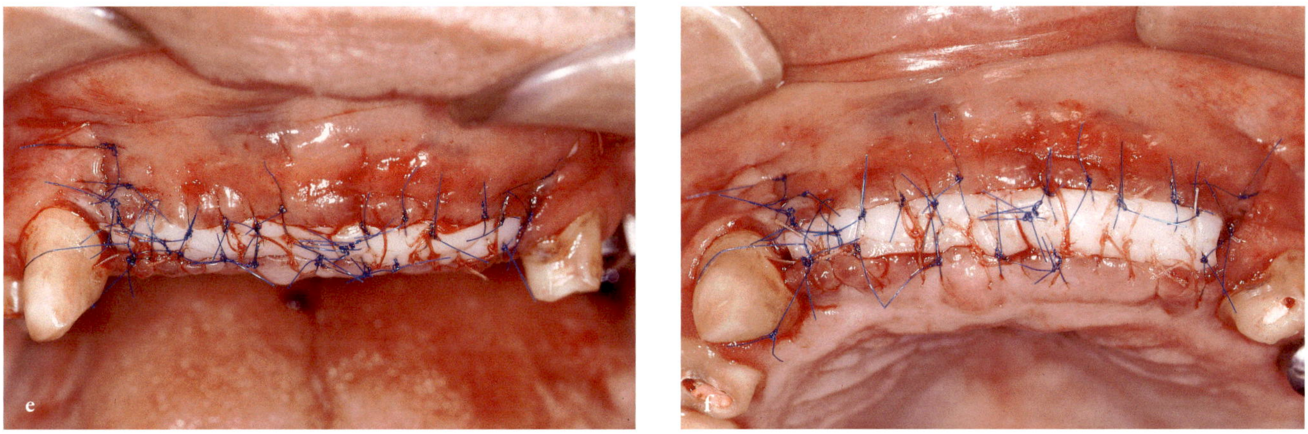

Figs 6-11e and 6-11f The keratinized tissue portion of the graft was positioned at the alveolar crest and sutured.

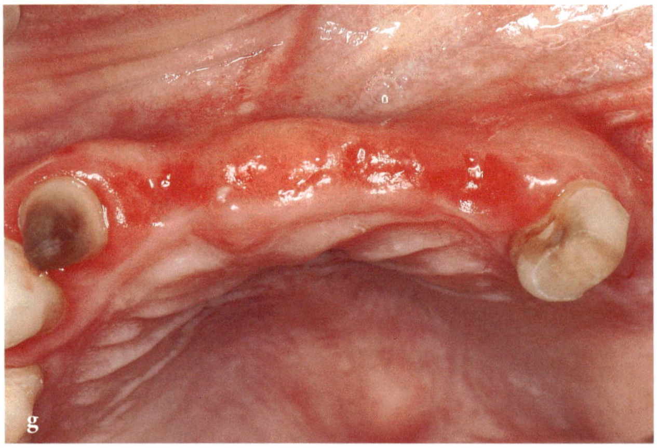

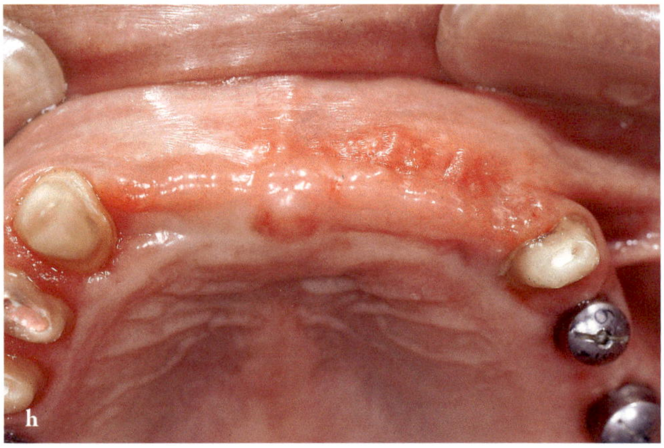

Figs 6-11g and 6-11h Before *(g)* and after *(h)* ridge augmentation.

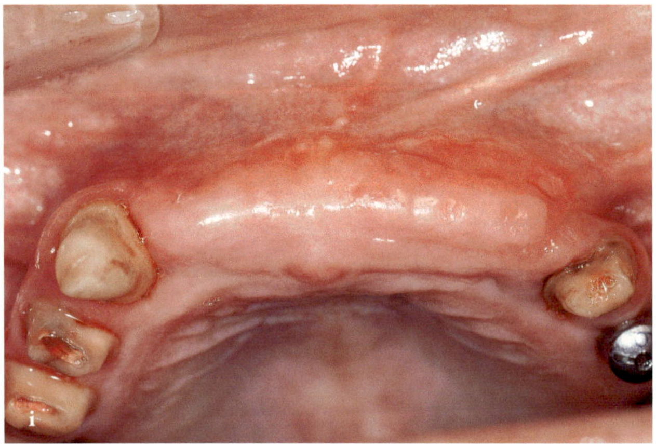

Fig 6-11i Occlusal view after soft tissue augmentation. The soft tissue profile was improved, and the amount of keratinized tissue was increased.

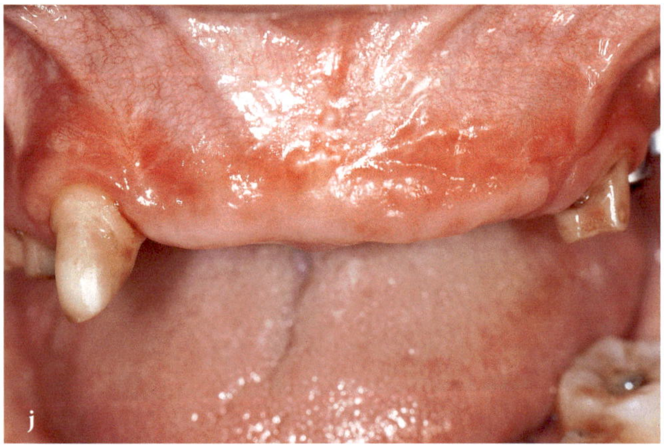

Fig 6-11j Facial view after soft tissue augmentation. An esthetic soft tissue profile will be created through tissue sculpting with provisional restorations.

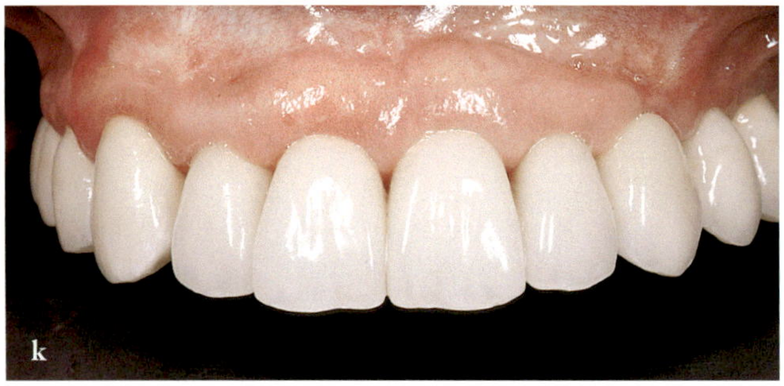

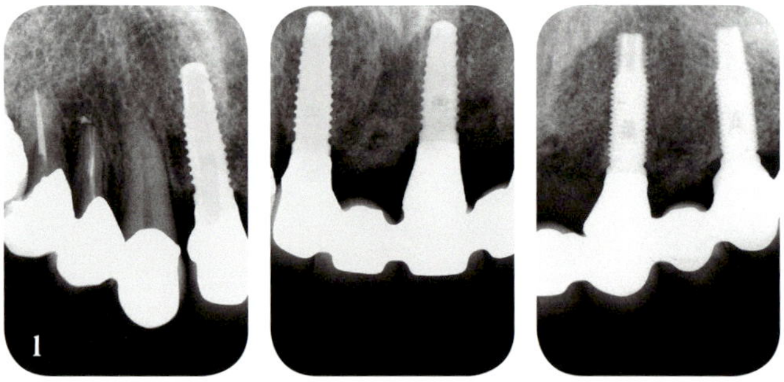

Figs 6-11k and 6-11l Facial view *(k)* and radiographs *(l)* of definitive restorations. An esthetic soft tissue profile and adequate keratinized tissue were established.

Pedicle connective tissue graft

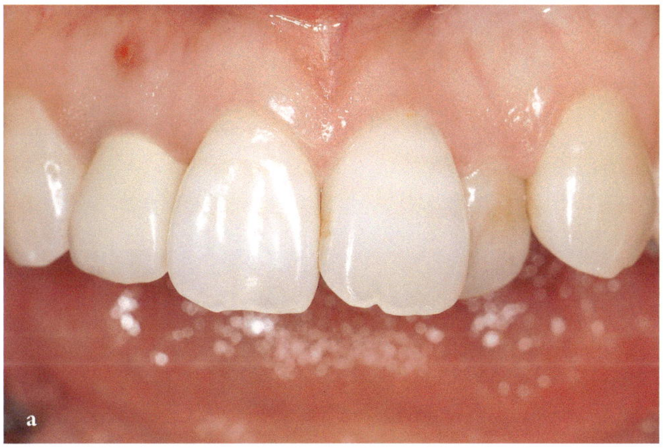

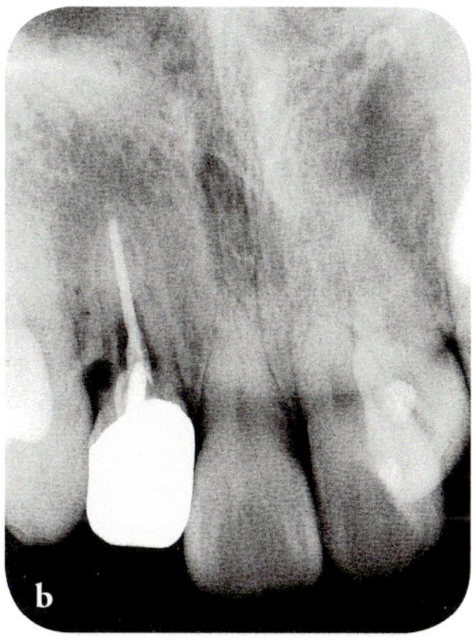

Figs 6-12a and 6-12b Internal resorption of the right lateral incisor was observed at the initial examination.

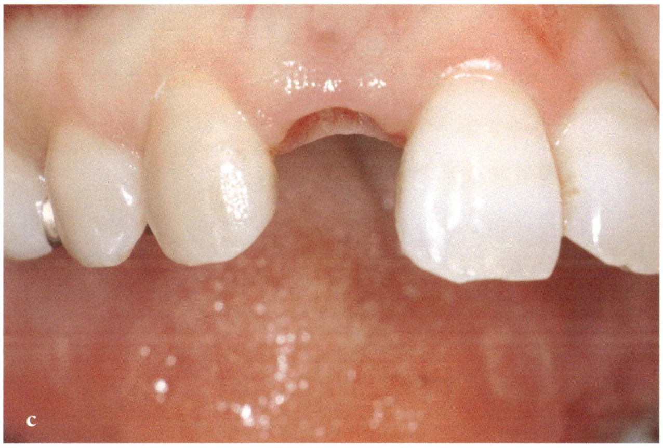

Fig 6-12c Two months after extraction.

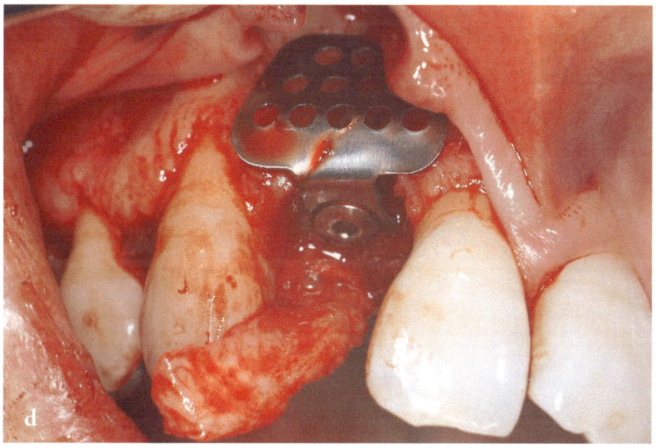

Fig 6-12d Implant placement with an FT wing.

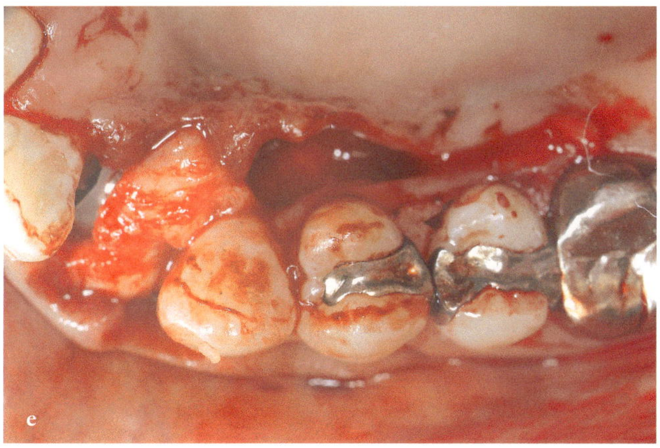

Fig 6-12e A pedicle connective tissue graft was harvested.

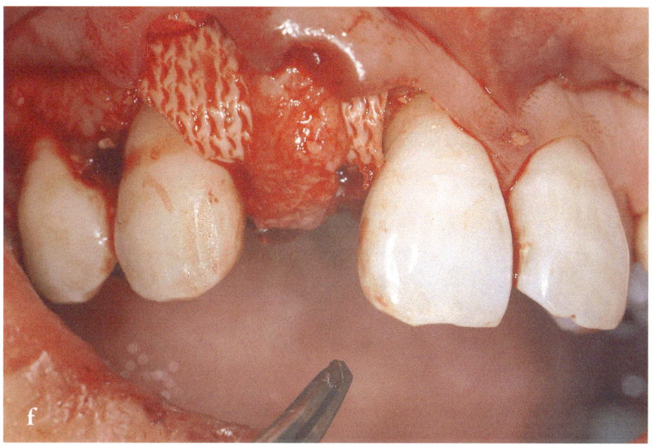

Fig 6-12f The pedicle connective tissue graft was placed over the bone graft, and a resorbable membrane was positioned.

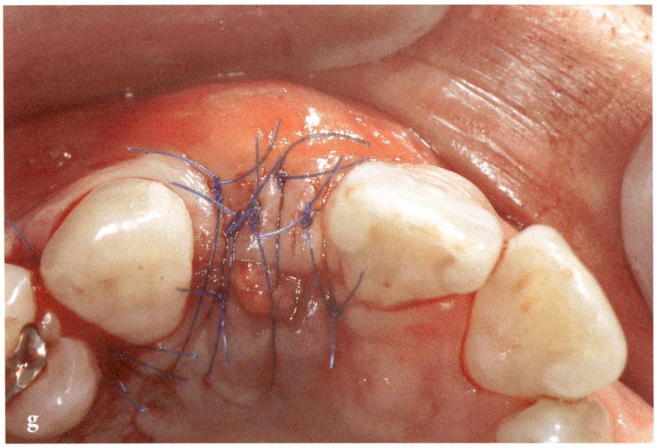

Fig 6-12g Occlusal view after suturing.

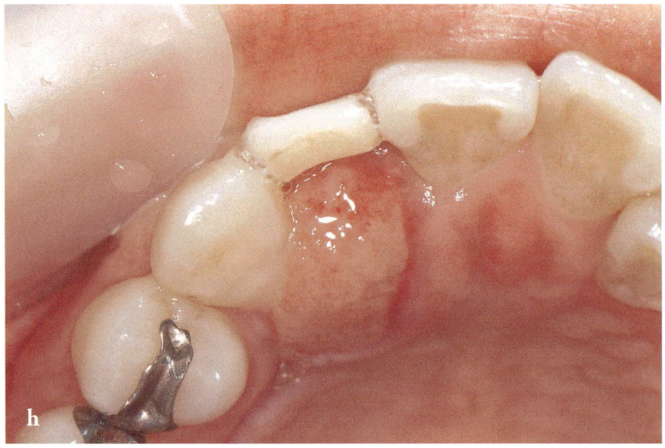

Fig 6-12h Two-week follow-up.

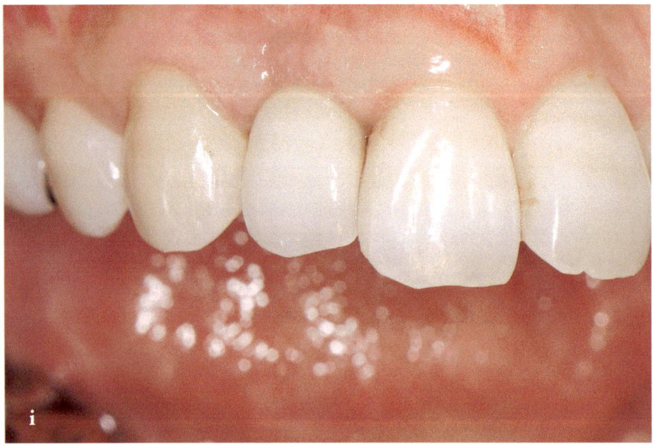

Fig 6-12i Facial view of definitive restoration. Prior to placement of the definitive restoration, after 6 months of healing, stage-two surgery was performed. Soft tissue profile was created with tissue sculpting.

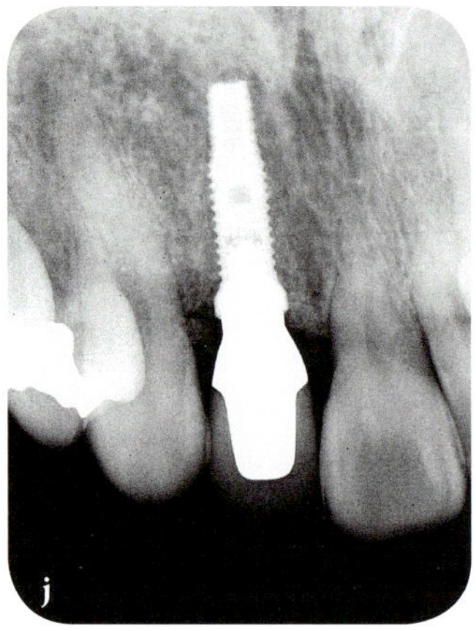

Fig 6-12j Periapical radiograph of the definitive restoration.

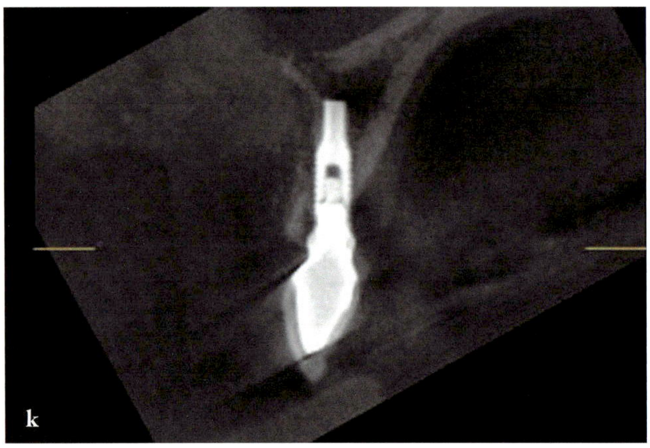

Fig 6-12k Computed tomographic evaluation.

Laterally positioned flap

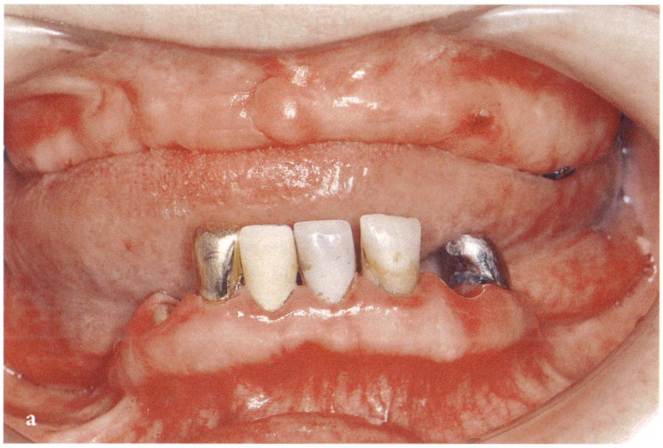

Fig 6-13a Facial view at initial examination.

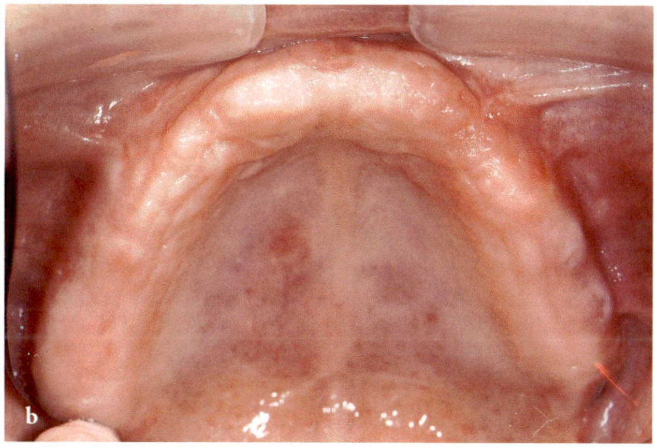

Fig 6-13b Occlusal view before stage-two surgery.

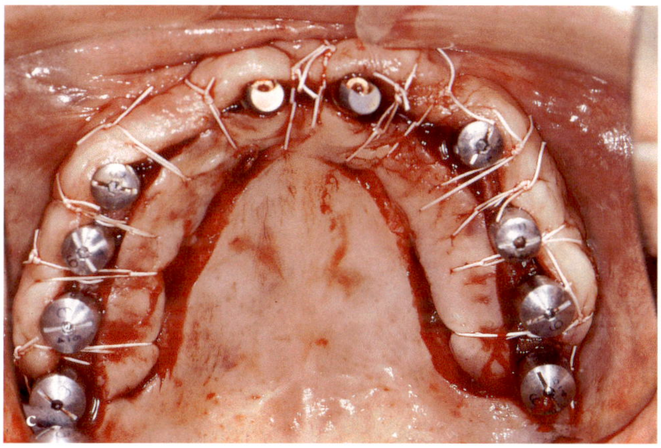

Fig 6-13c After laterally positioned flap procedure. A full-thickness flap was elevated from 5 mm palatal to the mucogingival junction, where the soft tissue thickness was 4 to 6 mm. The flap was moved buccally and sutured to the temporary healing abutments. When the buccal flap thickness was insufficient (less than 3 mm), connective tissue harvested from the palate was placed inside of the buccal flap, then sutured.

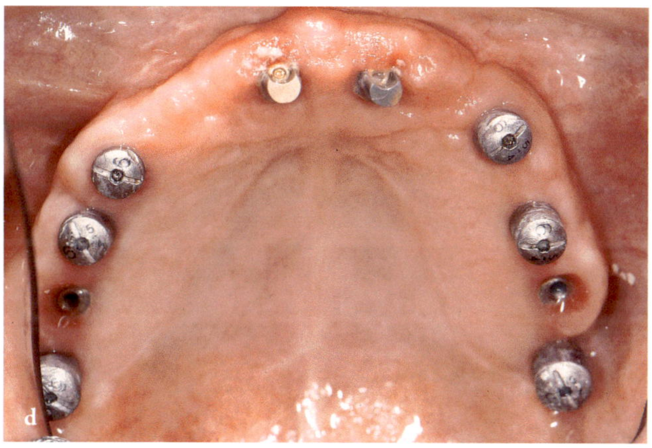

Fig 6-13d After 2 months of healing. Keratinized tissue with sufficient thickness was obtained, except around the most distal implants.

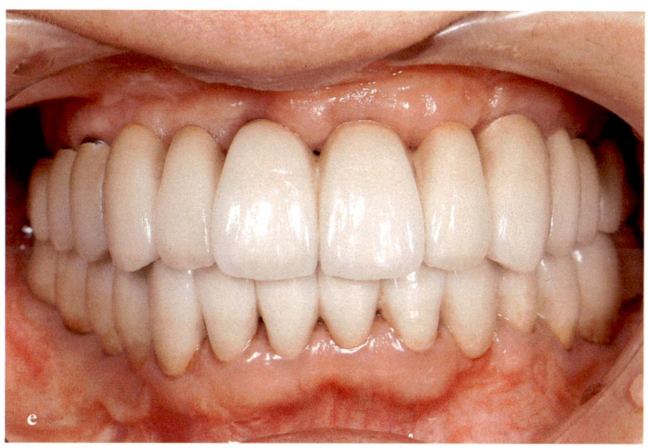

Fig 6-13e Facial view at the 1-year follow-up.

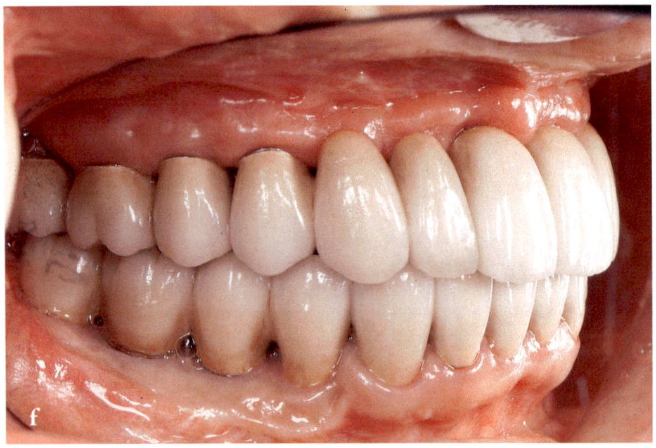
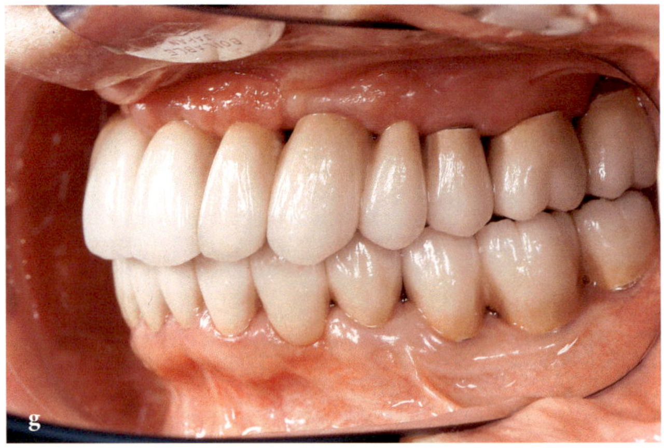

Figs 6-13f and 6-13g Lateral views at the 1-year follow-up. Sufficient buccal soft tissue augmentation was maintained.

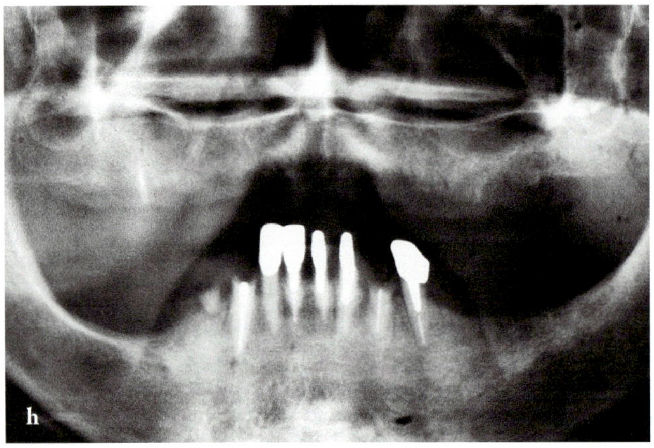
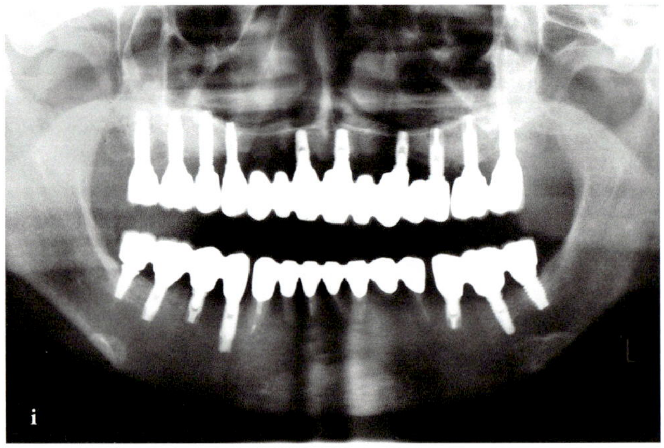

Figs 6-13h and 6-13i Panoramic radiographs before *(h)* and after *(i)* treatment.

Laterally positioned flap + interpositional graft

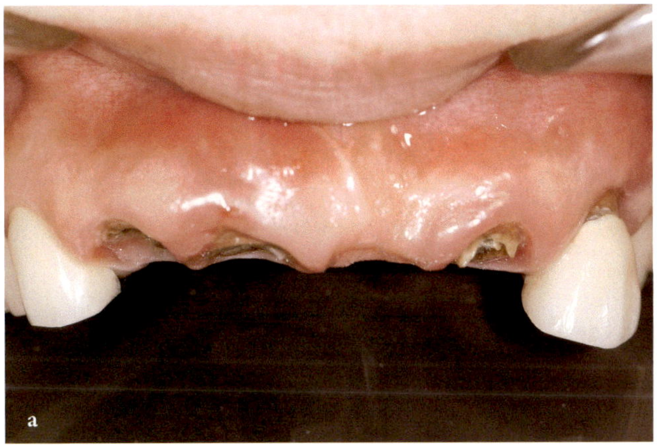

Fig 6-14a Same case as presented in Fig 4-6. Facial view at initial examination.

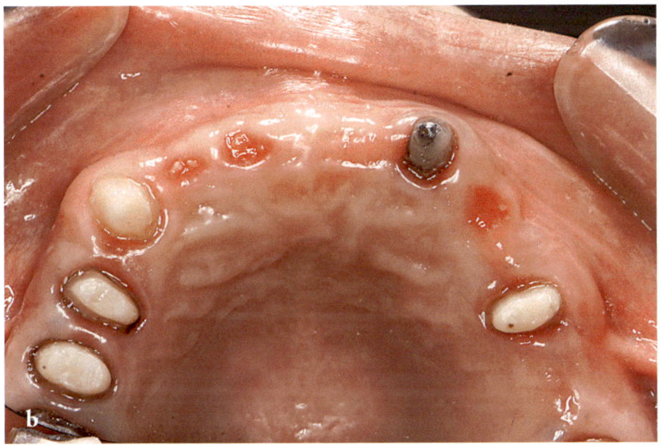

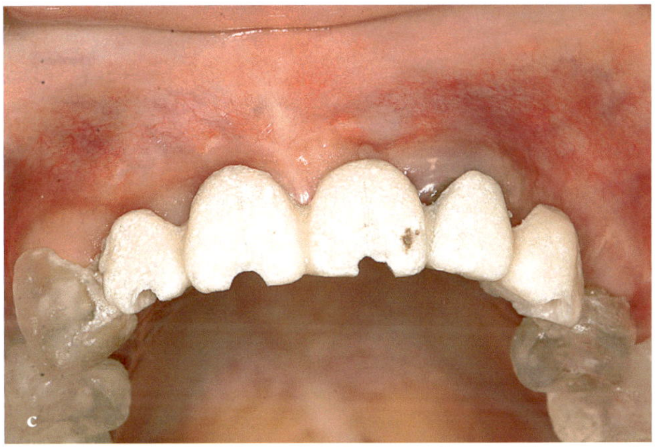

Figs 6-14b and 6-14c Occlusal views before soft tissue augmentation. An insufficient amount of keratinized tissue and soft tissue volume was observed.

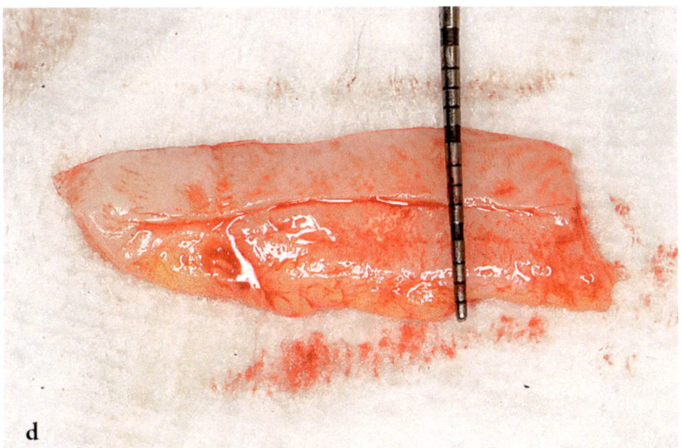

Fig 6-14d Connective tissue graft with 4 mm of keratinized tissue.

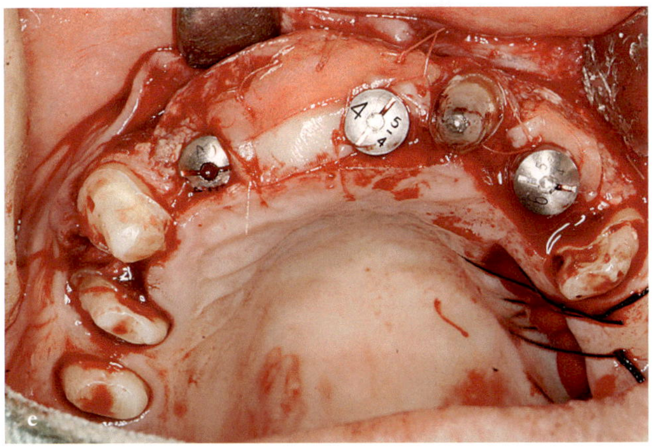

Fig 6-14e The keratinized tissue portion of the graft was trimmed and positioned in the future pontic site.

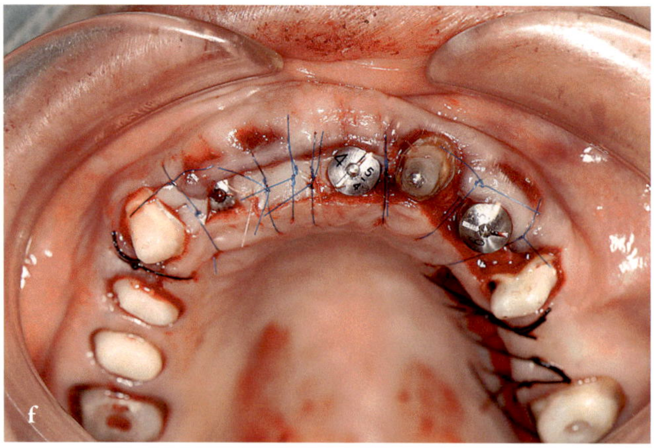

Fig 6-14f Occlusal view after suturing. A small amount of keratinized tissue was placed mesial to the right canine.

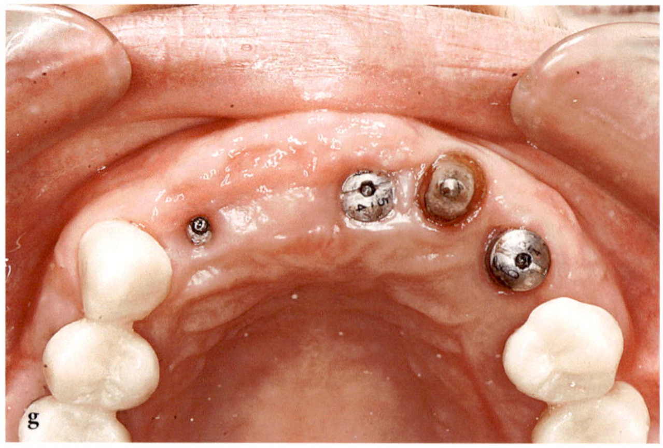

Fig 6-14g Occlusal view after 2 months of healing.

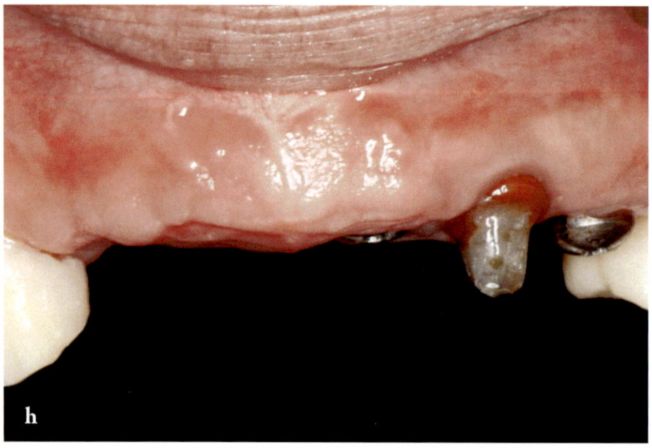

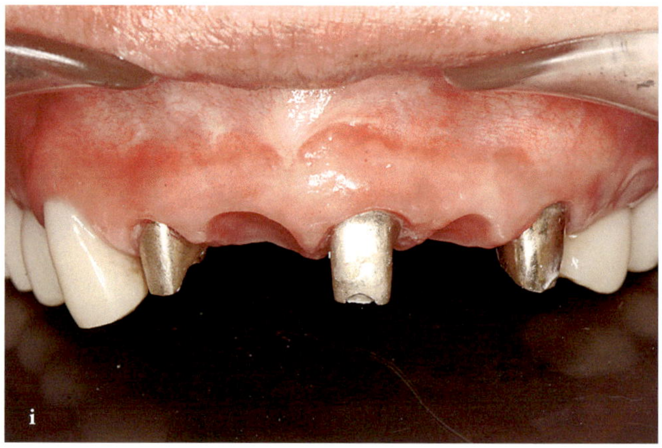

Figs 6-14h and 6-14i An esthetic soft tissue profile was established.

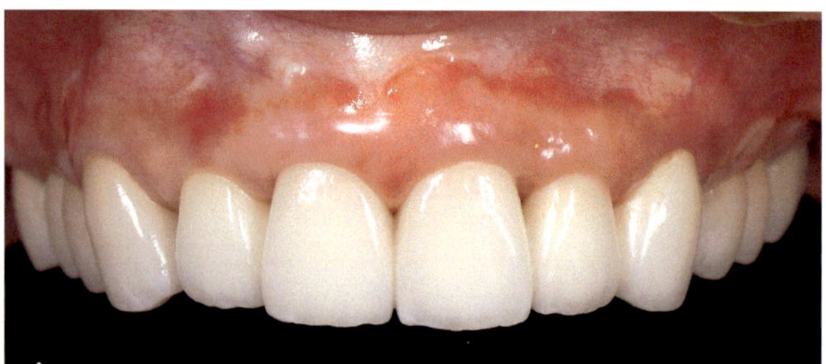

Fig 6-14j Facial view of the definitive restorations with an esthetic soft tissue profile.

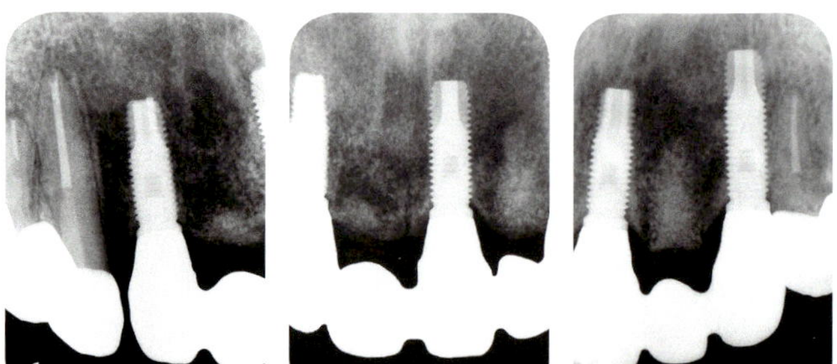

Fig 6-14k Radiographs of definitive restorations. Note the bone level of the pontic sites and the platform positions.

Tissue punch technique

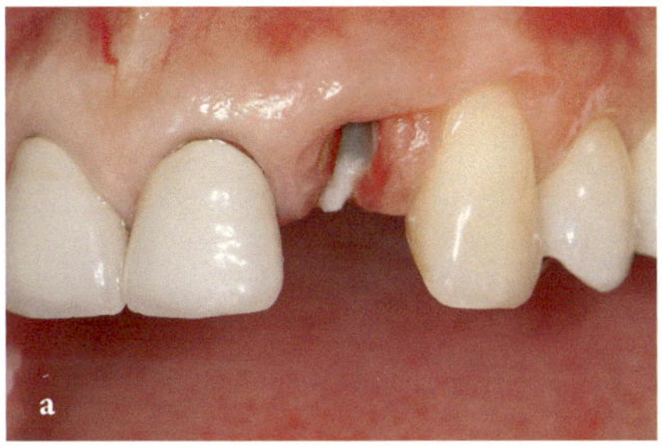

Fig 6-15a The left lateral incisor was diagnosed as hopeless.

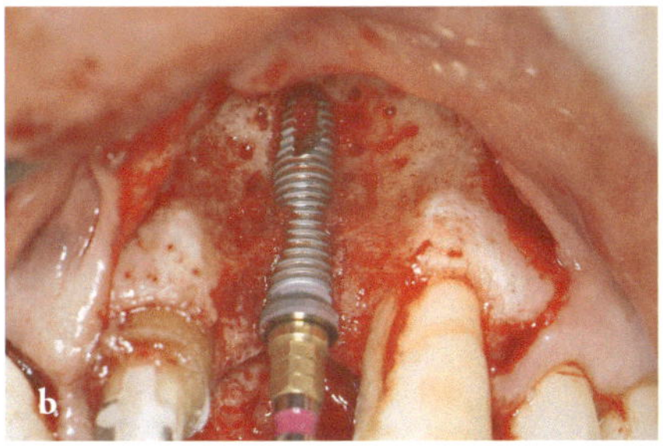

Fig 6-15b Two months following extraction, implant placement and GBR were performed.

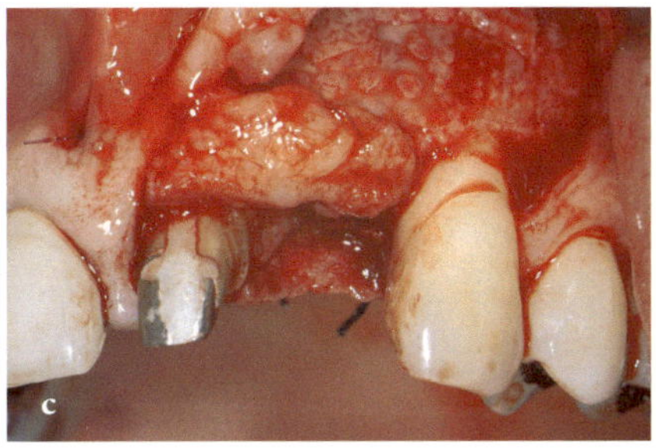

Fig 6-15c Six months after implant placement and GBR, a connective tissue graft was performed.

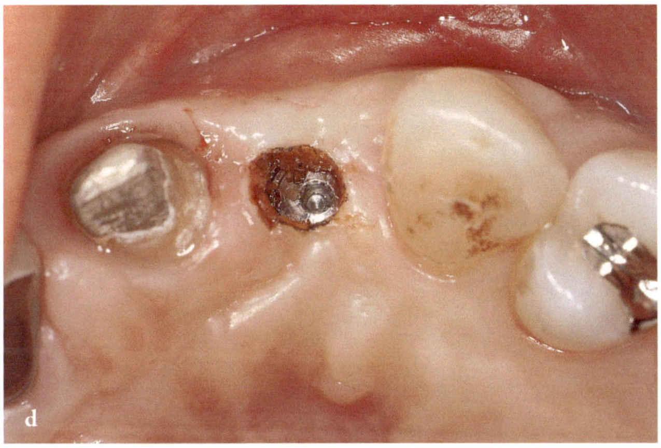

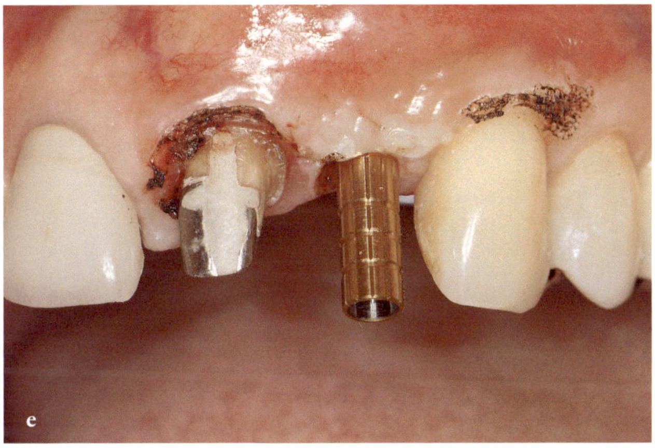

Figs 6-15d and 6-15e Two months after connective tissue grafting, the tissue punch technique was carried out with a CO_2 laser.

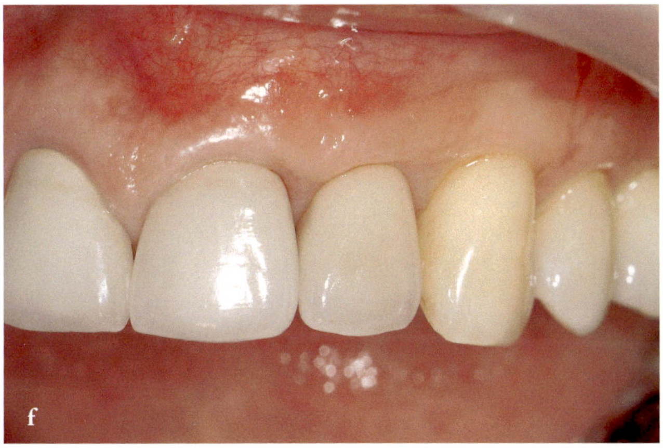

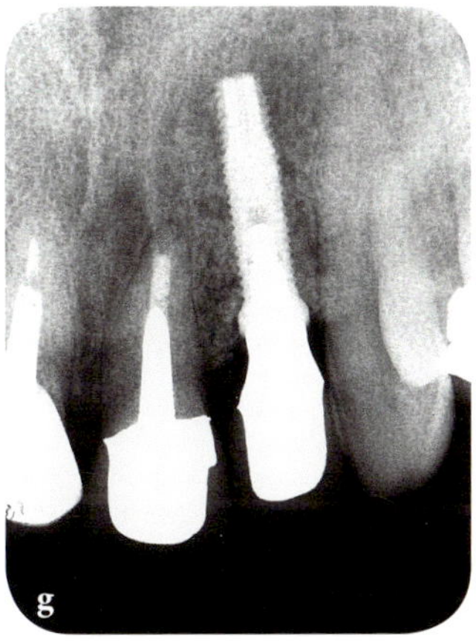

Figs 6-15f and 6-15g Lateral view *(f)* and periapical radiograph *(g)* of definitive restoration.

Summary

Although soft tissue augmentation procedures may seem complex, a proper understanding of soft tissue graft technique options, their indications, and the timing of the procedures increases treatment predictability and reduces the overall treatment period. When setting treatment goals, it is also important to understand the hard and soft tissue requirements and limitations for supporting an esthetic implant final restoration. Tissue sculpting with a provisional restoration is an important part of soft tissue management (see clinical cases in chapter 8).

References

1. Berglundh T, Lindhe J, Ericsson I, Marinello CP, Liljenberg B, Thomsen P. The soft tissue barrier at implants and teeth. Clin Oral Implants Res 1991;2(2):81–90.
2. Hermann JS, Buser D, Schenk RK, Schoolfield JD, Cochran DL. Biologic Width around one- and two-piece titanium implants. Clin Oral Implants Res 2001;12:559–571.
3. Cochran DL, Hermann JS, Schenk RK, Higginbottom FL, Buser D. Biologic width around titanium implants. A histometric analysis of the implanto-gingival junction around unloaded and loaded nonsubmerged implants in the canine mandible. J Periodontol 1997;68:186–198.
4. Berglundh T, Lindhe J, Jonsson K, Ericsson I. The topography of the vascular systems in the periodontal and peri-implant tissues in the dog. J Clin Periodontol 1994;21(3):189–193.
5. Tarnow D, Elian N, Fletcher P, et al. Vertical distance from the crest of bone to the height of the interproximal papilla between adjacent implants. J Periodontol 2003;74:1785–1788.
6. Nevins M, Mellonig JT, Fiorellini JP. Implant Therapy: Clinical Approaches and Evidence of Success, vol 2. Chicago: Quintessence, 1998.
7. Berglundh T, Lindhe J. Dimension of the periimplant mucosa. Biological width revisited. J Clin Periodontol 1996;23:971–973.
8. Kois J. Altering gingival levels: The restorative connection. Part 1: Biological variables. J Esthet Dent 1994;6:3–9.
9. Weisgold AS, Arnoux JP, Lu J. Single-tooth anterior implant: A word of caution. Part I. J Esthet Dent 1997;9:225–233.
10. Kan JY, Rungcharassaeng K, Umezu K, Kois JC. Dimensions of peri-implant mucosa: An evaluation of maxillary anterior single implants in humans. J Periodontol 2003;74:557–562.
11. Salama H, Salama M, Garber D, Adar P. The interproximal height of bone: A guidepost to predictable aesthetic strategies and soft tissue contours in anterior tooth replacement. Pract Periodontics Aesthet Dent 1998;10:1131–1141.
12. Funato A, Salama MA, Ishikawa T, Garber DA, Salama H. Timing, positioning, and sequential staging in esthetic implant therapy: A four-dimensional perspective. Int J Periodontics Restorative Dent 2007;27:313–323.
13. Funato A. Soft tissue management around implants. In: Miyamoto Y, Yoshie H. Technique and Science of Regenerative Dentistry, Periodontology, Esthetic Dentistry, and Implantology [in Japanese]. Tokyo: Quintessence, 2005:148–159.
14. Raetzke RB. Covering localized areas of root exposure employing the "envelope" technique. J Periodontol 1985;56:397–402.
15. Allen AL. Use of the supraperiosteal envelope in soft tissue grafting for root coverage. II. Clinical results. Int J Periodontics Restorative Dent 1994;14:302–315.
16. Nemcovsky CE, Moses O. Rotated palatal flap. A surgical approach to increase keratinized tissue width in maxillary implant uncovering: Technique and clinical evaluation. Int J Periodontics Restorative Dent 2002;22:607–612.
17. Mathews DP. The pediculated connective tissue graft: A technique for improving unaesthetic implant restorations. Pract Proced Aesthet Dent 2002;14:719–724.
18. Nemcovsky CE, Artzi Z, Moses O, Gelernter I. Healing of dehiscence defects at delayed-immediate implant sites primarily closed by a rotated palatal flap following extraction. Int J Oral Maxillofac Implants 2000;15:550–558.
19. Nemcovsky CE, Moses O, Artzi Z, Gelernter I. Clinical coverage of dehiscence defects in immediate implant procedures: Three surgical modalities to achieve primary soft tissue closure. Int J Oral Maxillofac Implants 2000;15:843–852.
20. Chen ST, Dahlin C. Connective tissue grafting for primary closure of extraction sockets treated with an osteopromotive membrane technique: Surgical technique and clinical results. Int J Periodontics Restorative Dent 1996;16:348–355.
21. Landsberg CJ. Socket seal surgery combined with immediate implant placement: A novel approach for single-tooth replacement. Int J Periodontics Restorative Dent 1997;17:140–149.
22. Tinti C, Benfenati SP. The ramp mattress suture: A new suturing technique combined with a surgical procedure to obtain papillae between implants in the buccal area. Int J Periodontics Restorative Dent 2002;22:63–69.
23. Nemcovsky CE, Artzi Z. Split palatal flap. I. A surgical approach for primary soft tissue healing in ridge augmentation procedures: Technique and clinical results. Int J Periodontics Restorative Dent 1999;19:175–181.

Chapter 7

Treatment Planning

for Single- and Multiple-Tooth Implant Cases

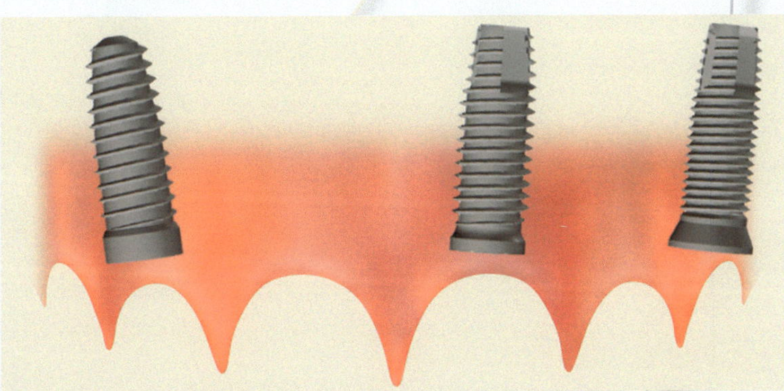

The significance of applying the four-dimensional (4D) concept in esthetic implant therapy was demonstrated in chapters 1 through 6. The purpose of the 4D concept for esthetic implant therapy is to show that the timing of the treatment sequence is just as important as bone and soft tissue requirements and the traditional three-dimensional (3D) management of implant position. The key points of the 4D concept were discussed in detail: the timing of implant placement (immediate, early, and delayed implant placement), the socket preservation technique, the root submergence technique, 3D ridge augmentation, and soft tissue management. In this chapter, application of the 4D concept for esthetic implant therapy is demonstrated through the presentation of clinical cases.

Strategies and Principles of Esthetic Implant Therapy

The treatment planning and sequencing strategies and principles of the 4D concept for esthetic implant therapy are summarized in Box 7-1.

Single-Tooth Implant Cases

Evaluation of tooth targeted for extraction

The tooth targeted for extraction must be carefully assessed, taking into account the necessity of orthodontic tooth extrusion and the timing of extraction, implant placement, ridge augmentation, and soft tissue management. The tooth targeted for extraction can serve an important function prior to extraction.

Evaluation of future implant location

A single-tooth implant in the esthetic region can be treated successfully (Fig 7-1). However, if a single-tooth implant is placed next to another implant (Fig 7-2), it cannot be expected to have an esthetic result because of the unpredictable nature of creating a papilla between two implants. Moreover, when single implants are used to replace adjacent missing teeth, definitive restorations generally do not resemble the natural dentition. Adjoining implant placement in the esthetic region is the most challenging treatment performed today and should be avoided whenever possible.

Evaluation of the natural teeth adjacent to the future implant site

Management of the natural teeth is critical in implant therapy in the esthetic region. The proximal alveolar bone level of the natural teeth adjacent to the future implant site must be carefully evaluated because it determines the papilla height between the implant and the natural tooth. This alveolar bone level also determines the vertical goal or limitation of ridge augmentation. Today, orthodontic tooth extrusion is the only predictable option to increase the proximal alveolar bone level.

Box 7-1 Strategies and principles of esthetic implant therapy

1. Consider immediate implant placement when possible.
2. Perform 3D preservation and augmentation of peri-implant tissue.
3. Allow as much distance as possible between neighboring implants.
4. Insert pontic whenever possible in esthetic area.
5. Consider platform switching when possible.
6. Place implants in native bone when possible.
7. Reduce abutment disconnection.

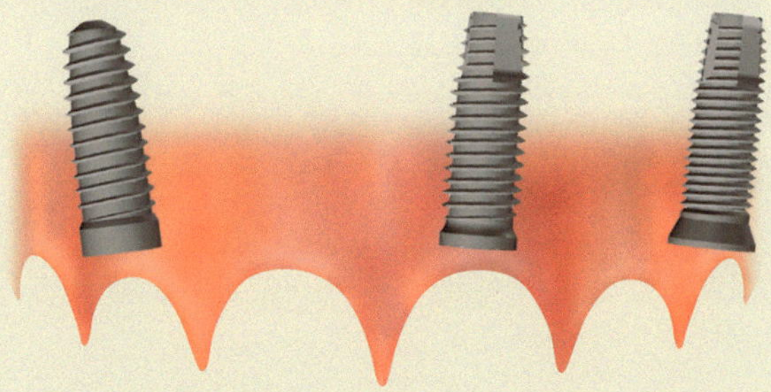

Single-tooth implant case 1: Nonadjoining implants

Application of 4D concept to this case

1. Consider immediate implant placement when possible.
2. Perform 3D preservation and augmentation of peri-implant tissue.
3. Allow as much distance as possible between neighboring implants.
4. Insert pontic whenever possible in esthetic area.
5. Consider platform switching when possible.
6. Place implants in native bone when possible.
7. Reduce abutment disconnection.

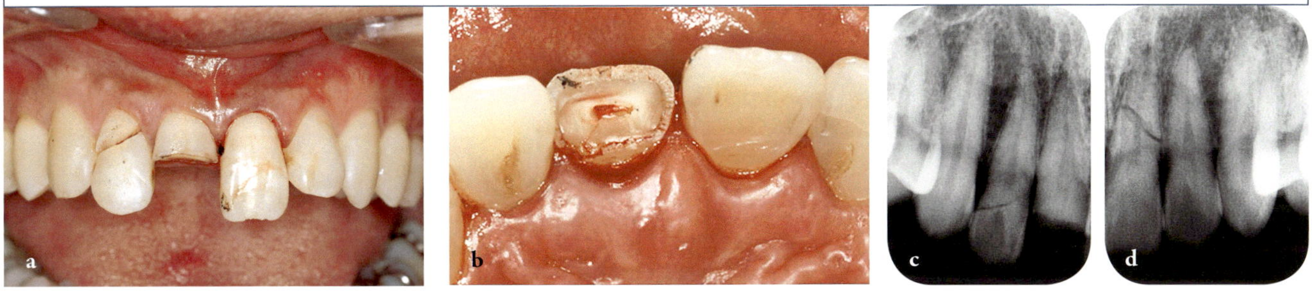

Figs 7-1a to 7-1d A 41-year-old man presented with mobility and fracture of his anterior teeth. The right lateral incisor had a deep subgingival fracture; the right central incisor had a supragingival fracture; and the left central incisor had a root fracture. Implant placement in the right lateral and left central incisor sites and a crown for the right central incisor were planned.

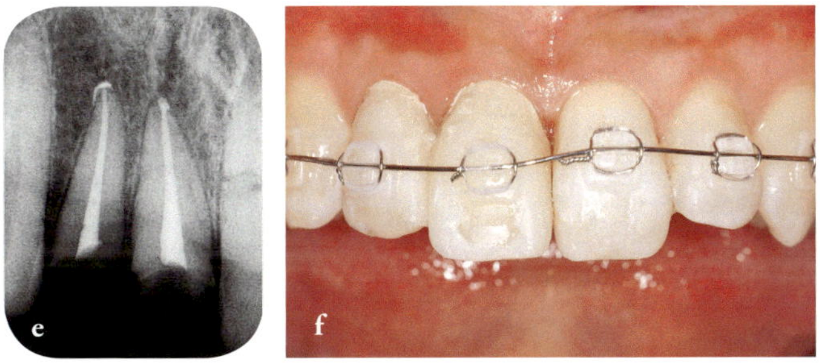

Figs 7-1e to 7-1g Orthodontic extrusion of the right lateral and central incisors was initiated after root canal treatment. The left central incisor was maintained until a gingival abscess began to form around the root fracture area, at which point it was extracted.

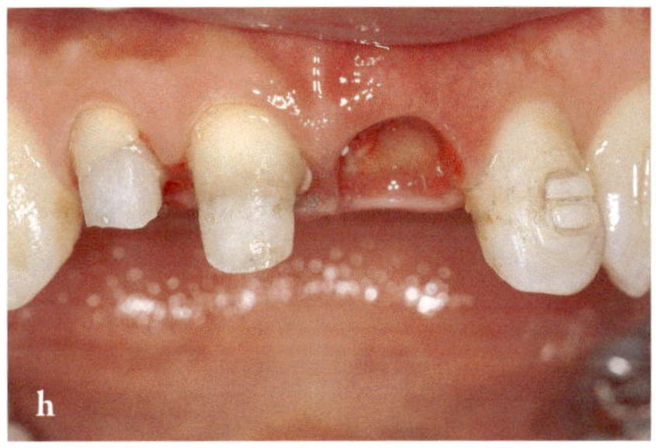

Fig 7-1h Two months after extraction of the left central incisor.

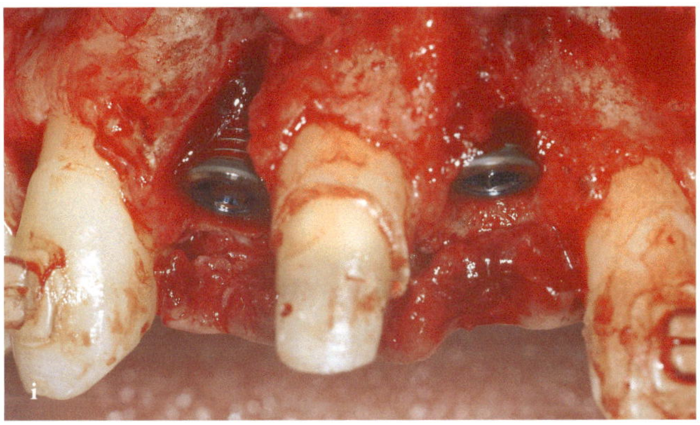

Fig 7-1i Immediate implant placement was performed for the right lateral incisor, which was Class 3 (see Fig 3-10). Buccal dehiscence was observed, but the implant was placed within the alveolar housing.

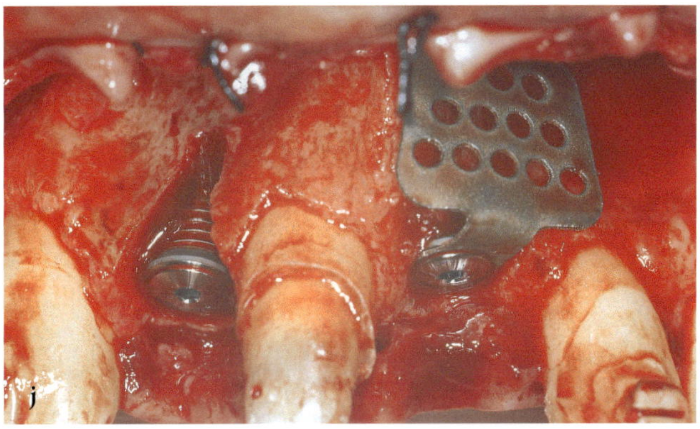

Fig 7-1j An FT wing was stabilized over the left central incisor implant only because the soft tissue primary closure at the extraction site was less predictable.

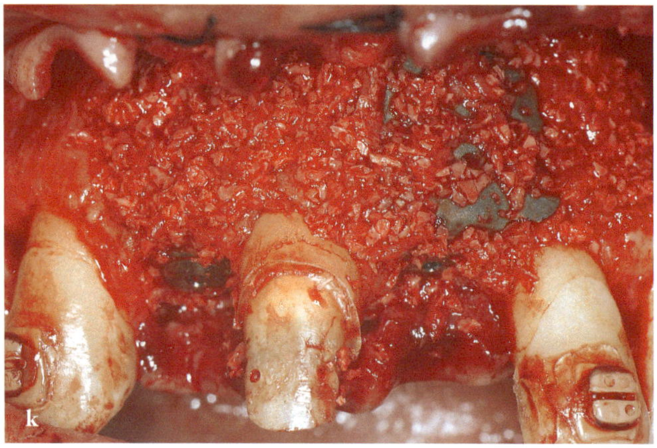

Fig 7-1k Autogenous bone and xenograft mixture was placed and subsequently covered with a collagen membrane.

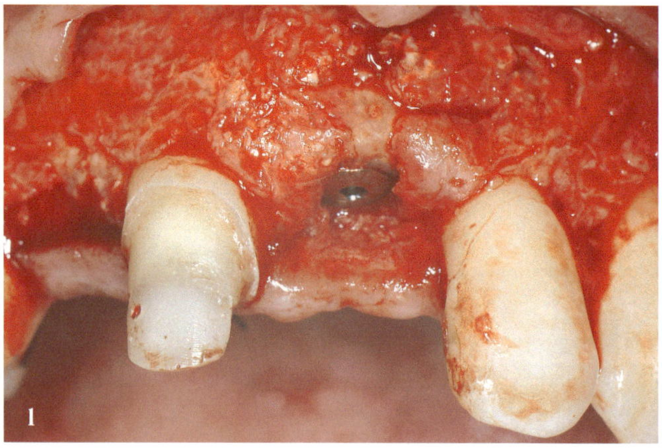

Fig 7-1l The FT wing was removed 6 months later. Sufficient buccal bone was observed at both implant sites.

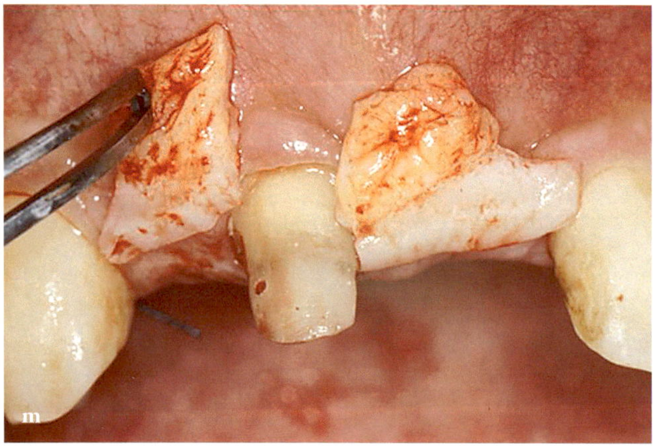

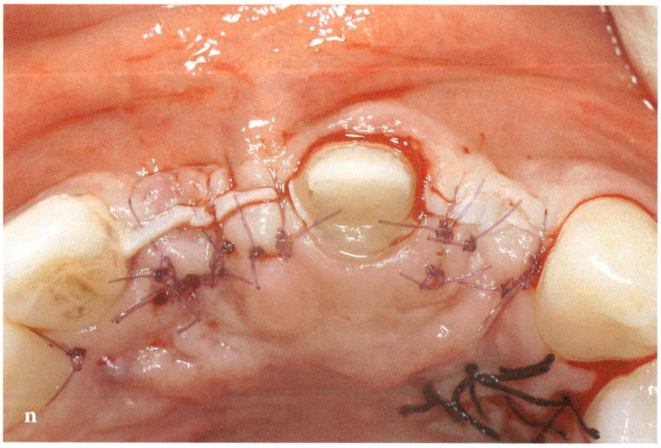

Figs 7-1m and 7-1n Connective tissue grafting was performed.

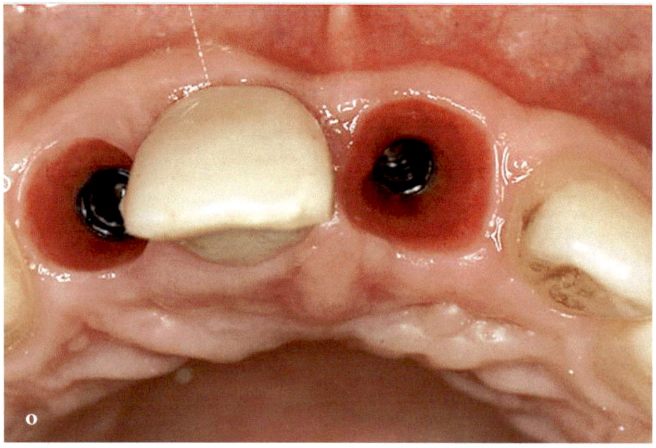

Fig 7-1o Two months later, the tissue punch technique was performed.

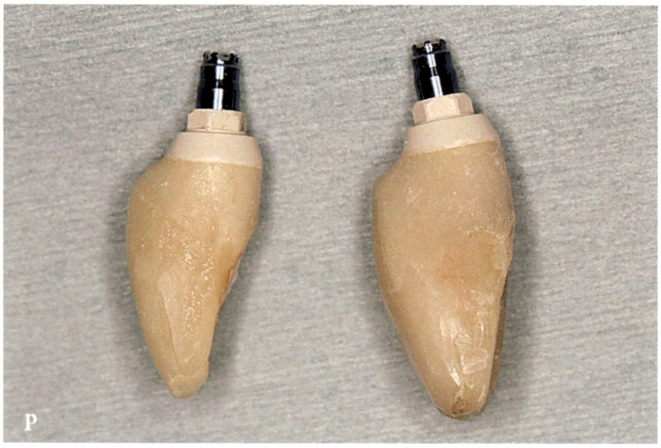

Fig 7-1p Soft tissue sculpting was performed using the screw-retained provisional restorations.

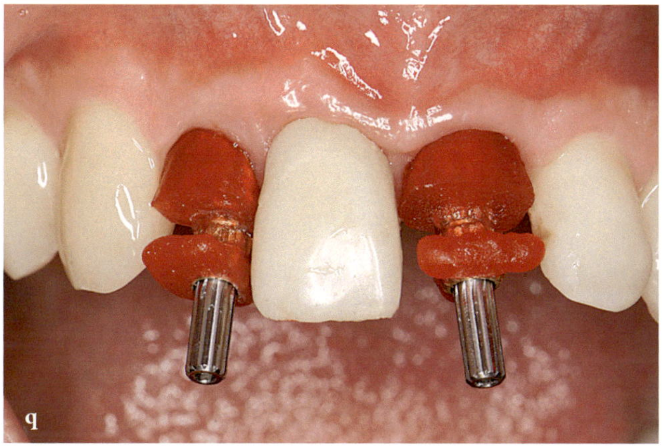

Fig 7-1q Final impressions were taken with custom impression copings.

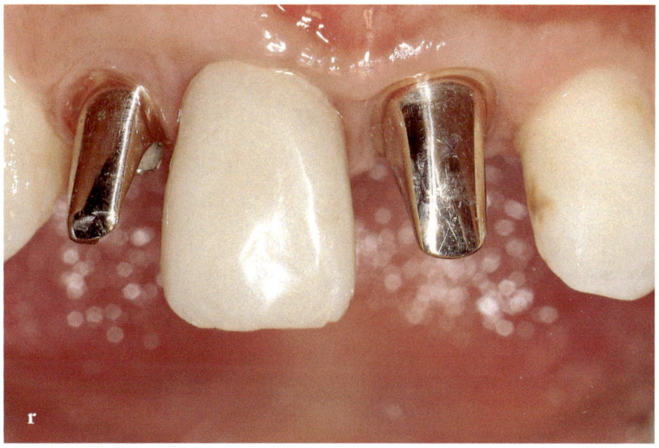

Fig 7-1r Gold UCLA abutments were fabricated.

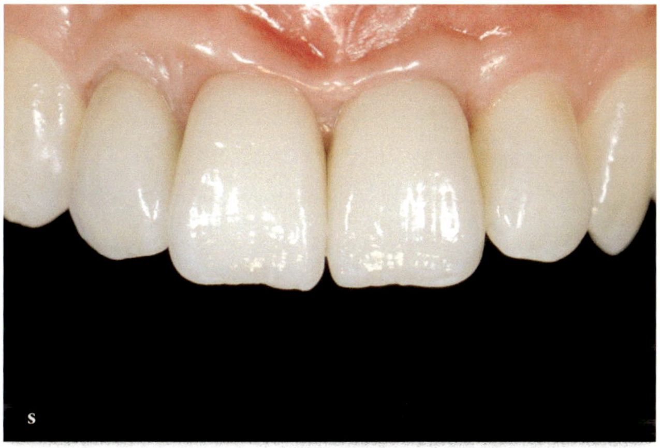

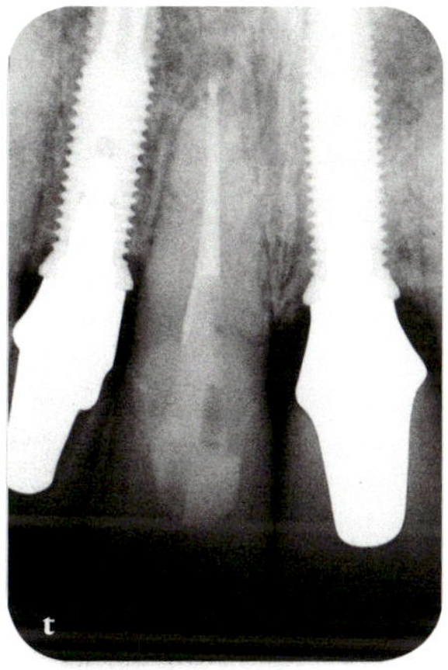

Figs 7-1s and 7-1t Facial view *(s)* and periapical radiograph *(t)* of the definitive restorations at the 1-year follow-up.

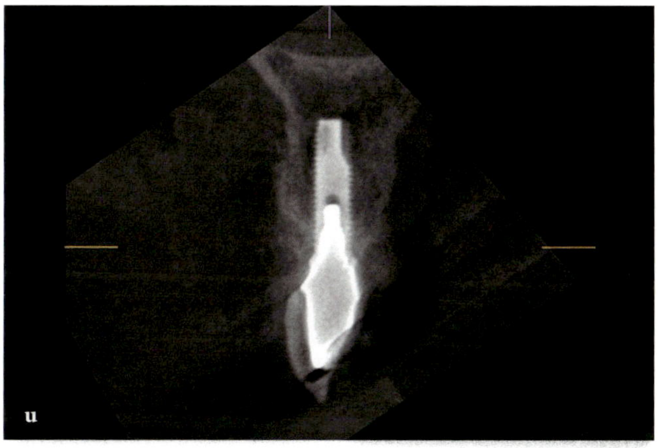

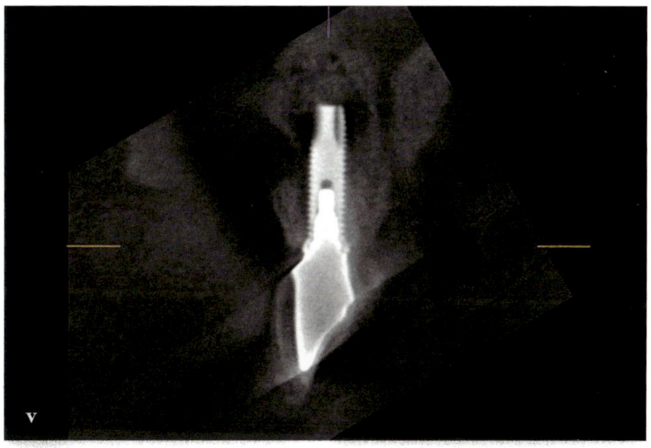

Figs 7-1u and 7-1v One-year computed tomographic evaluation.

Single-tooth implant case 2: Adjoining implants

Application of 4D concept to this case

1. Consider immediate implant placement when possible.
2. Perform 3D preservation and augmentation of peri-implant tissue.
3. Allow as much distance as possible between neighboring implants.
4. Insert pontic whenever possible in esthetic area.
5. Consider platform switching when possible.
6. Place implants in native bone when possible.
7. Reduce abutment disconnection.

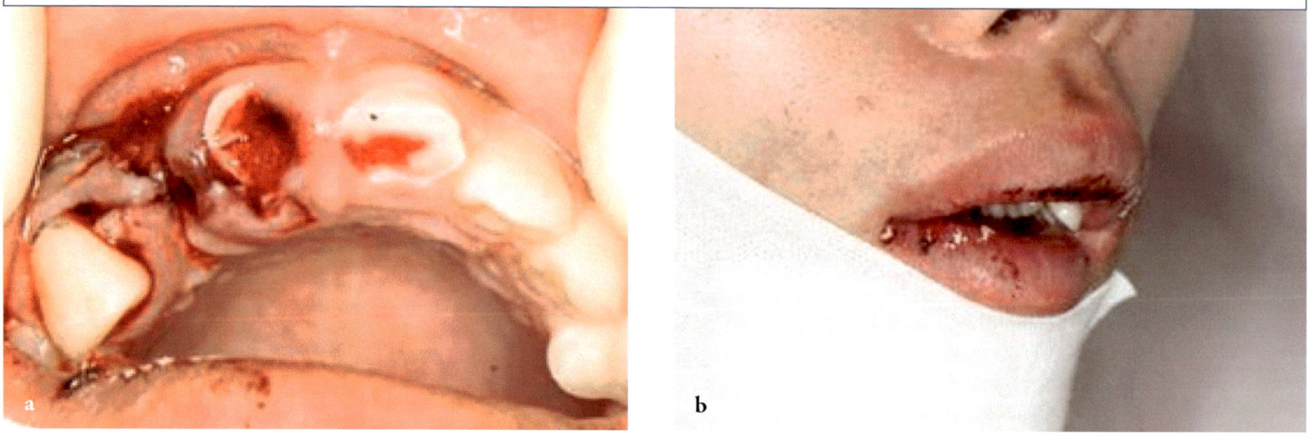

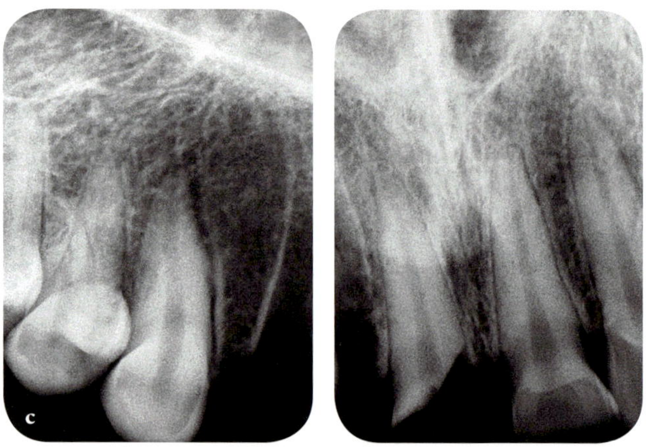

Figs 7-2a to 7-2c Same case as shown in Fig 1-2. The patient was a 20-year-old man who needed to replace teeth that had been damaged in an accident. The right lateral incisor and its entire surrounding buccal bone was lost. The right central incisor had a subgingival fracture and could be restored with orthodontic extrusion and crown lengthening, but the definitive crown would not match the left central incisor. The treatment plan was to place implants in the right lateral and central incisors sites and a crown on the left central incisor.

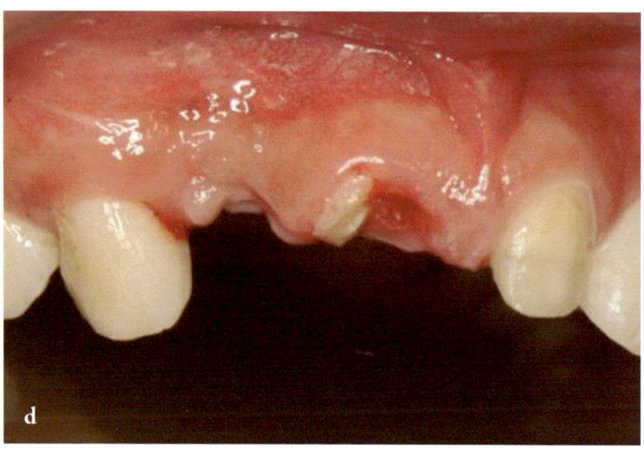

Fig 7-2d Clinical view after 6 months of healing and before surgery.

Two options for treatment planning and sequencing this case

Option A

- Extract the right central incisor. Allow 6 to 8 weeks for soft tissue healing.
- Perform implant placement and simultaneous guided bone regeneration (GBR) at the right central and lateral incisor sites. Allow 6 months for healing.
- Perform soft tissue augmentation.
- Stage-two surgery.

Advantage

- Predictable 3D bone augmentation with GBR

Disadvantage

- Greater surgical trauma due to the large amount of bone augmentation

Option B

- Perform implant placement and simultaneous GBR at the right lateral incisor site.
- Augment the soft tissue, and take an impression at the right lateral incisor implant site while removing the membrane.
- Stage-two surgery: Place the custom abutment and provisional restoration.
- Orthodontically extrude the right central incisor.
- Extract the right central incisor, and perform immediate implant placement with GBR buccally.
- After 2 months, place provisional restoration on the right central incisor implant.
- Place definitive restorations after 6 months of observation.

Advantages

- A small amount of augmentation and more predictable GBR at the right lateral incisor site with retention of the right central incisor.
- Orthodontic extrusion of the right central incisor and immediate implant placement will better preserve the interproximal bone and soft tissue.
- Minimize potential need for soft tissue augmentation.
- Predictable staged soft tissue sculpting.

Disadvantages

- Longer treatment period.
- Buccal bone volume of the right central incisor is unpredictable because of immediate implant placement.

Option B was selected in this case to preserve and augment existing tissue and to reduce surgical trauma.

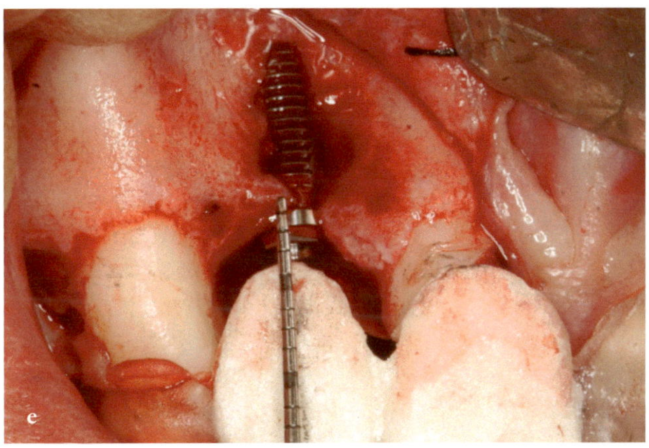

Fig 7-2e An implant was placed 2 to 3 mm apical to the free gingival margin, more than 1.5 mm from the adjacent teeth, and with ideal inclination of the long axis of the implant.

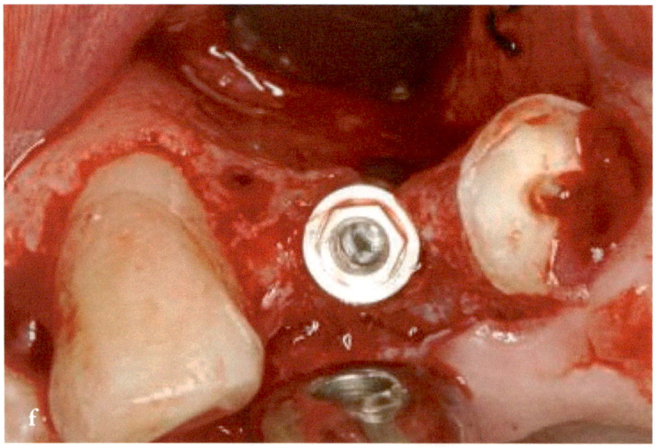

Fig 7-2f Occlusal view. No buccal bone was present at the implant platform level.

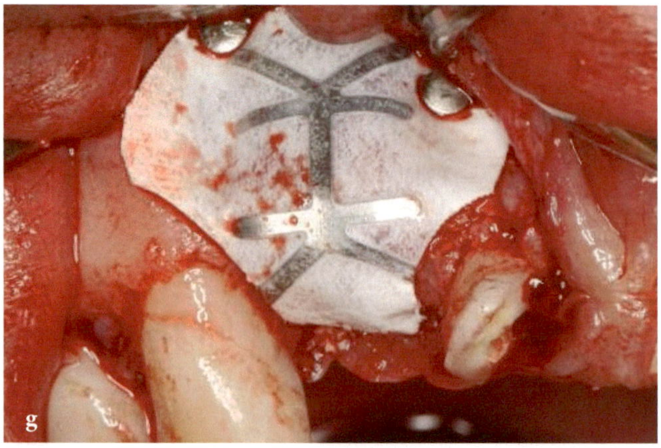

Fig 7-2g 3D space maintenance with a titanium-reinforced membrane.

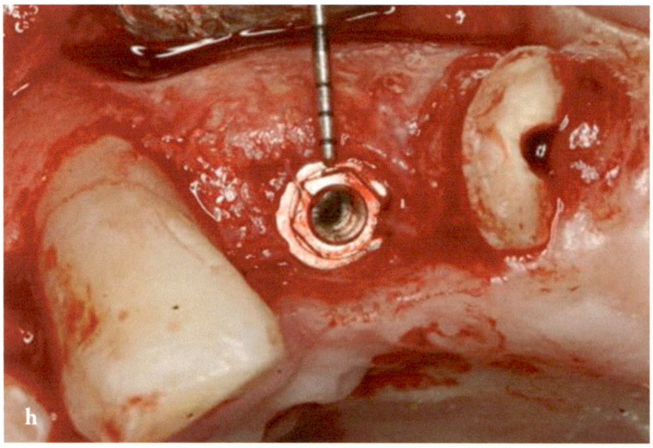

Fig 7-2h At membrane removal, 5 months later, 3 mm of buccal bone had been regenerated at the implant platform level.

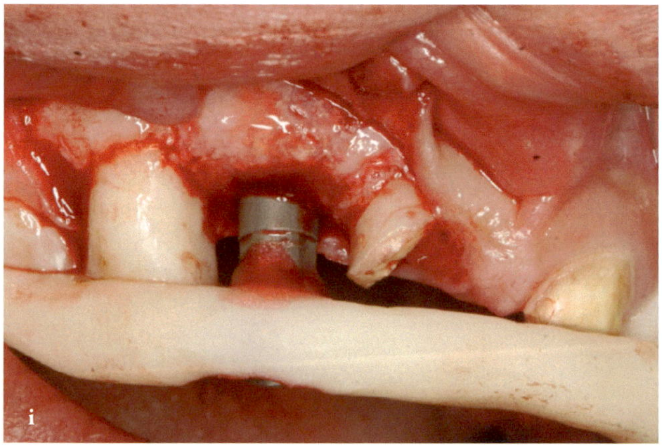

Fig 7-2i An implant index was taken.

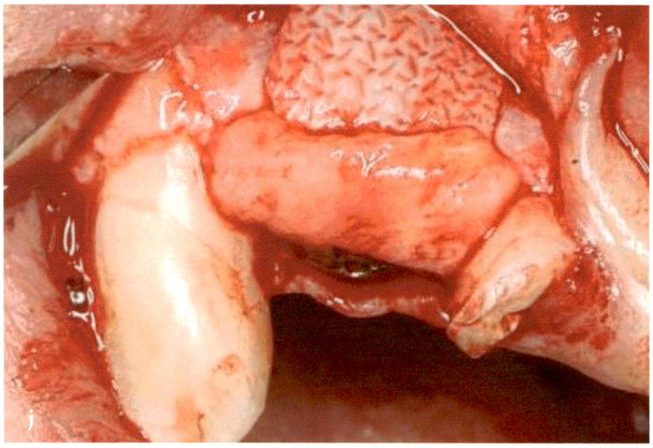

Fig 7-2j A 2-mm temporary healing abutment was placed over the implant and then submerged with connective tissue grafting.

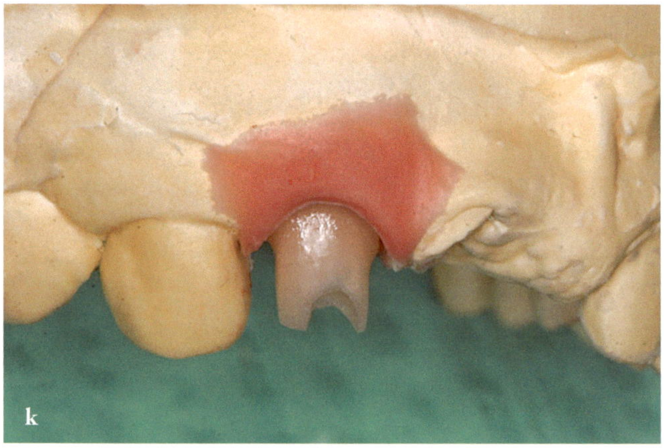

Fig 7-2k A custom abutment was fabricated.

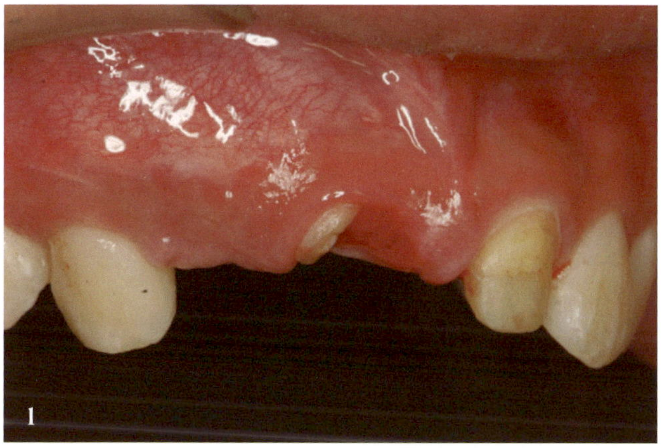

Fig 7-2l Two months after connective tissue grafting. An ideal alveolar ridge form and soft tissue quality were established.

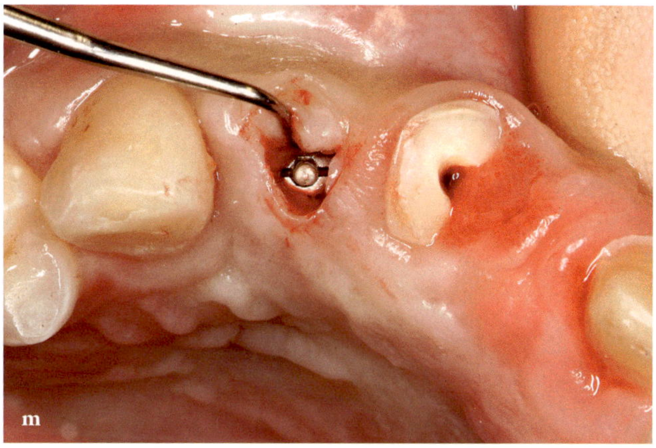

Fig 7-2m Tissue punch was performed to connect the custom abutment, and tissue sculpting was initiated.

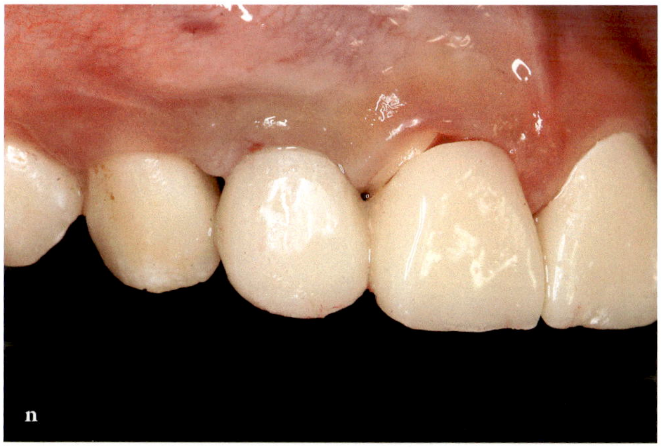

Fig 7-2n Facial view of the right lateral incisor with a provisional restoration.

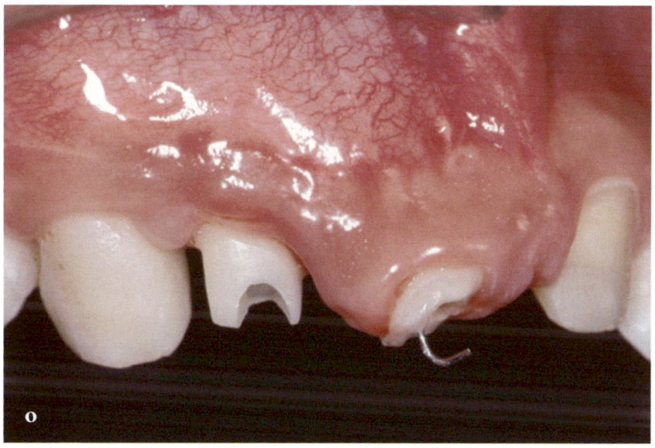

Fig 7-2o The right central incisor was extruded 5 mm and retained for 4 weeks.

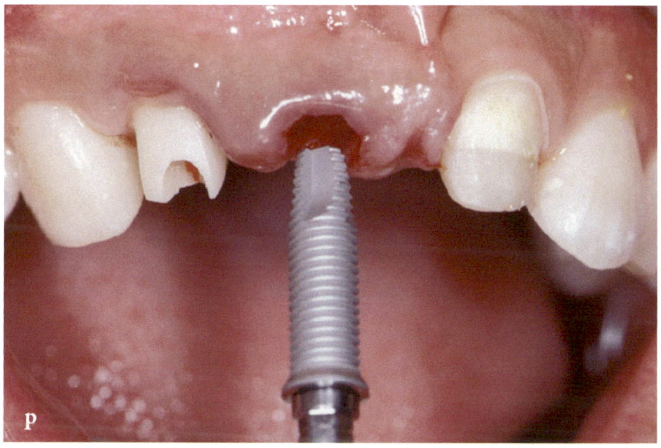

Fig 7-2p Immediate implant placement was performed at the right central incisor site, which was Class 1 (see Fig 3-10). An implant with a platform-switching feature was selected to maintain bone height between implants.

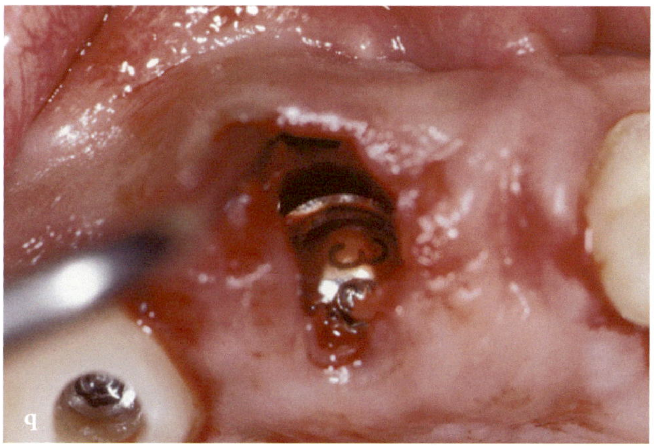

Fig 7-2q A buccal envelope flap was created at the extraction socket. Bone graft was placed inside and outside of the extraction socket.

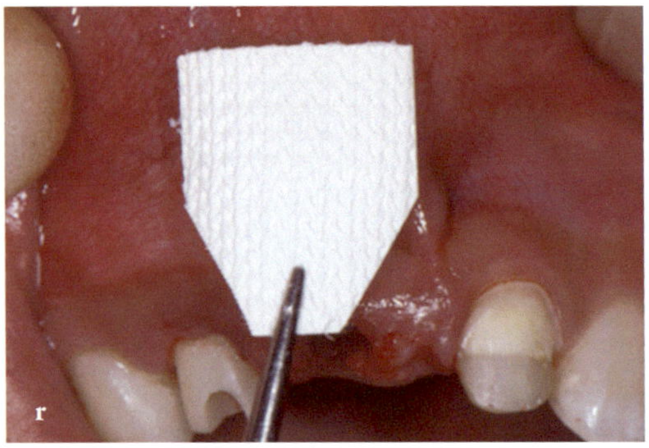

Fig 7-2r A cross-linked collagen membrane was placed between the flap and the bone graft.

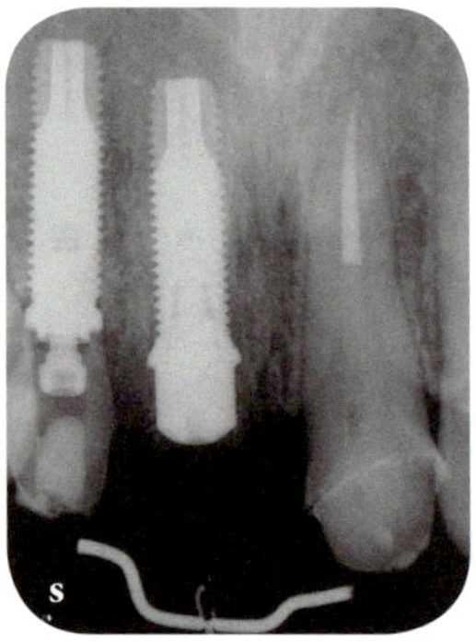

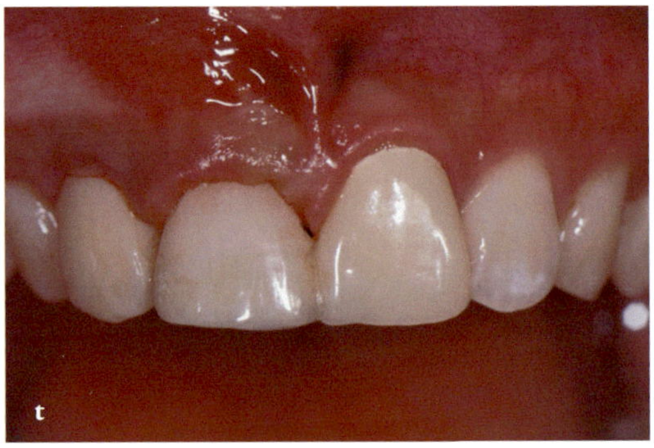

Figs 7-2s and 7-2t The extraction socket was sealed with an ovate pontic.

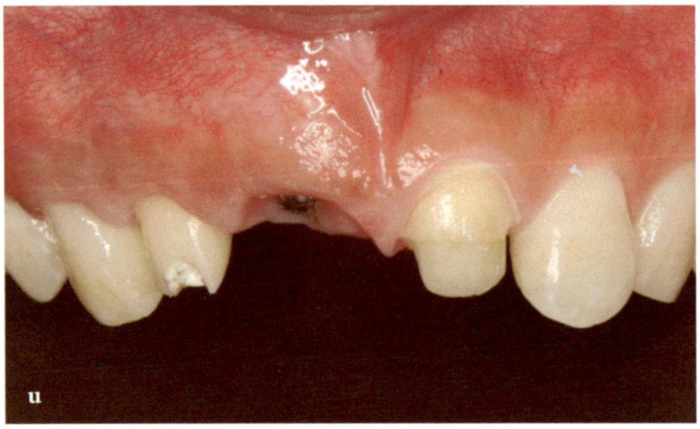

Fig 7-2u Facial view 2 months later.

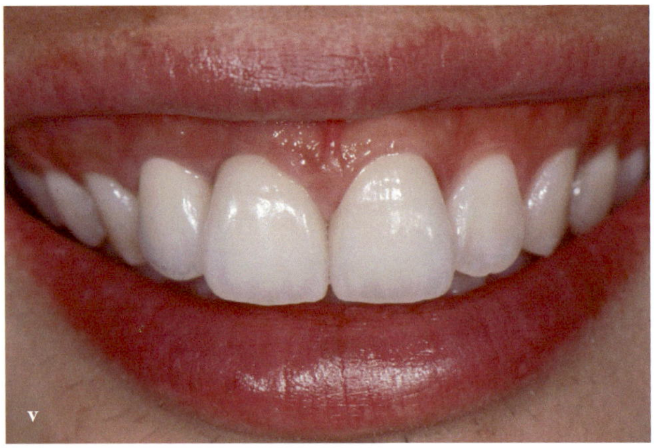

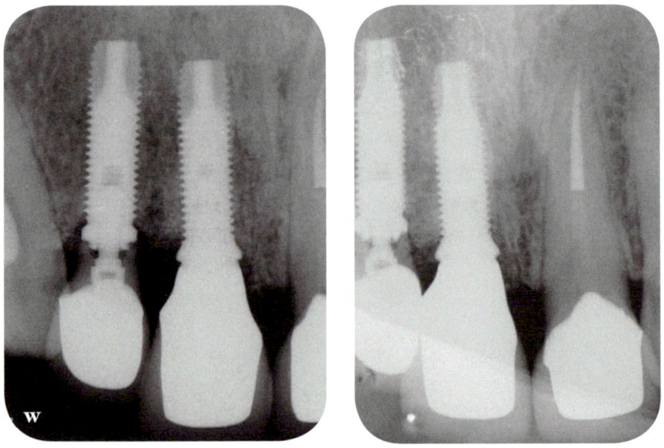

Figs 7-2v and 7-2w Facial view *(v)* and periapical radiographs *(w)* of the definitive restoration. With careful consideration of the timing of implant placement as well as bone and soft tissue augmentation and preservation, an acceptable result was obtained in a patient with a challenging high smile line.

Box 7-2 Abutment teeth

Roles of abutment teeth
- To support the provisional restoration
- To augment bone and soft tissue through orthodontic extrusion
- To maintain bone and soft tissue through the root submergence technique
- To serve as a reference point for the alveolar ridge augmentation goal
- To guide implant placement

Evaluation of abutment teeth
- Periodontal condition
- Endodontic condition
- Remaining tooth structure
- Tooth position
- Tooth arrangement

Multiple-Tooth Implant Cases

In multiple-tooth implant cases, creating definitive restorations that resemble the natural dentition remains a challenge. Existing dentition must be used effectively to maintain function and esthetics during the protracted treatment period. Cooperation between the patient and the treatment team is essential for a successful outcome. The clinician must be able to foresee potential challenges and create an appropriate treatment plan and sequence, then proficiently execute this treatment plan.

Stable posterior occlusal support is critical for assuring wound stability during bone and soft tissue management in the anterior region. If implant placement in the posterior region is necessary to establish posterior occlusal support, it must be performed prior to the treatment of the anterior region.

The provisional restoration to be supported by the remaining dentition will dictate treatment planning and sequence and therefore must be carefully designed. In addition to supporting the provisional restoration, the abutment teeth must maintain the functions listed in Box 7-2.

Case 1: Strategic selection of abutment teeth

For the case shown in Fig 7-3, the number of implants and their locations were determined based on the criteria presented in Box 7-1. In this case, adjoining implants could have been avoided by placing implants in the right first molar, first premolar, and lateral incisor and in the left central incisor and canine positions. However, to avoid implant placement in the left central incisor site, which had a severe alveolar bone defect, the right first molar, first premolar, canine, and central incisor and the left canine were selected as implant sites. The left central and lateral incisors were selected as pontic sites. Staged implant placement was planned for the adjoining implants at the right first premolar and canine sites to maintain the interproximal tissue.

The right first molar and first premolar and the left central incisor, lateral incisor, and canine were extracted. The provisional restorations were supported by the remaining teeth (see Fig 7-3d). During the postextraction healing period, periodontal and orthodontic treatment in the mandible was initiated.

Multiple-tooth implant case 1: Strategic selection of abutment teeth

Application of 4D concept to this case

1. Consider immediate implant placement when possible.
2. Perform 3D preservation and augmentation of peri-implant tissue.
3. Allow as much distance as possible between neighboring implants.
4. Insert pontic whenever possible in esthetic area.
5. Consider platform switching when possible.
6. Place implants in native bone when possible.
7. Reduce abutment disconnection.

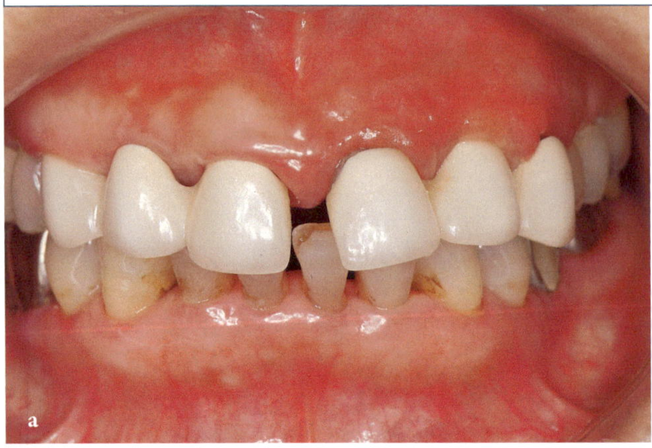

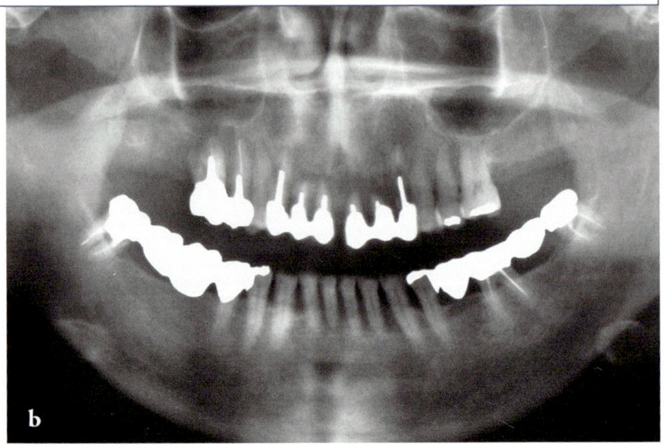

Figs 7-3a and 7-3b Facial view *(a)* and panoramic radiograph *(b)* at the initial examination. Abutment tooth selection, provisional restoration design, and determination of implant number and location were performed.

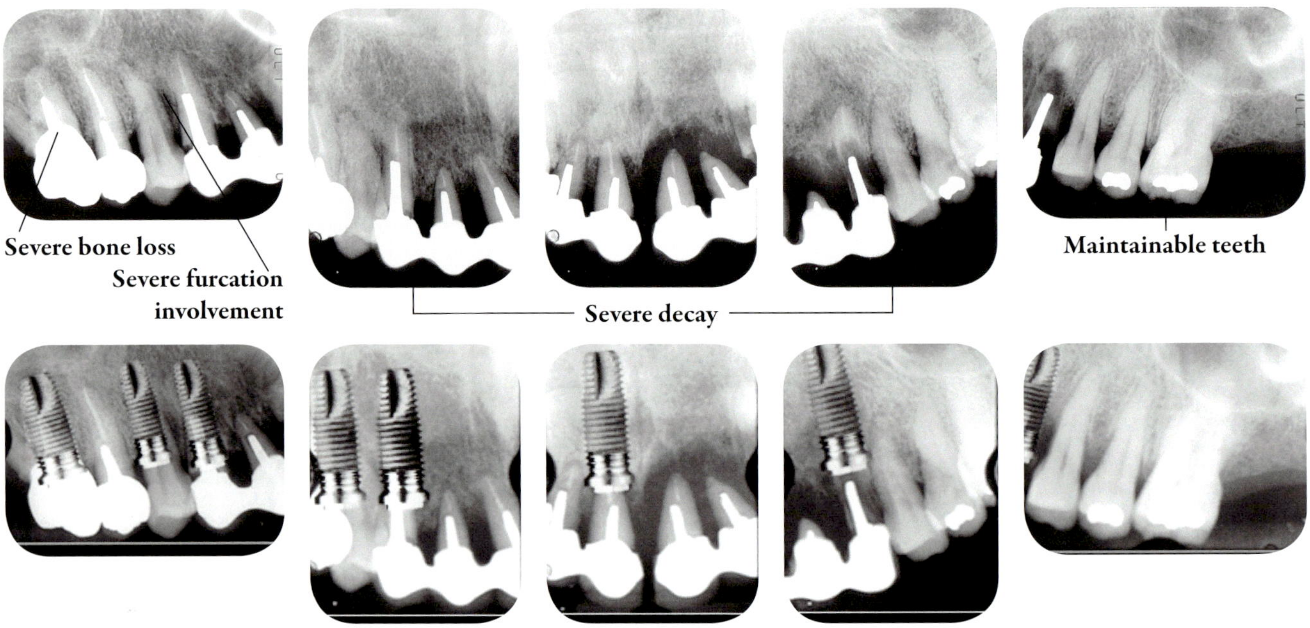

Fig 7-3c Implant locations were selected based on the amount of existing bone and the criteria presented in Box 7-1. The right first molar, first premolar, canine, and central incisor as well as the left canine were selected.

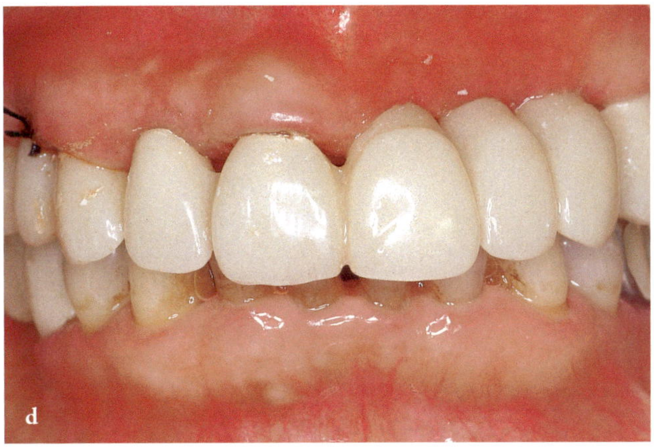

Fig 7-3d Provisional restoration at 3 months. It was supported by the right second premolar, canine, and central incisor and the left first premolar through first molar.

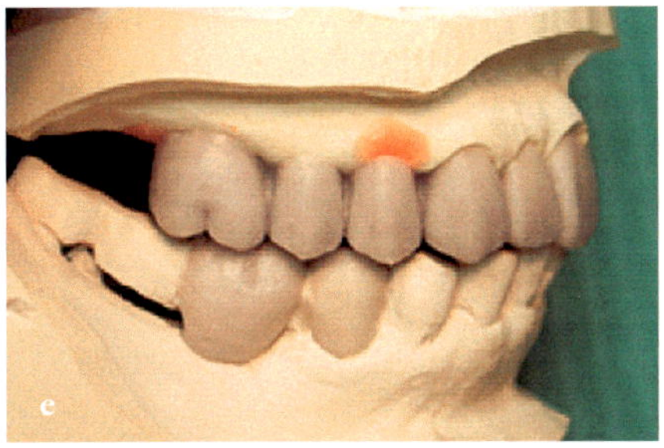

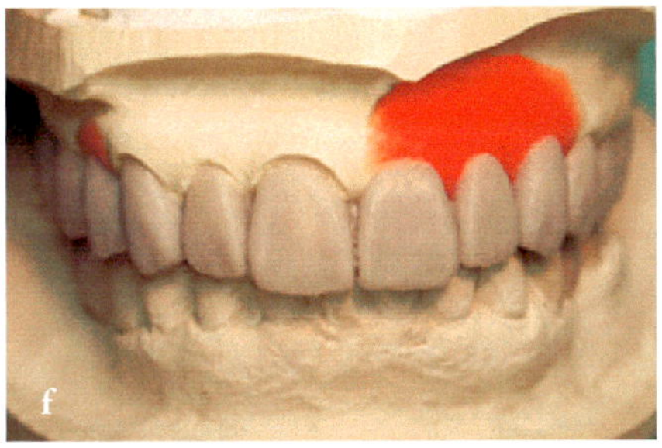

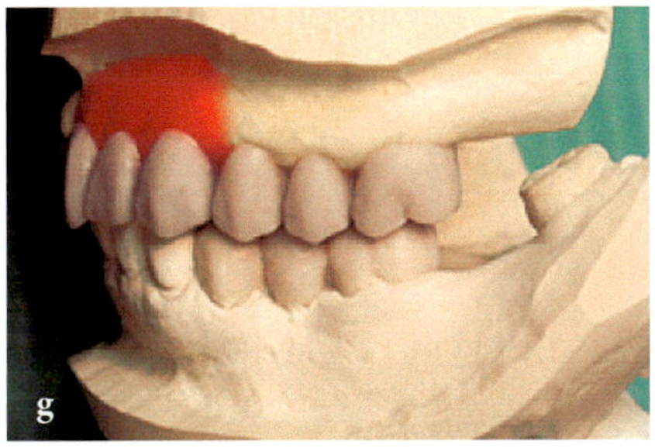

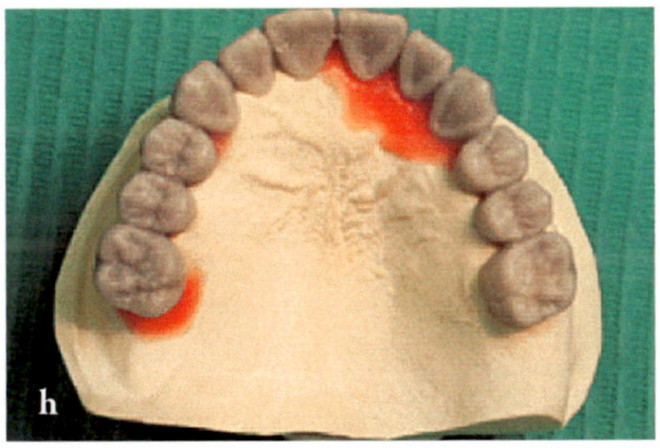

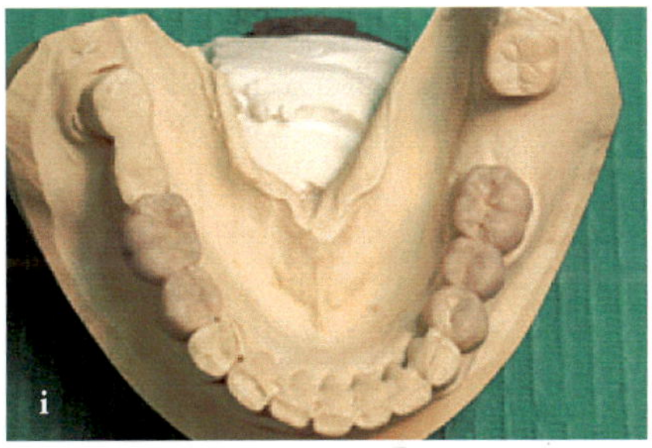

Figs 7-3e to 7-3i Diagnostic wax-up at 8 months, after orthodontic retraction of the mandibular anterior teeth, which was performed while the maxillary tissues were healing following extraction.

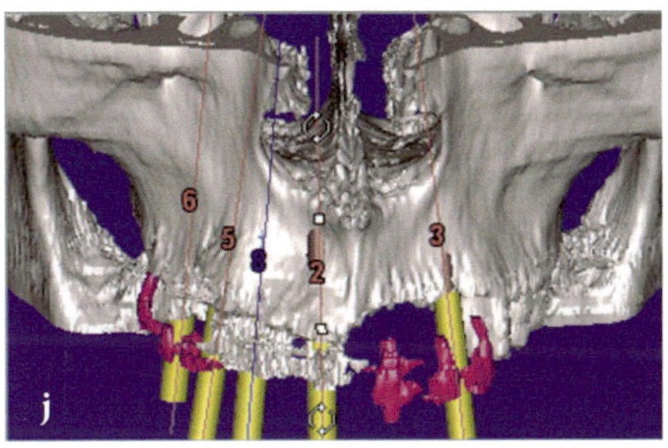

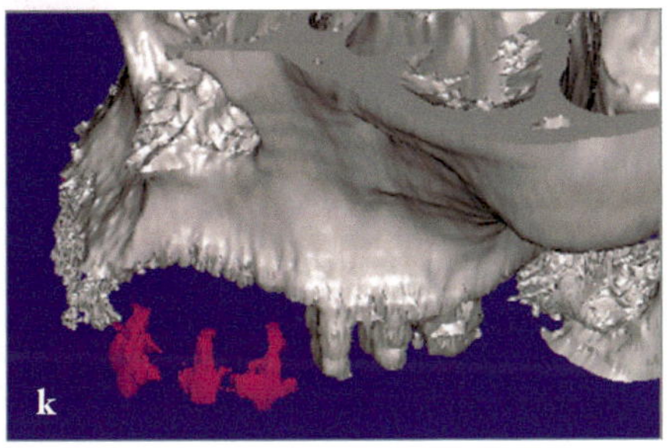

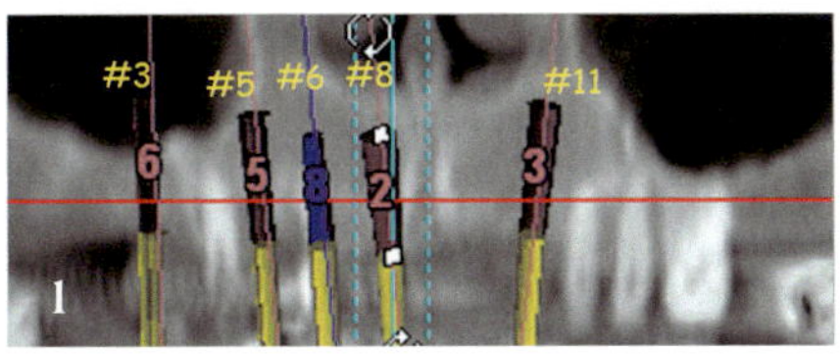

Figs 7-3j to 7-3l Implant treatment simulation in 3D imaging software at 9 months.

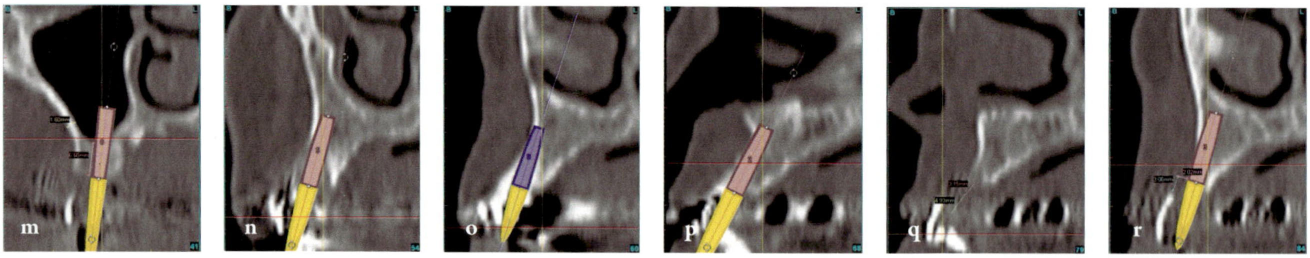

Figs 7-3m to 7-3r Cross-sectional images of the right first molar *(m)*, first premolar *(n)*, canine *(o)*, and central incisor *(p)* and the left lateral incisor *(q)* and canine *(r)*.

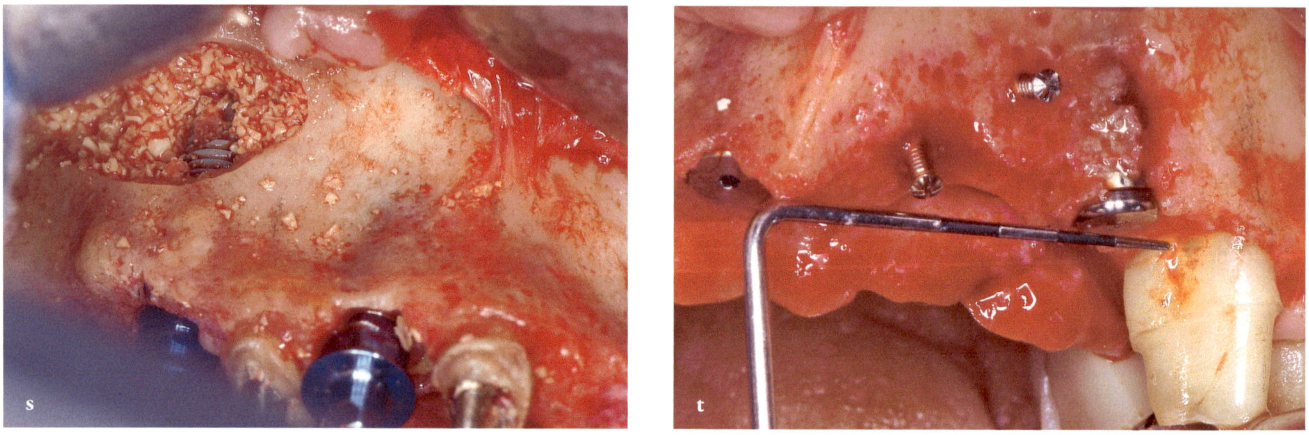

Figs 7-3s and 7-3t Right sinus lift and implant placement in the right first molar, first premolar, and central incisor and the left canine at 10 months. Immediate implant placement was performed at the right central incisor.

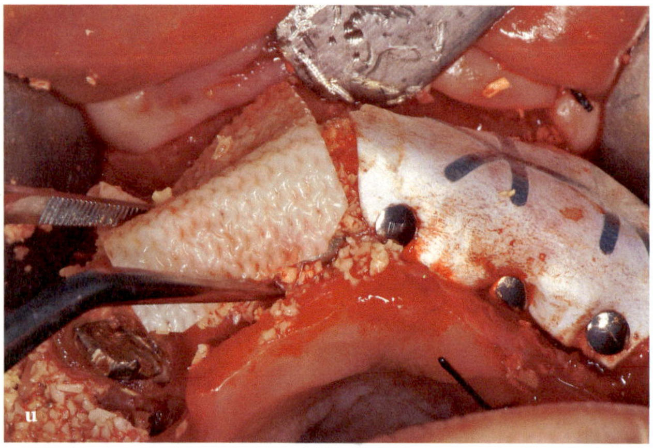

Fig 7-3u Vertical bone augmentation was performed with a titanium-reinforced membrane, while a cross-linked collagen membrane was used for horizontal bone augmentation. Bone graft was placed outside of the right central incisor extraction socket.

Step 1

Right maxillary sinus lift, implant placement in the right first molar and first premolar and left canine sites, and immediate implant placement in the right central incisor were performed simultaneously (see Figs 7-3s and 7-3t).

Vertical bone augmentation in the left central incisor to canine area with a titanium-reinforced membrane and horizontal bone augmentation for the right central and lateral incisor sites were performed next (see Fig 7-3u). Buccal bone augmentation of the right canine site should have been done at this time to aid the planned immediate implant placement.

Step 2

After 7 months of healing, the membrane was removed, and further bone as well as soft tissue augmentation was performed (see Figs 7-3v to 7-3dd).

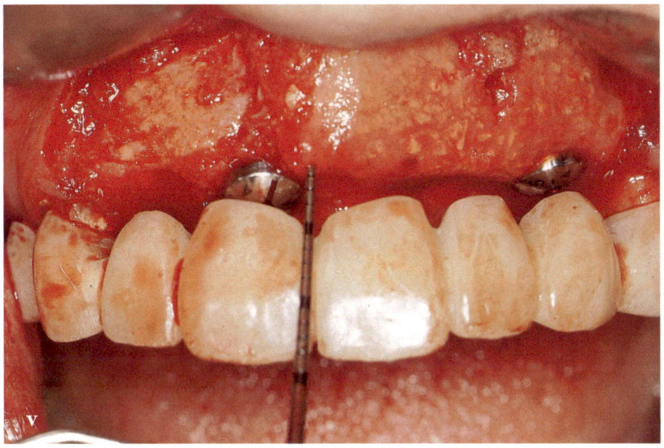

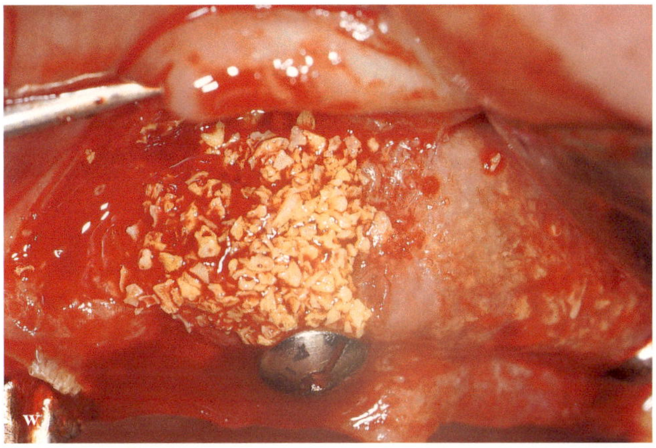

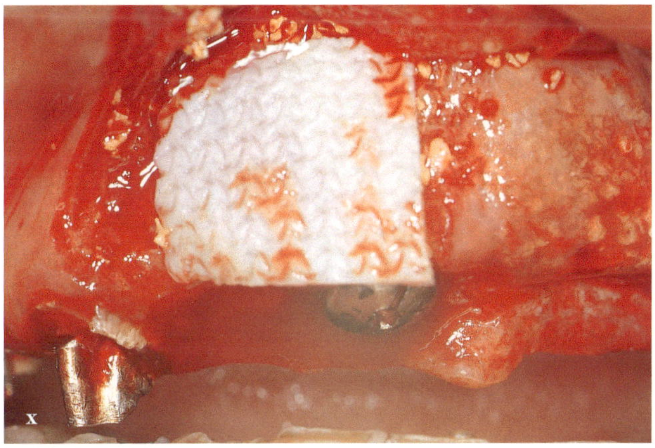

Fig 7-3v At 1 year 5 months (7 months after augmentation), the interproximal bone is Class 1 (see Fig 2-5).

Figs 7-3w and 7-3x Additional horizontal bone augmentation was carried out for the right central incisor.

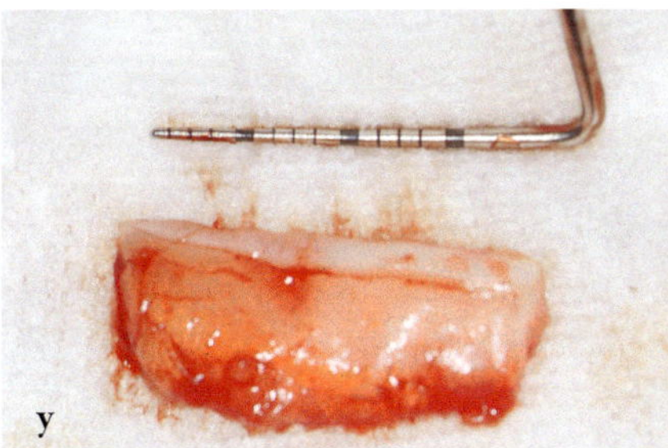

Fig 7-3y Connective tissue grafting was performed in the left lateral incisor and canine area.

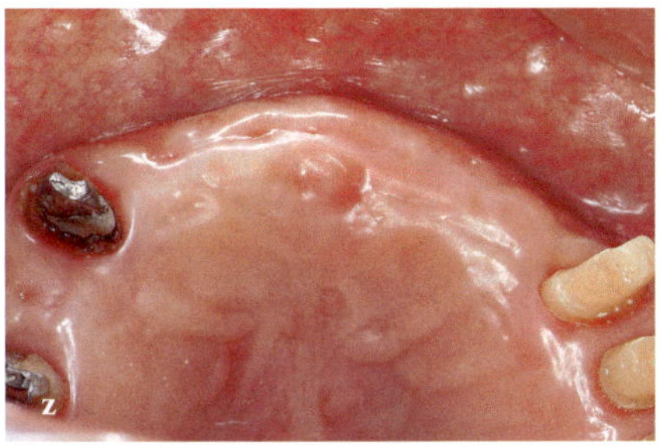

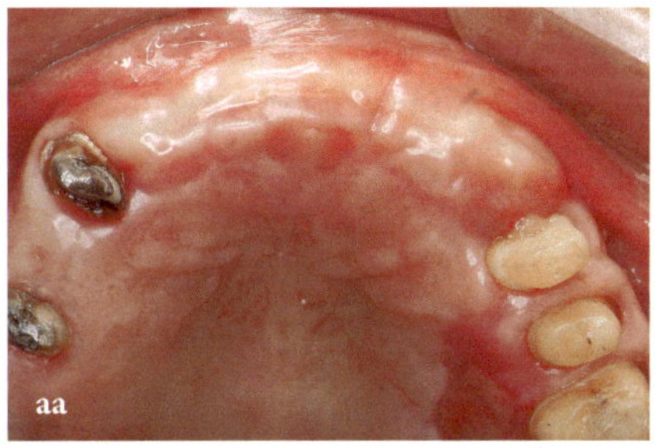

Figs 7-3z and 7-3aa Comparison of occlusal view before *(z)* and after *(aa)* implant placement and bone and soft tissue grafting.

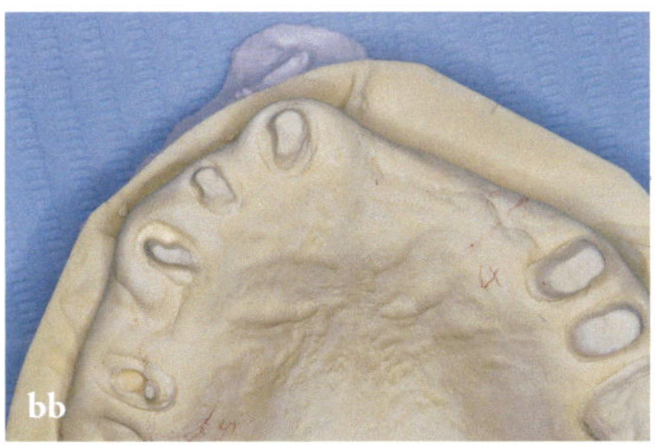

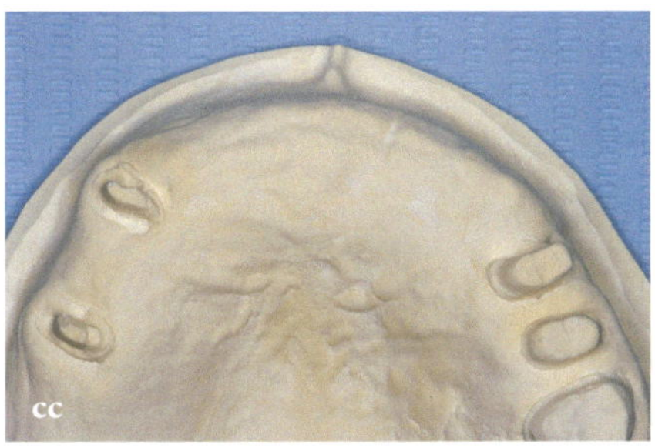

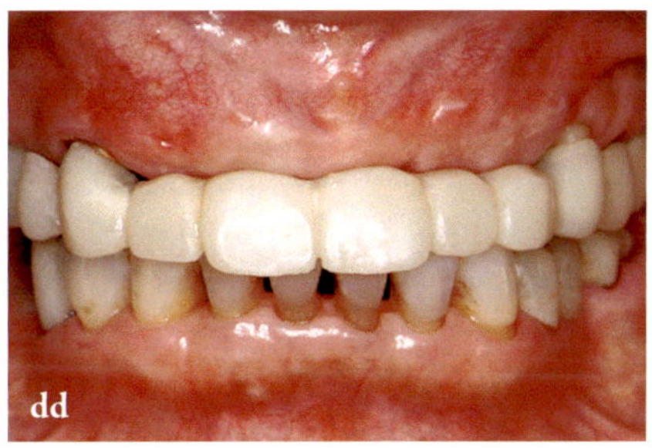

Figs 7-3bb to 7-3dd Comparison of diagnostic casts before *(bb)* and after *(cc)* implant placement and bone and soft tissue grafting as well as the clinical facial view *(dd)* show that favorable arch form and adequate vertical height of the alveolar ridge was achieved.

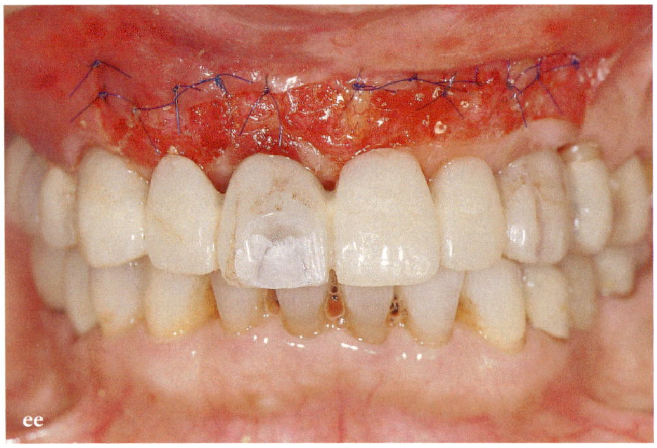

Fig 7-3ee At 2 years 1 month, an apically positioned flap was performed to increase the zone of keratinized tissue.

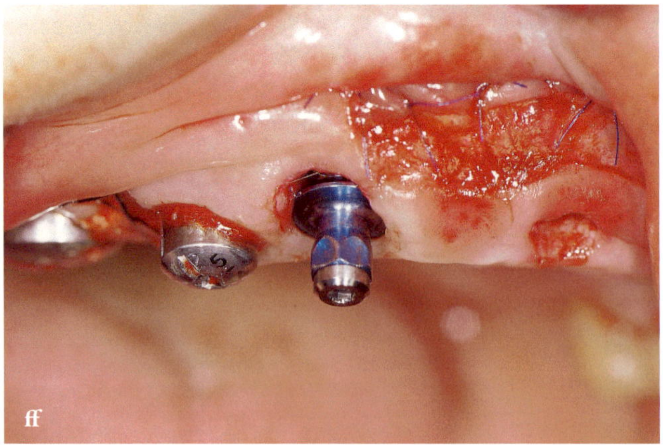

Fig 7-3ff Immediate implant placement was performed at the right canine site, which was Class 1 (see Fig 3-10).

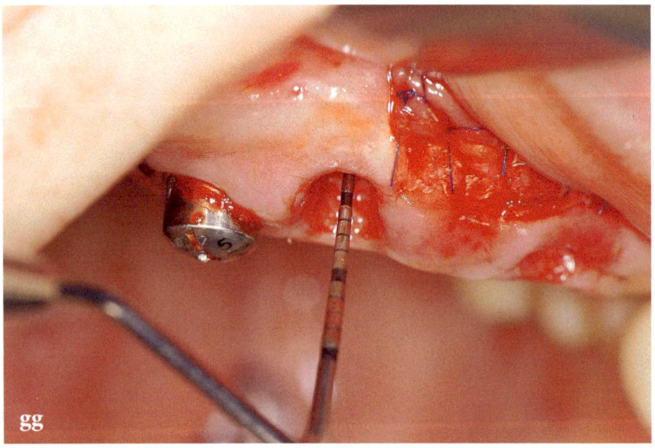

Fig 7-3gg The implant platform was positioned 3 mm apical of the free gingival margin.

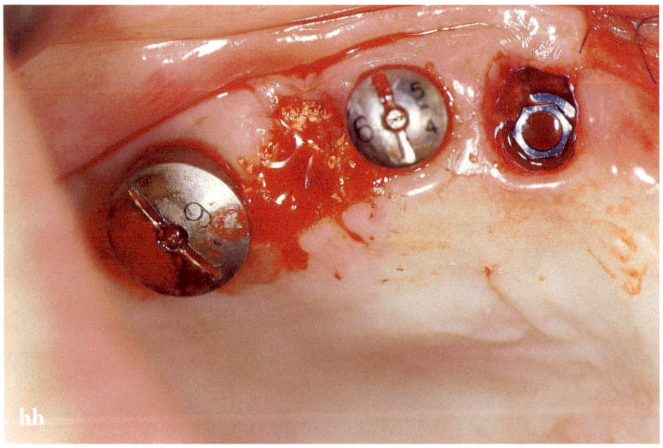

Fig 7-3hh Bone graft was placed into a gap between the implant and buccal bone. Socket preservation for the right second premolar pontic site was carried out. During this surgical procedure, temporary healing abutments were placed.

Step 3

After 2 months of healing, stage-two surgery was carried out, and soft tissue sculpting was initiated with a provisional restoration.

Step 4

When tissue sculpting was almost complete, an apically positioned flap was performed to increase keratinized tissue (see Fig 7-3ee). In addition, immediate implant placement at the right canine site and socket preservation at the right second premolar pontic site were performed (see Figs 7-3ff to 7-3hh).

Step 5

The definitive restorations were fabricated and placed (see Figs 7-3ii to 7-3nn). Retention of the right canine improved bone augmentation and preservation of the tissue between the implants in the right canine and first premolar sites.

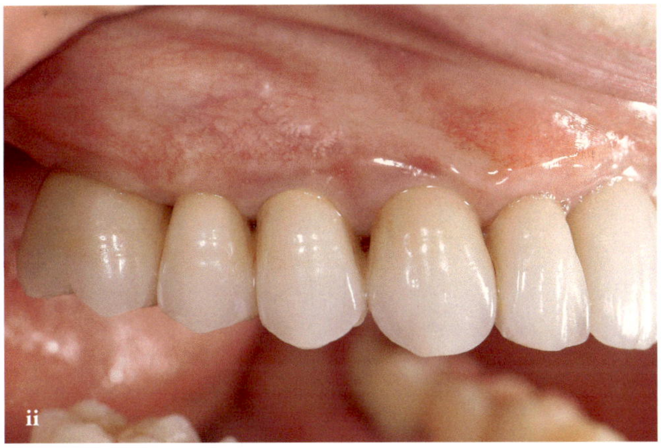

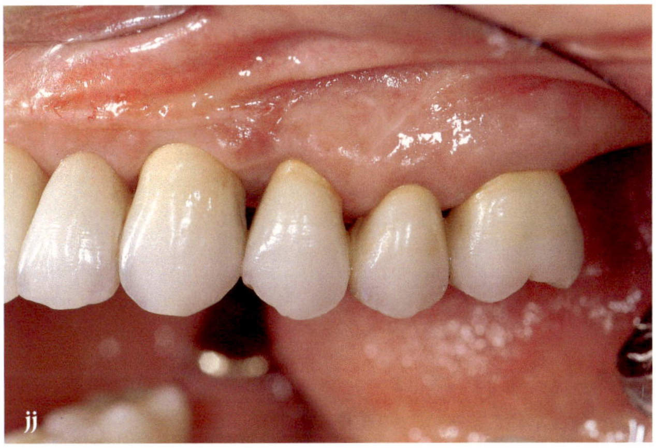

Figs 7-3ii to 7-3kk Definitive restorations at 3 years 9 months. *(ii)* Staged implant placement in the right first premolar and flapless immediate implant placement in the canine allowed for sufficient distance between the implants to create an adequate papilla. *(jj)* Papilla height between the left canine and first premolar is reduced because of the attachment loss on the mesial of the first premolar. *(kk)* Periapical radiographs of definitive restorations. Bone level is coronal to the implant platform level in the anterior region.

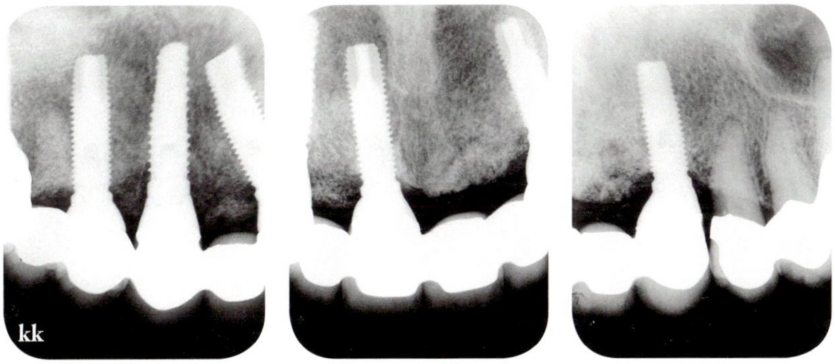

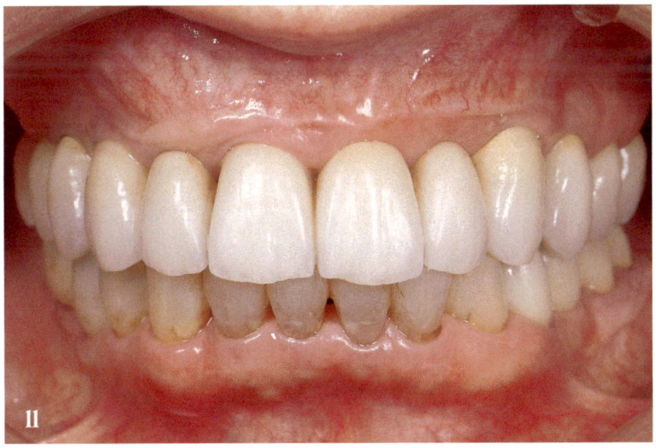

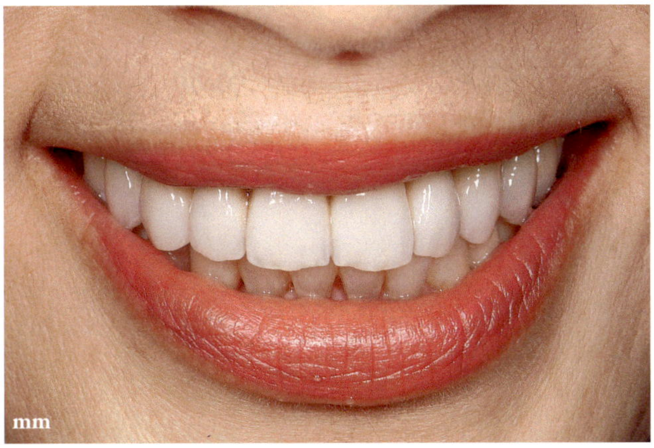

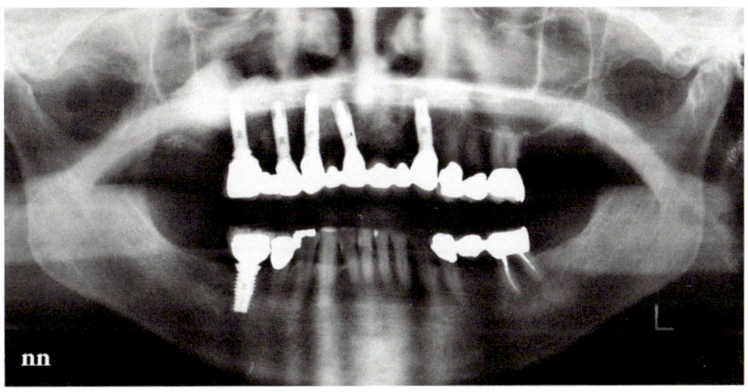

Figs 7-3ll to 7-3nn At 5 years 4 months. One-year follow-up of definitive restorations. A natural-looking smile was achieved.

Case 2: Staged bone and soft tissue management in the esthetic area

The patient shown in Fig 7-4 was a 50-year-old man who had periodontal and esthetic problems. He was a light smoker and had lost one of the central incisors and the left canine immediately before the initial examination. He presented with generalized advanced periodontal disease, a severe alveolar ridge defect, and occlusal collapse.

Goals of treatment

The patient and the clinician must collaborate to establish realistic treatment goals using a diagnostic wax-up and provisional restorations. In this case, the following treatment plan was developed and agreed upon by patient and clinician.

The right canine and first and second premolars were to be treated with splinted crowns after periodontal regenerative therapy. Implants were to be placed in the right first molar and lateral incisor sites as well as in the left central incisor, canine, second premolar, and first molar sites. The provisional restoration was to be supported by the right first and second premolars, canine, and lateral incisor and the left first premolar. The vertical goal of augmentation of the anterior maxilla was indicated by a line from the bone level of the right canine to that of the left first premolar (see Fig 7-4j, *yellow line*). The following sections outline the steps of the 3D ridge augmentation.

Multiple-tooth implant case 2: Staged bone and soft tissue management in the esthetic area

Application of 4D concept to this case

1. Consider immediate implant placement when possible.
2. Perform 3D preservation and augmentation of peri-implant tissue.
3. Allow as much distance as possible between neighboring implants.
4. Insert pontic whenever possible in esthetic area.
5. Consider platform switching when possible.
6. Place implants in native bone when possible.
7. Reduce abutment disconnection.

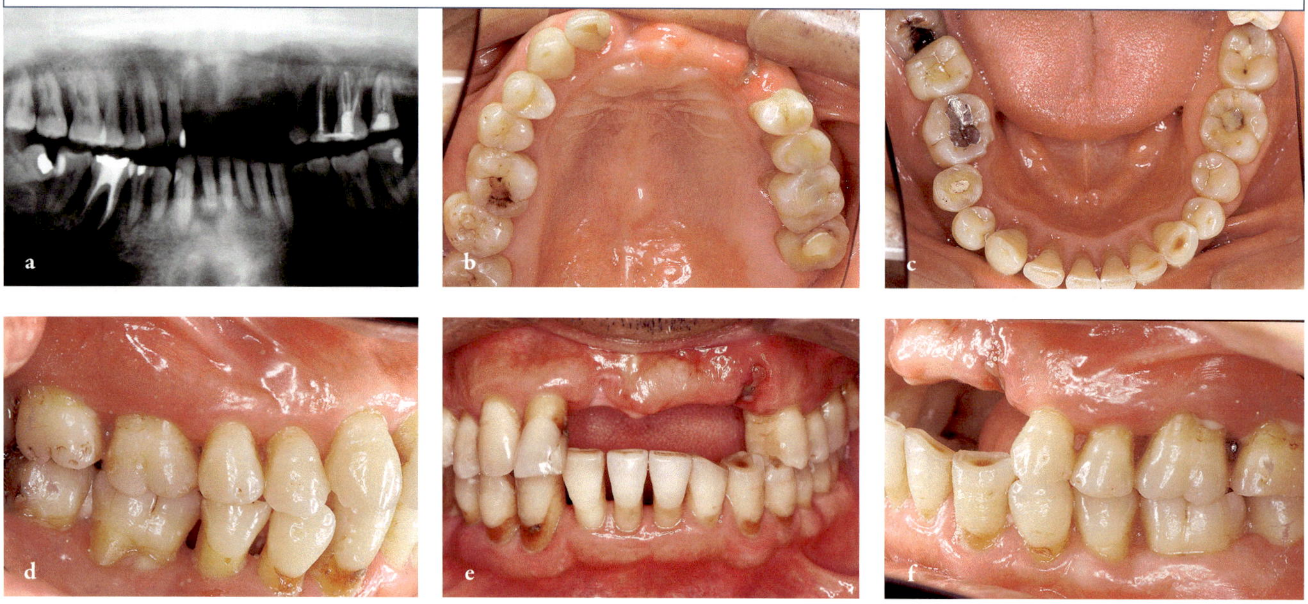

Figs 7-4a to 7-4f Initial examination. Pathological migration of teeth (ie, flare out of anterior maxilla and extrusion of anterior mandible), uneven occlusal plane, posterior bite collapse, and suppuration from most teeth were observed.

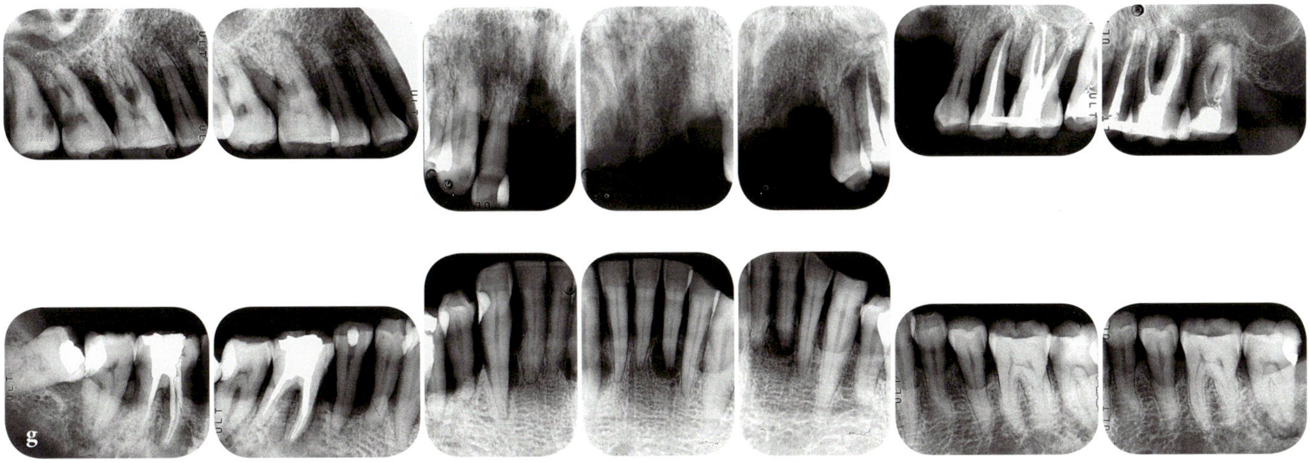

Fig 7-4g Periapical radiographs at the initial examination.

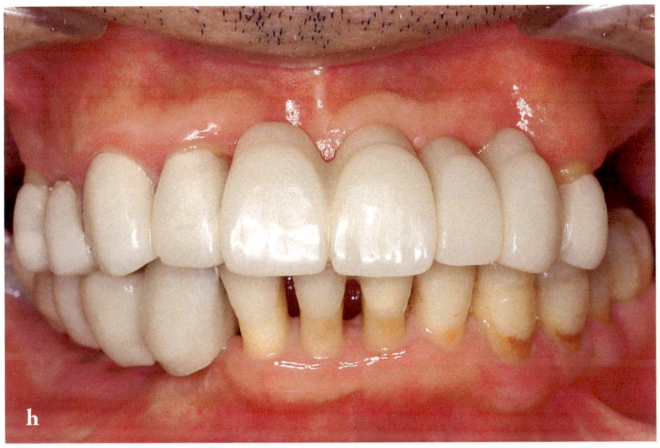

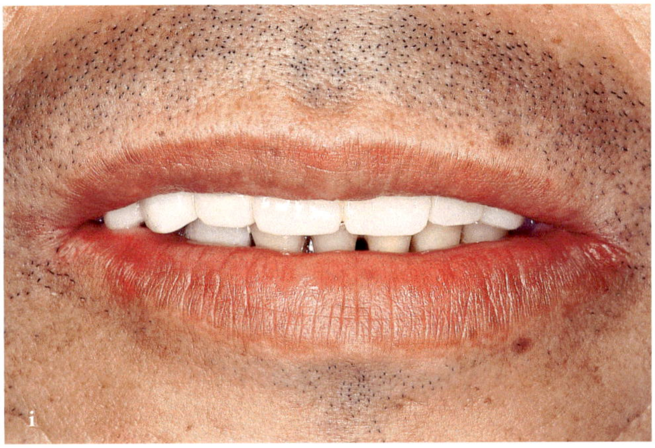

Figs 7-4h and 7-4i Initial set of provisional restorations.

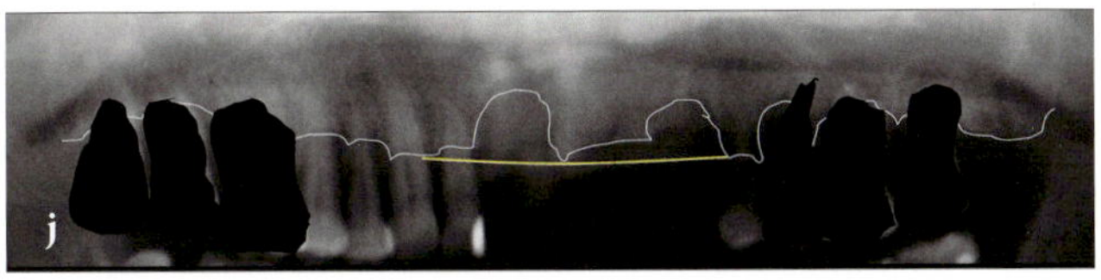

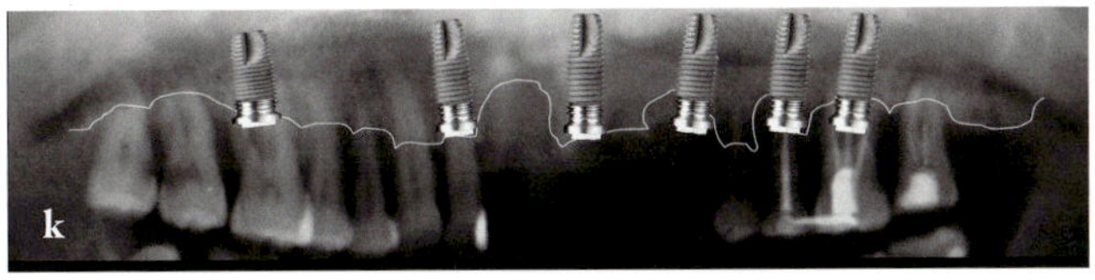

Figs 7-4j and 7-4k Goal for vertical ridge augmentation *(j, yellow line)* and proposed implant sites *(k)*.

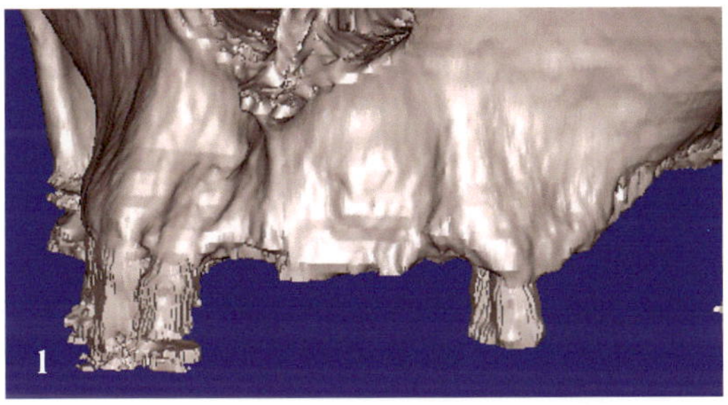

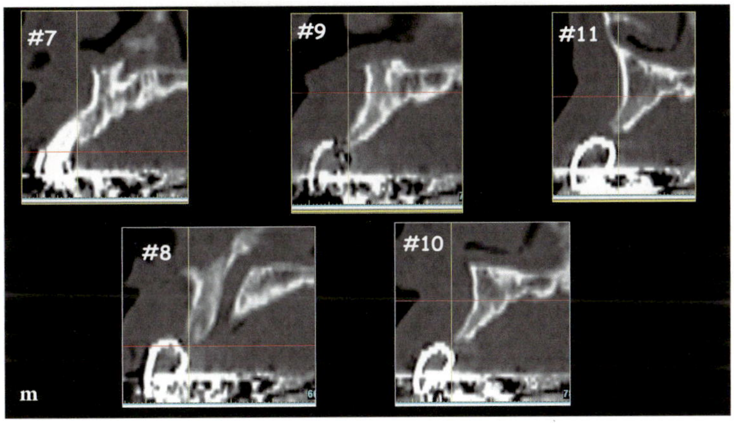

Figs 7-4l and 7-4m Computed tomographic evaluation. An advanced ridge defect was observed.

Step 1

Implant placement and horizontal guided bone regeneration (GBR) with a titanium-reinforced membrane and bone graft were performed at the left canine site (see Figs 7-4n and 7-4o). In addition, implant placement and simultaneous sinus lift were carried out at the left second premolar and first molar sites.

Step 2

Immediate implant placement was performed in the right lateral incisor site (see Fig 7-4q). Vertical GBR with bone graft and cross-linked collagen membrane was completed, and a temporary healing abutment (4 mm in height) was placed on the left canine implant to aid vertical augmentation (see Figs 7-4r to 7-4t).

Step 1

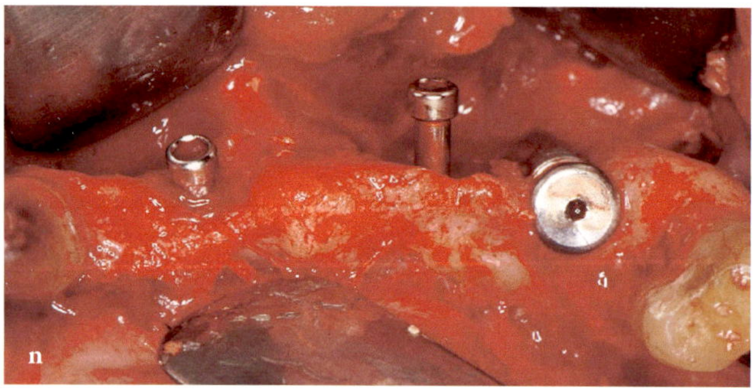

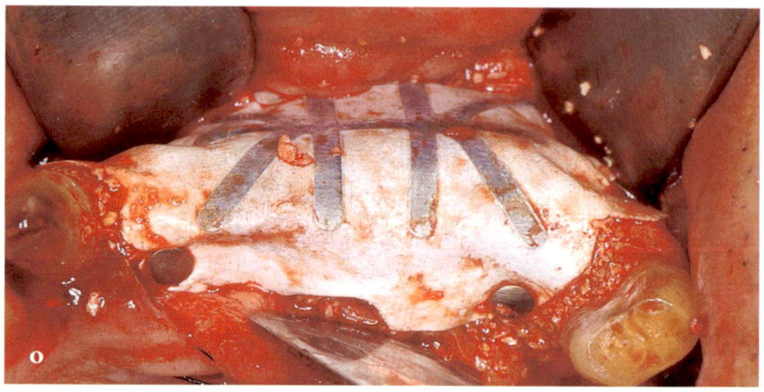

Figs 7-4n and 7-4o Horizontal GBR with a titanium-reinforced membrane.

Step 2

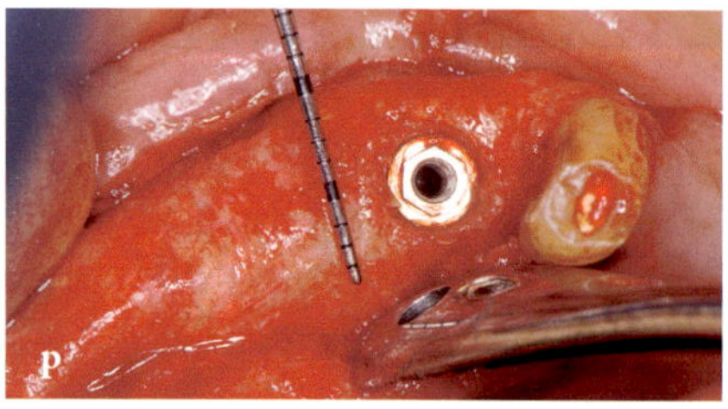

Fig 7-4p Three months later, more than 2 mm of buccal bone was regenerated.

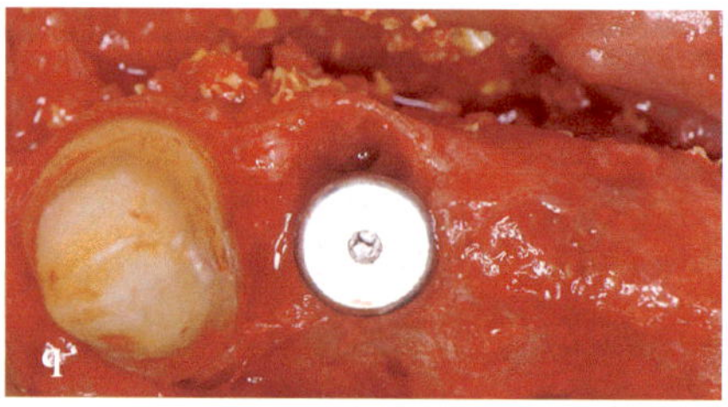

Fig 7-4q Immediate implant placement in the right lateral incisor.

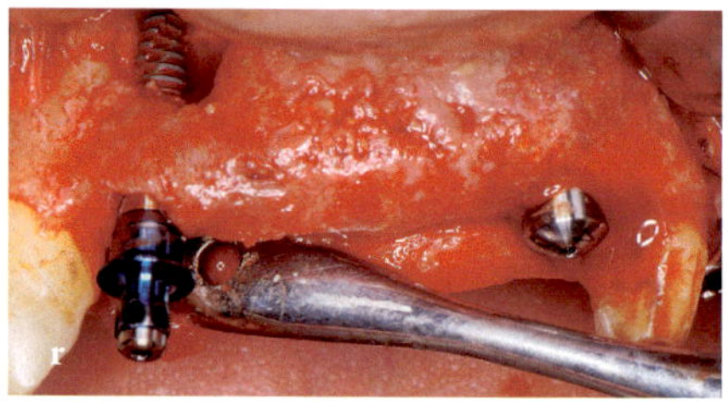

Fig 7-4r A 4-mm temporary healing abutment was placed on the left canine.

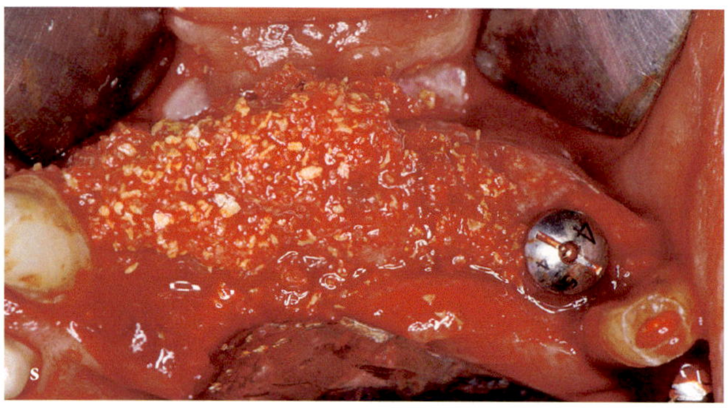

Fig 7-4s Additional ridge augmentation with bone graft and cross-linked collagen membrane was performed.

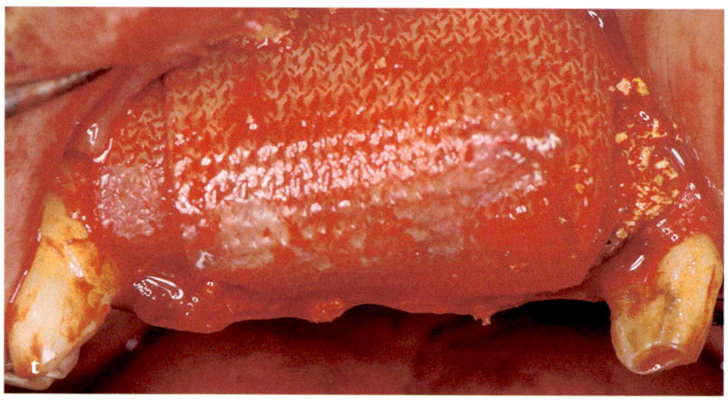

Fig 7-4t Two layers of cross-linked collagen membrane were placed.

Step 3

An implant was placed in the left central incisor site, and soft tissue grafting was performed to enhance the buccal bone width (see Figs 7-4u and 7-4v).

Step 3

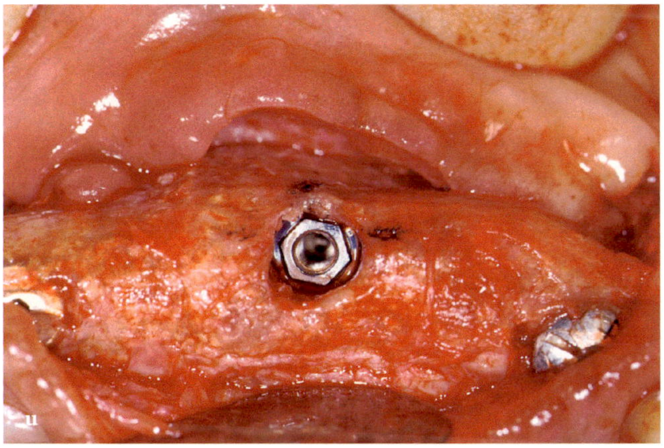

Fig 7-4u Implant placement was in the ideal position for the left central incisor, but the buccal bone was not sufficient. Soft tissue augmentation with connective tissue grafting was performed at this time.

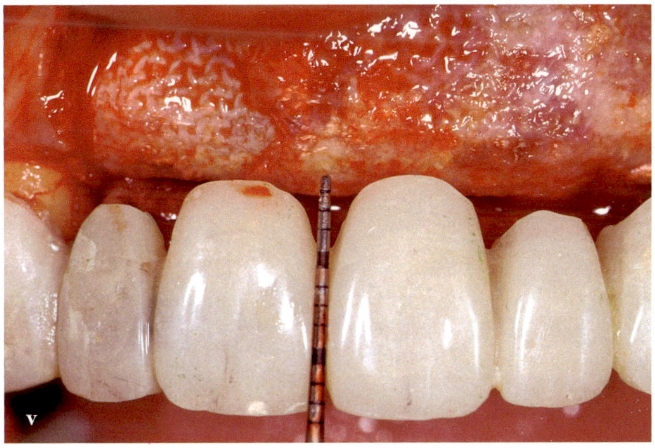

Fig 7-4v The alveolar ridge was augmented to 4 mm from the contact point of the surgical stent.

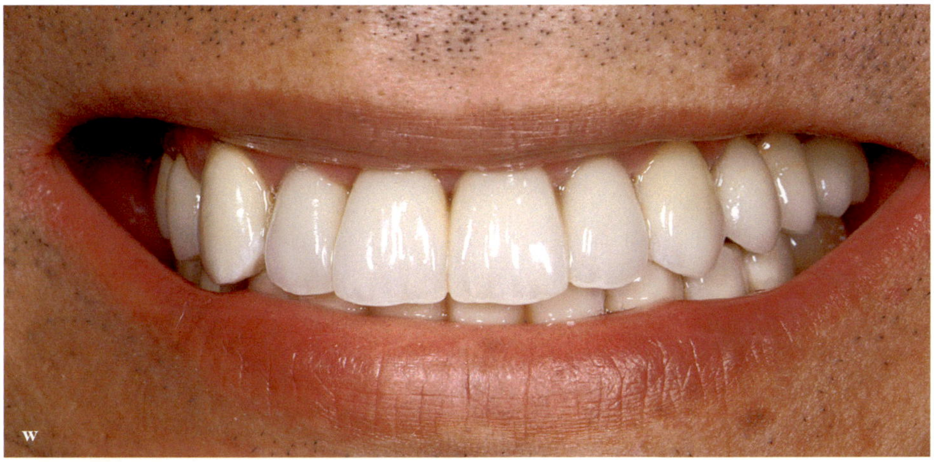

Fig 7-4w Facial view with definitive restorations. The patient's smile, definitive restoration, and soft tissue profile are in harmony.

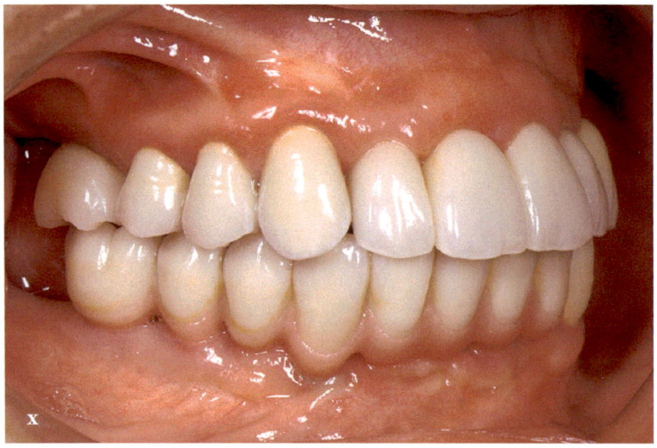

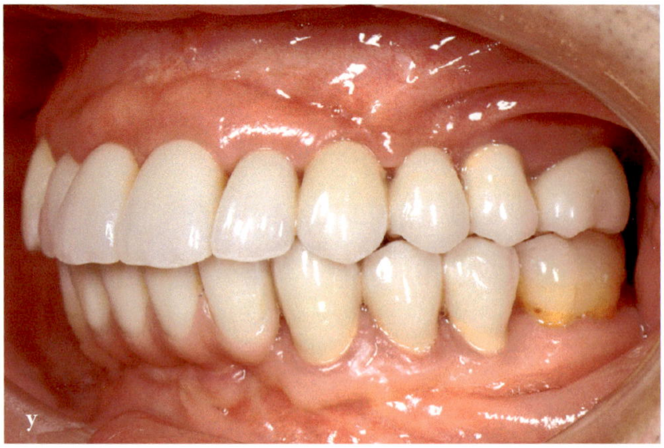

Figs 7-4x and 7-4y Lateral views with definitive restoration. Adequate tissue volume was established.

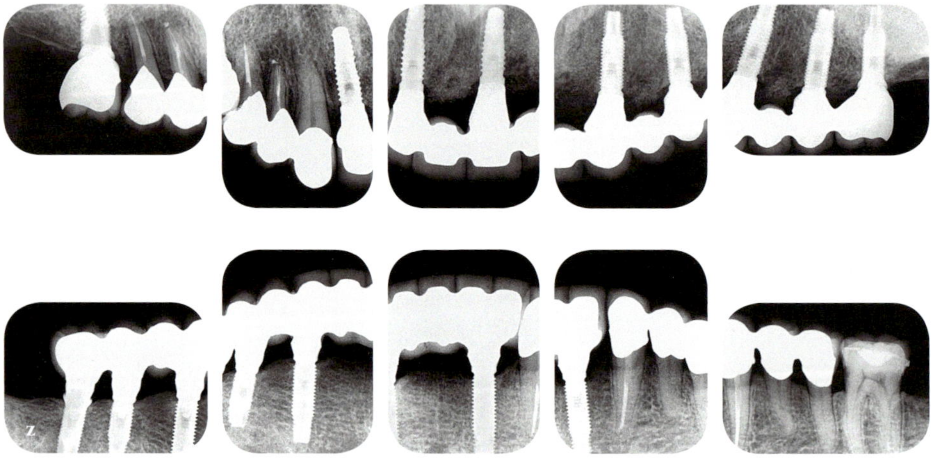

Fig 7-4z Periapical radiographs with definitive restorations.

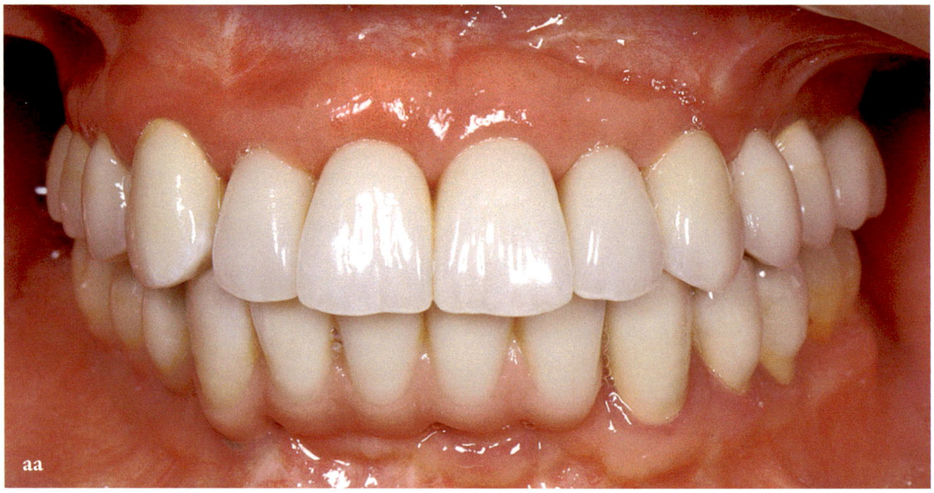

Fig 7-4aa Facial view at 2-year follow-up.

Case 3: Establishing posterior occlusal support

In the case shown in Fig 7-5, most of the patient's teeth were diagnosed as hopeless (see Figs 7-5a to 7-5c). Treatment planning and sequence were critical for achieving an esthetic final result.

Bone augmentation and preservation

Successful horizontal and vertical bone augmentation in the maxillary anterior area was critical for an esthetic final result. The diagnostic wax-up suggested that the alveolar ridge in the posterior mandible had excess vertical height. The anterior alveolar ridge of the mandible would be preserved after extraction of the hopeless teeth.

Occlusal support

Successful anterior bone and soft tissue augmentation was assured with fixed provisional restorations supported by posterior implants.

Treatment plan and sequence

Implants were placed in the maxillary right and left premolars and first molars (see Fig 7-5d). Stage-two surgery and extraction of the remaining teeth were performed 4 months later (see Fig 7-5f). The fixed provisional restoration was supported by posterior implants. Additional implants were placed in both maxillary lateral incisor sites (see Figs 7-5m and 7-5n) to allow insertion of pontics for an esthetic final result (see Figs 7-5z and 7-5aa).

Multiple-tooth implant case 3: Establishing posterior occlusal support

Application of 4D concept to this case

1. Consider immediate implant placement when possible.
2. Perform 3D preservation and augmentation of peri-implant tissue.
3. Allow as much distance as possible between neighboring implants.
4. Insert pontic whenever possible in esthetic area.
5. Consider platform switching when possible.
6. Place implants in native bone when possible.
7. Reduce abutment disconnection.

☞ Key clinical points

- Implant placement in posterior region at an early stage
- Provisional restoration in maxilla supported by posterior implants
- GBR in anterior maxilla
- Implant placement in posterior mandible and ridge preservation following extraction of remaining teeth

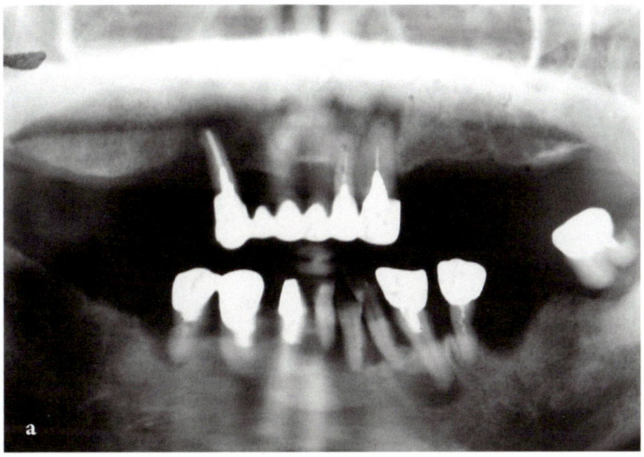

Fig 7-5a Panoramic radiograph at initial examination.

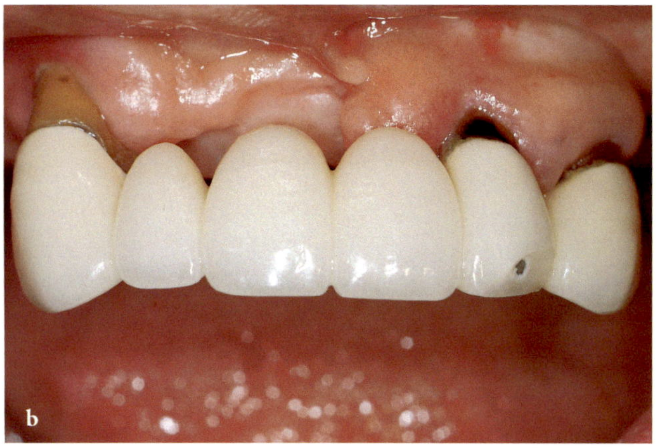

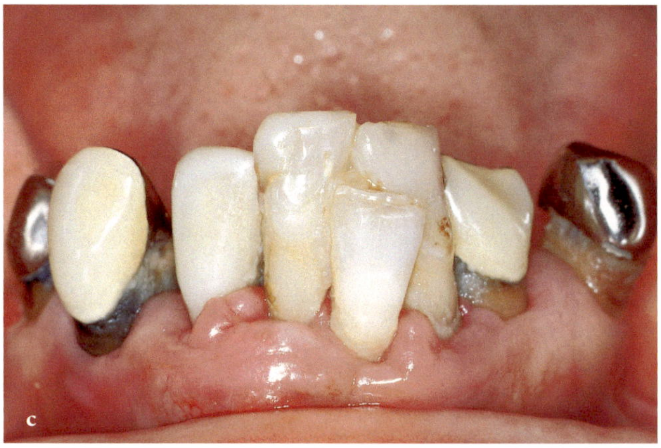

Figs 7-5b and 7-5c Maxillary *(b)* and mandibular *(c)* facial views at initial examination. Patient presented with tooth mobility and requested esthetic implant treatment.

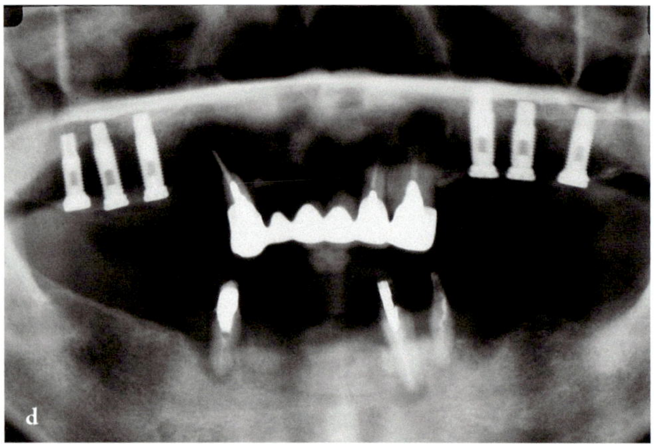

Fig 7-5d At 2 months implants were placed in the posterior maxilla on both sides.

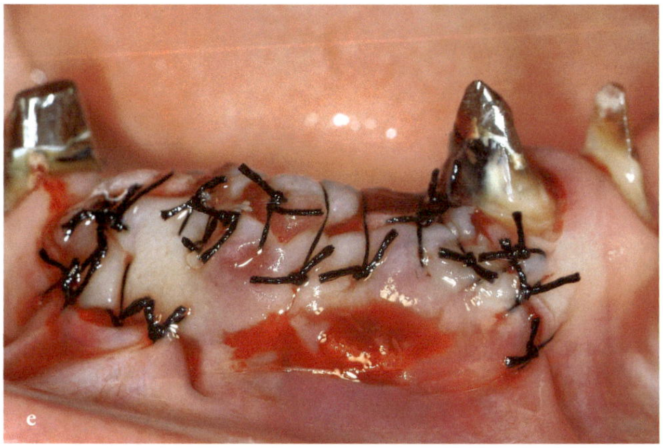

Fig 7-5e Socket preservation was performed following extraction of the teeth in the anterior mandible.

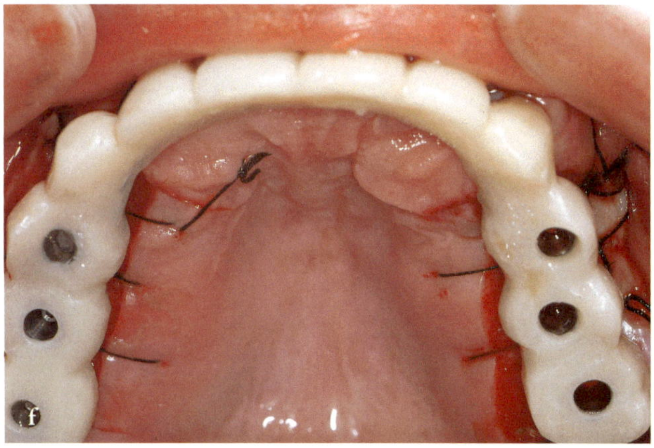

Fig 7-5f At 6 months, stage-two surgery was performed, and a fixed provisional restoration, supported by the maxillary posterior implants, was placed. The anterior teeth were extracted.

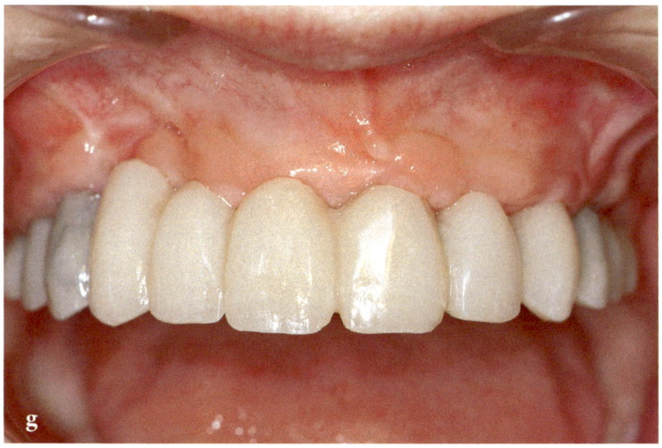

Fig 7-5g Facial view of the provisional restoration 2 months after extraction of the maxillary anterior teeth.

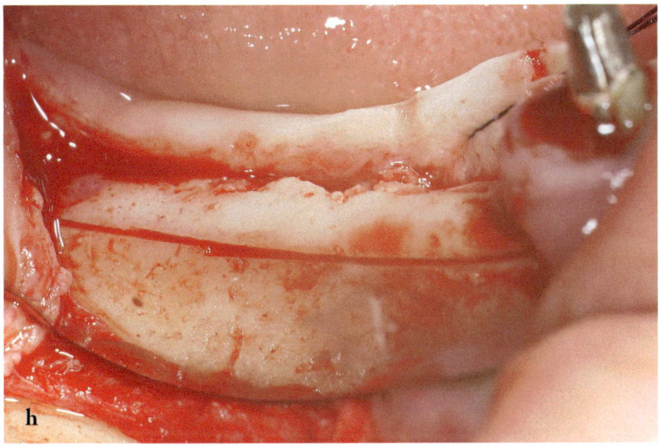

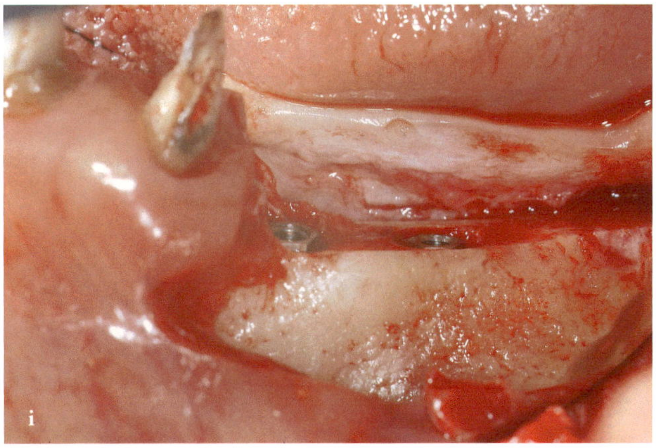

Figs 7-5h and 7-5i Excess alveolar bone in the posterior mandible was sectioned, and implants were placed in the second premolar and first molar sites on both sides. Sectioned bone was used as an autogenous block bone graft in the maxilla.

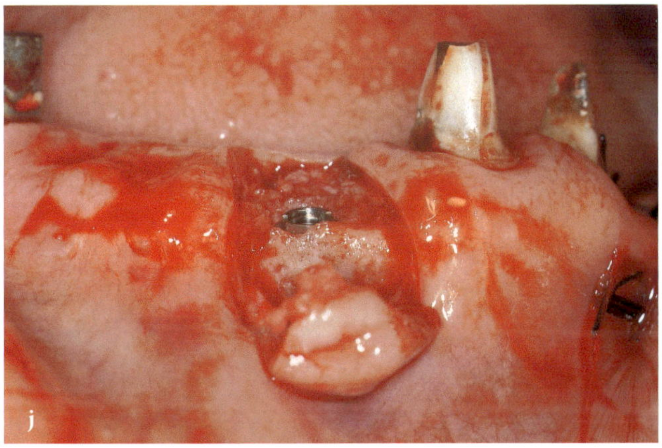

Fig 7-5j An implant was placed in the mandibular left central incisor site.

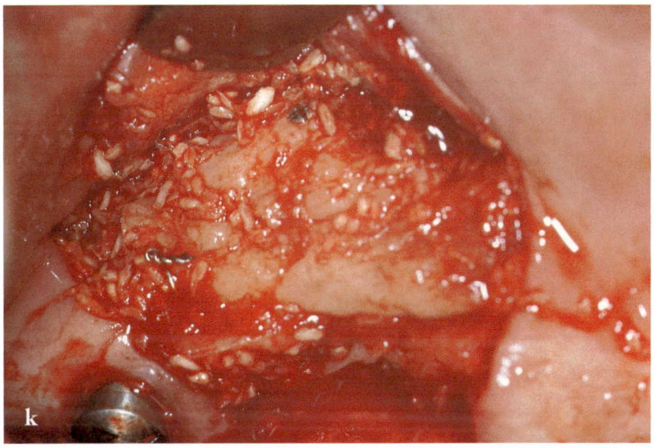

Fig 7-5k An autogenous block bone graft was stabilized with screws and metal wire. Particulate bone graft was used to fill in around the block graft.

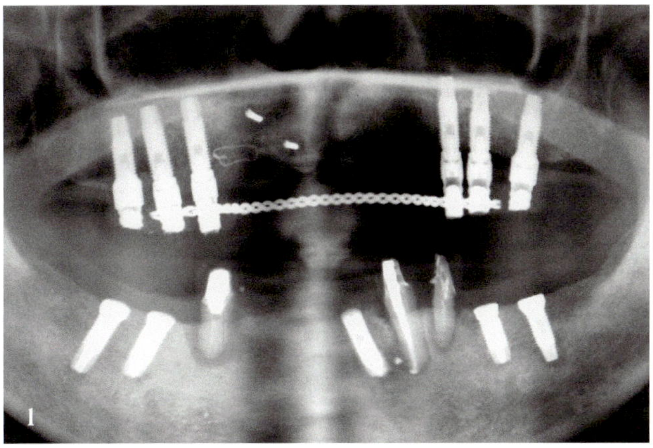

Fig 7-5l Panoramic radiograph after placement of implants and bone graft.

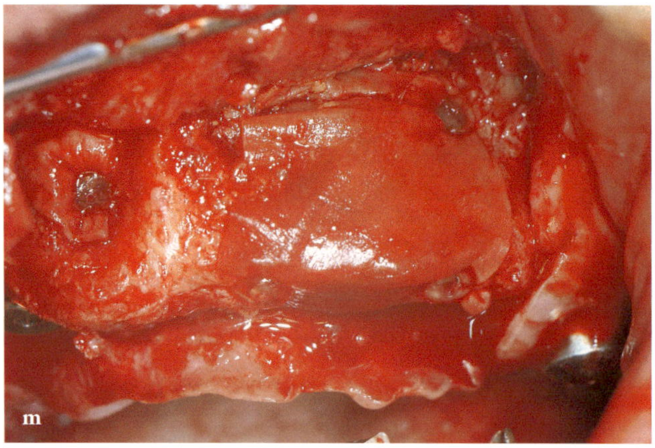

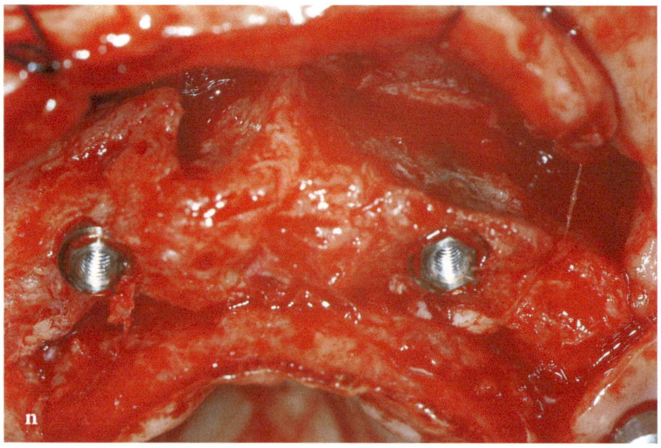

Figs 7-5m and 7-5n At 11 months, 3 months after placement of the autogenous block bone graft, implants were placed in both maxillary lateral incisor sites. Additional GBR was performed.

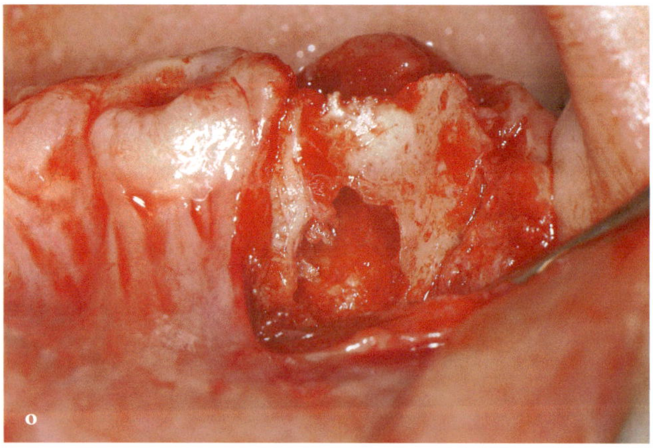

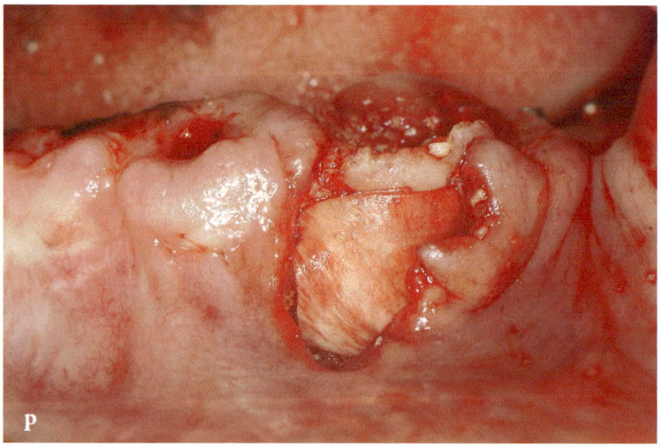

Figs 7-5o and 7-5p Socket preservation in the mandible.

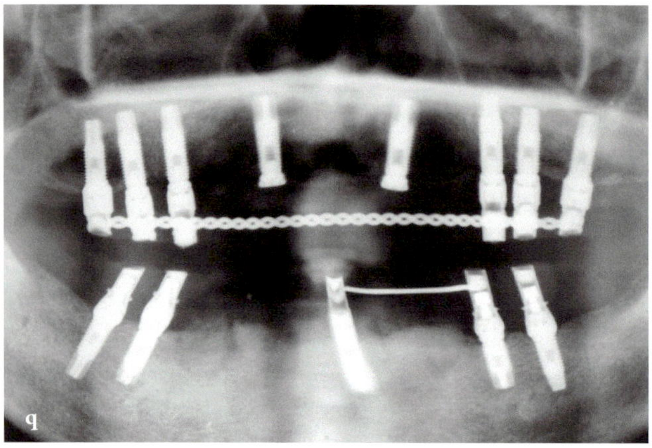

Fig 7-5q Panoramic radiograph after surgery.

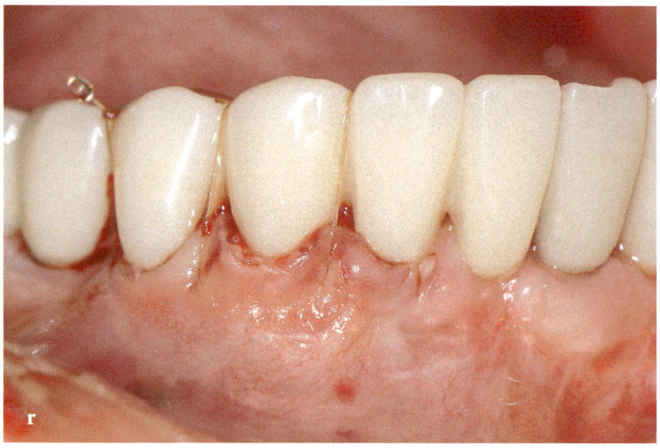

Fig 7-5r A provisional restoration was placed in the mandible.

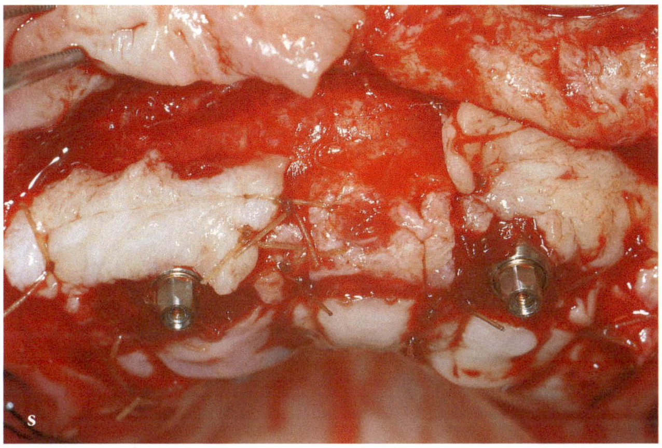

Fig 7-5s At 1 year 3 months, stage-two surgery with connective tissue grafting was performed at the maxillary lateral incisor sites.

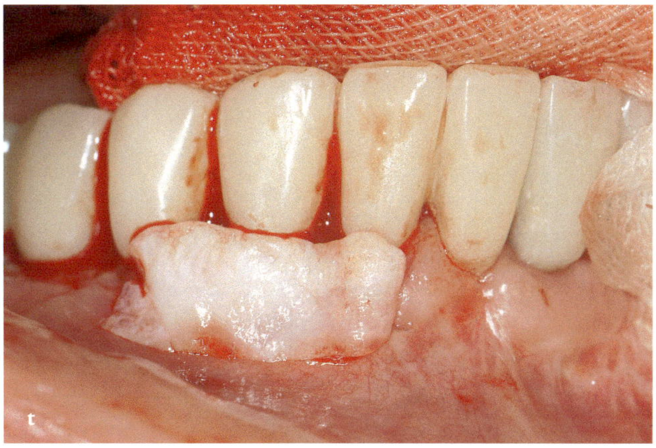

Fig 7-5t A connective tissue graft was placed at the future mandibular right canine implant site.

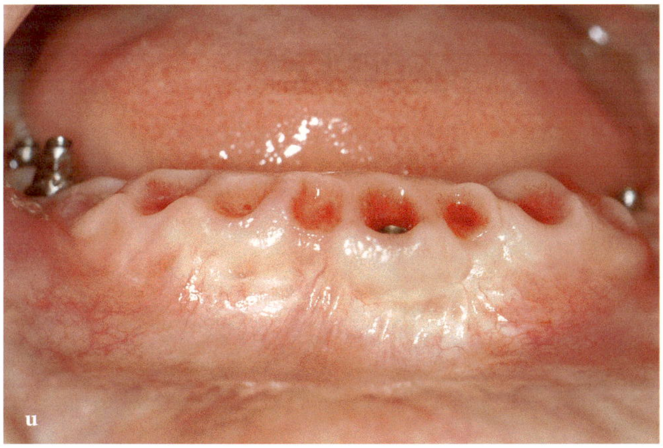

Fig 7-5u At 1 year 8 months, tissue sculpting was completed with a provisional restoration.

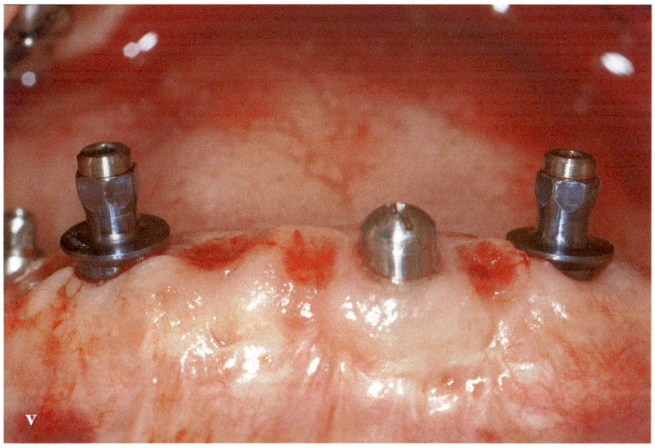

Fig 7-5v Implants were placed in the mandibular canine sites using a flapless technique.

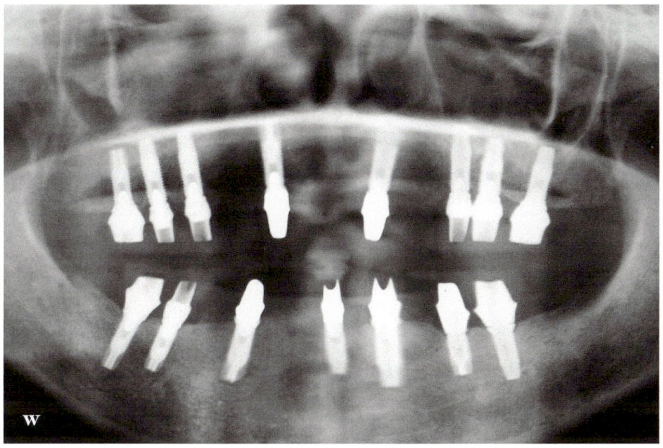

Fig 7-5w Panoramic radiograph after implant placement.

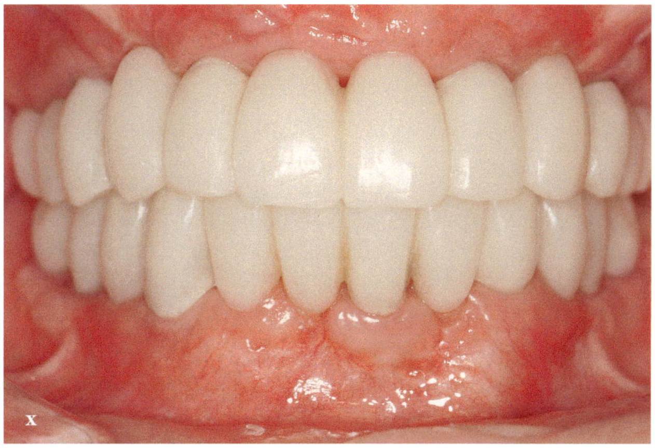

Fig 7-5x The provisional restoration supported by definitive abutments.

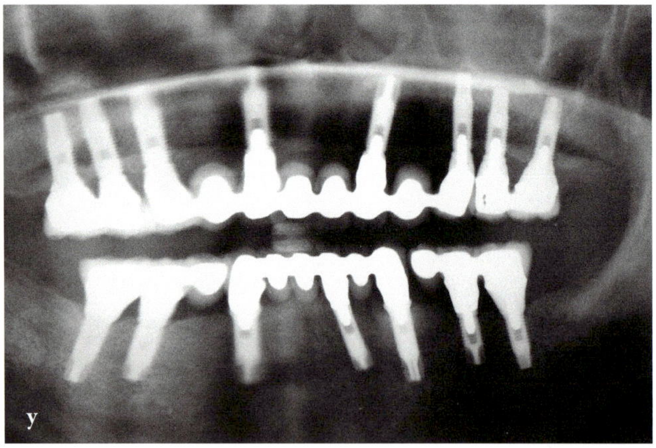

Fig 7-5y At 2 years 6 months. Panoramic radiograph with definitive restoration. The definitive restoration was sectioned as central incisor–first premolar and second premolar–first molar on both sides of the maxilla and as central incisor–canine and first premolar–first molar on both sides of the mandible.

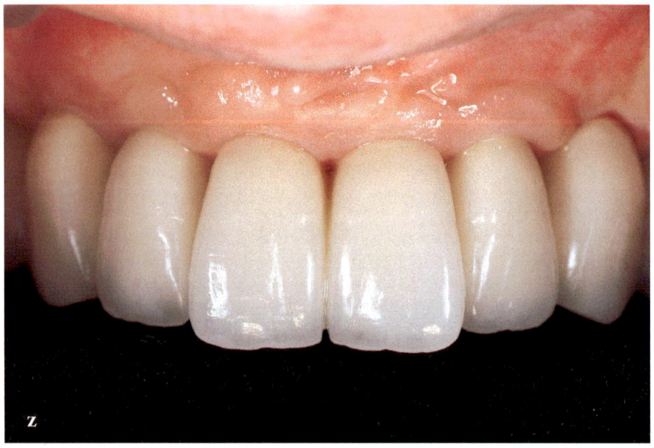

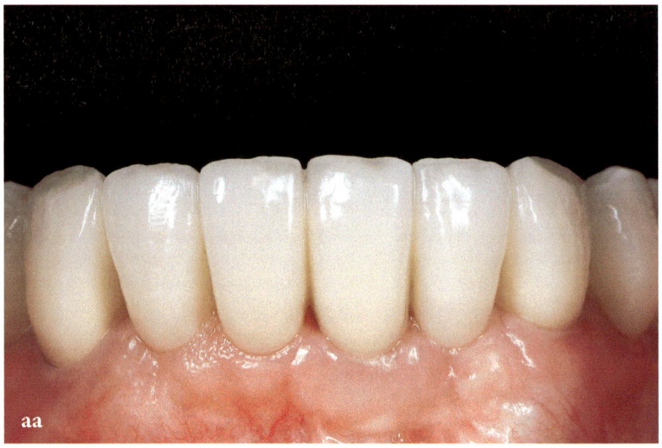

Figs 7-5z and 7-5aa At 4 years 6 months. Two-year follow-up with definitive restoration. An esthetic result was maintained through application of the 4D concept.

Case 4: Platform switching

In the case shown in Fig 7-6, implants were placed in the maxillary right first molar to first premolar sites with an osteotome (see Figs 7-6f and 7-6g). Implant placement and GBR were performed in the mandibular right first molar site (see Fig 7-6i). After stage-two surgery, occlusal rehabilitation was achieved with a provisional restoration.

An implant was placed in the mandibular left first molar site. Implants were also placed in both maxillary canine as well as the left central incisor sites with autogenous bone graft harvested from the left mandibular ramus (see Figs 7-6k to 7-6s).

After stage-two surgery for the maxillary anterior implants (see Figs 7-6v and 7-6w), implants were placed in the left posterior maxilla (see Fig 7-6y).

Multiple-tooth implant case 4: Platform switching

Application of 4D concept to this case

1. Consider immediate implant placement when possible.
2. Perform 3D preservation and augmentation of peri-implant tissue.
3. Allow as much distance as possible between neighboring implants.
4. Insert pontic whenever possible in esthetic area.
5. Consider platform switching when possible.
6. Place implants in native bone when possible.
7. Reduce abutment disconnection.

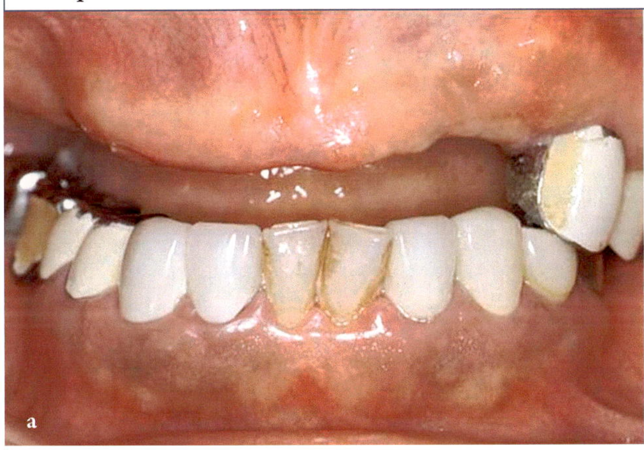

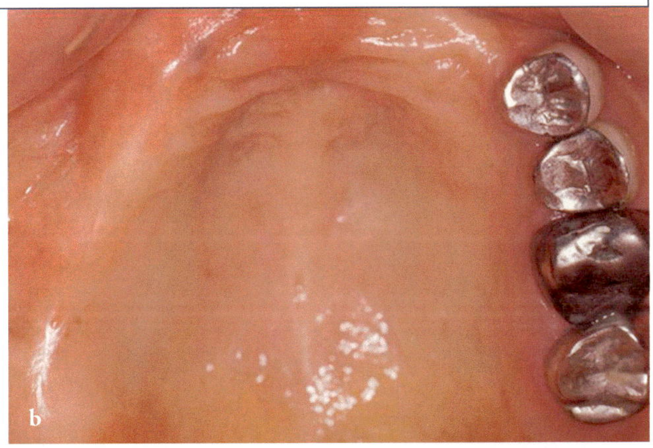

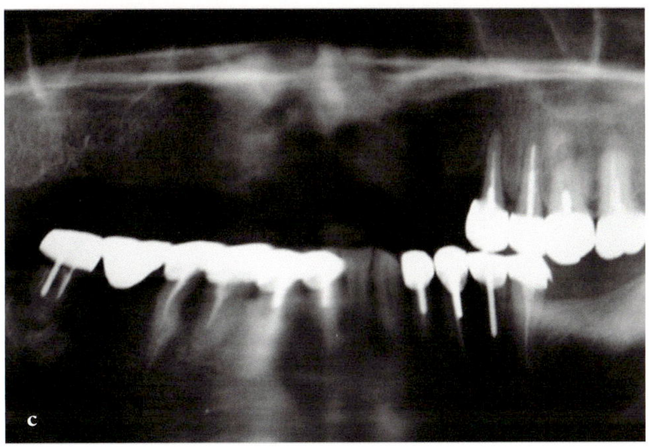

Figs 7-6a to 7-6c Facial *(a)*, occlusal *(b)*, and radiographic *(c)* view at initial examination. The patient requested esthetic implant treatment.

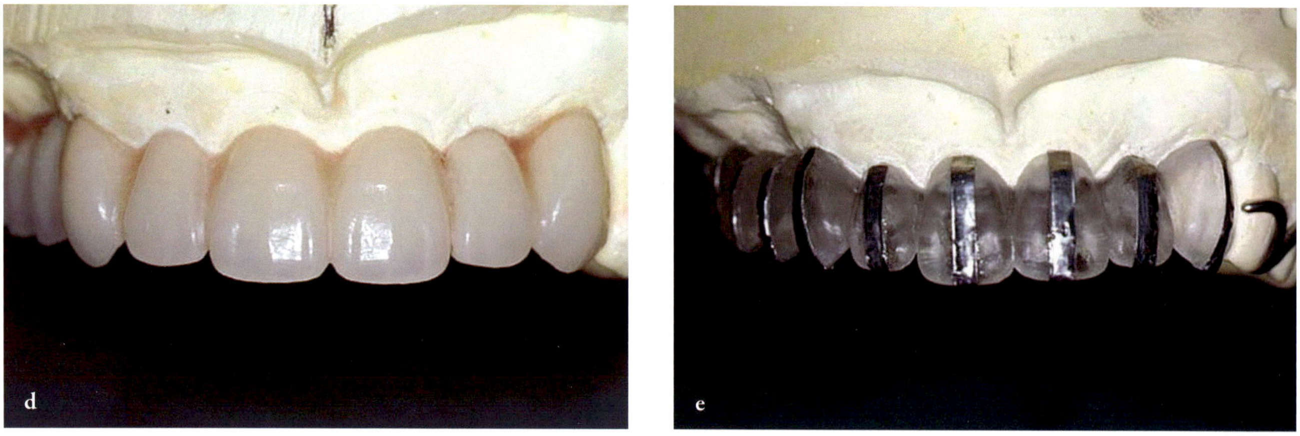

Figs 7-6d and 7-6e Diagnostic wax-up *(d)* and surgical stent *(e)*.

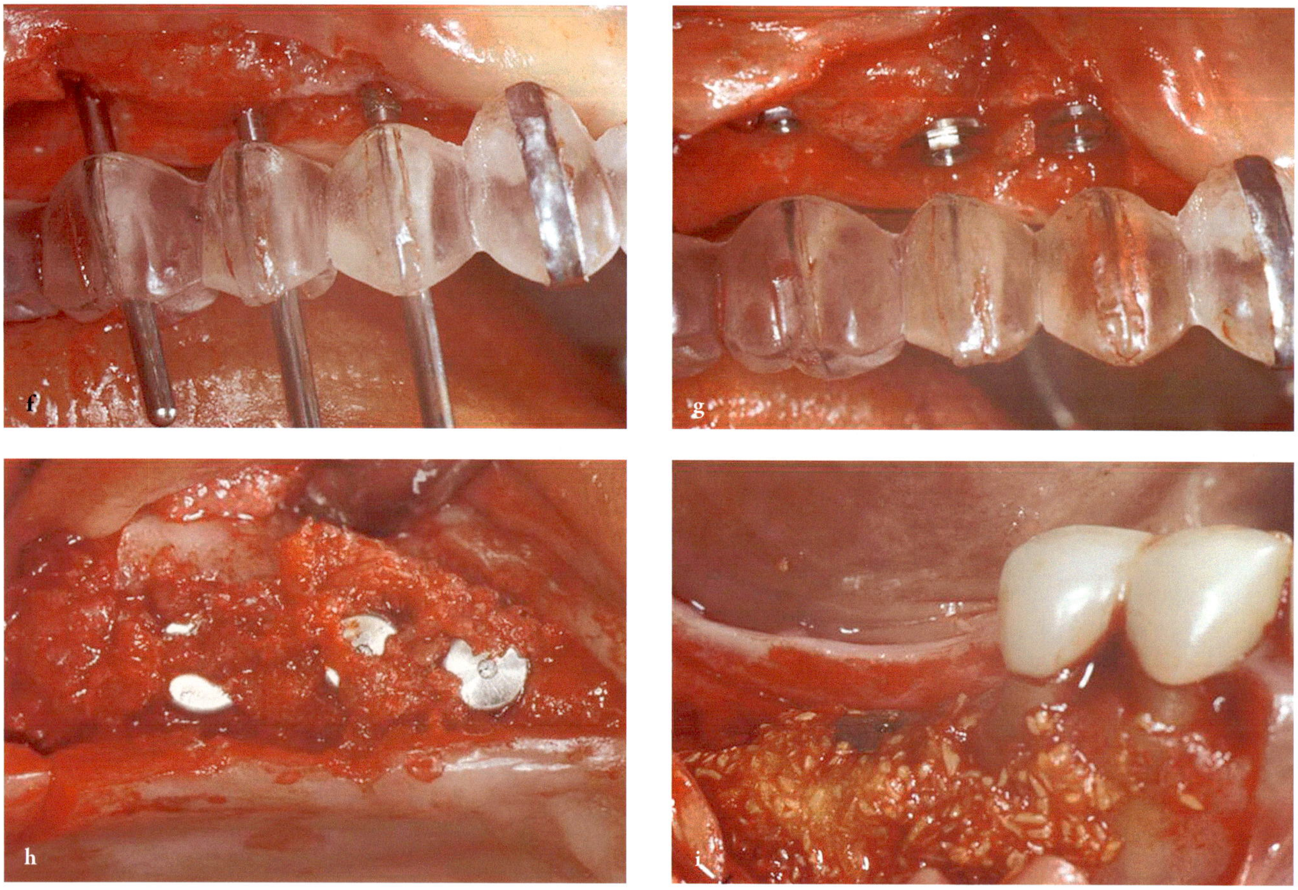

Figs 7-6f to 7-6i Implant placement in the maxillary right premolar and first molar sites with an osteotome sinus lift. Horizontal GBR was performed in that same area and at the mandibular right first molar.

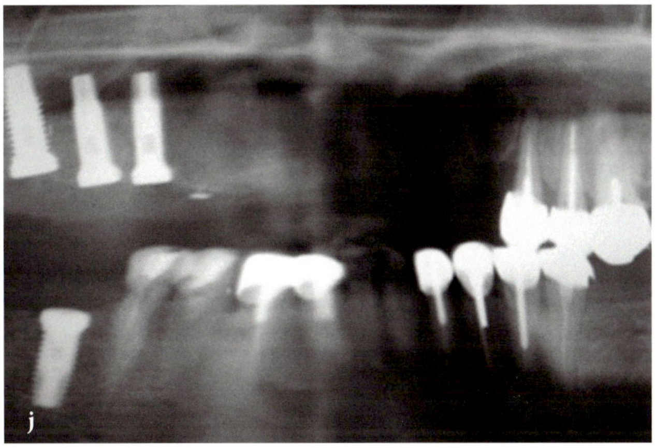

Fig 7-6j Panoramic radiograph after implant placement.

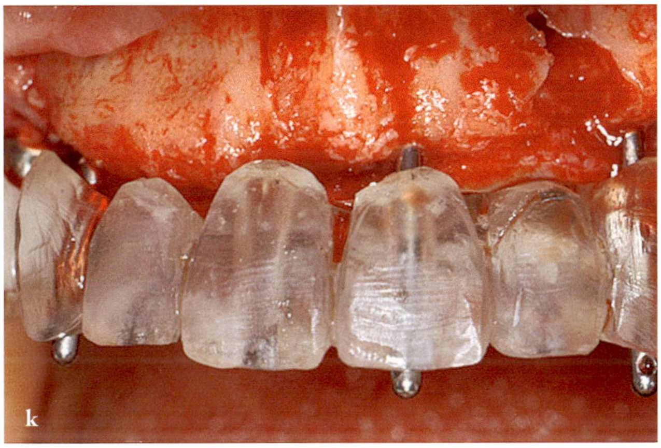

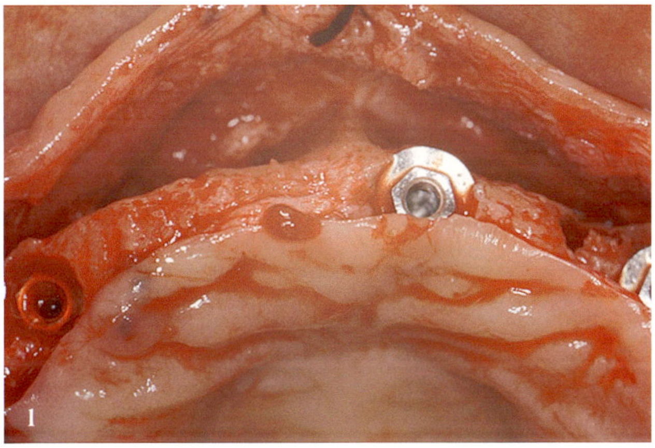

Figs 7-6k and 7-6l Ideal implant placement in both maxillary canines and the left central incisor with a 2710 bur. Immediate implant placement was used at the right canine.

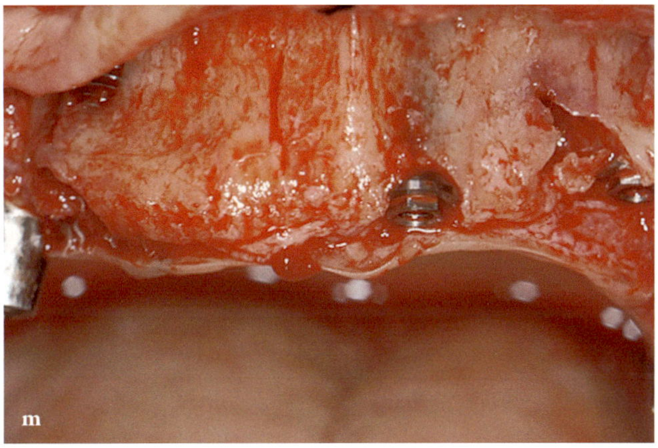

Fig 7-6m To support an esthetic soft tissue profile, at least 2 mm of buccal bone width and 2 to 3 mm of bone height augmentation were necessary.

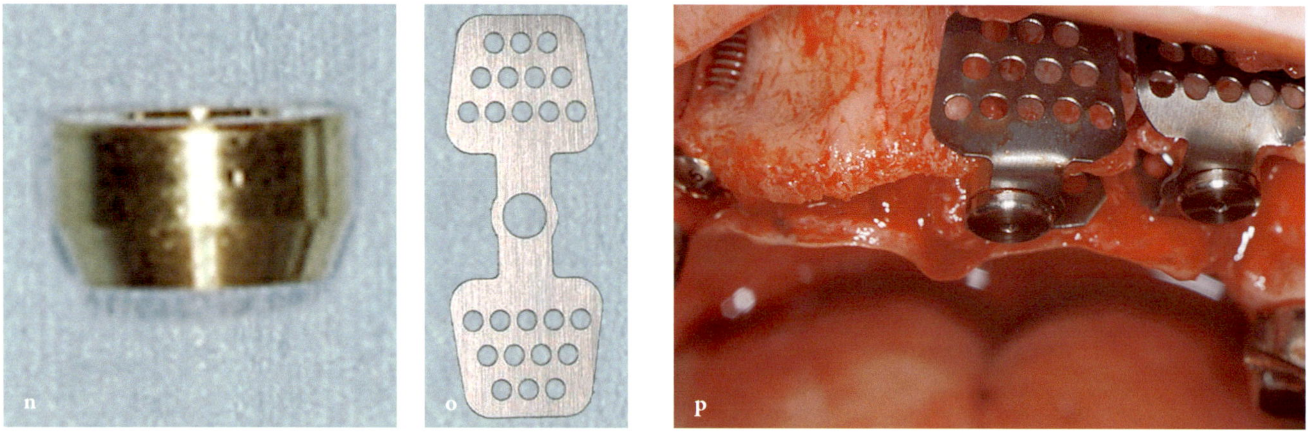

Figs 7-6n to 7-6p A 3-mm-height, pure gold FT abutment prototype and an FT wing were placed on the implants, then stabilized with cover screws.

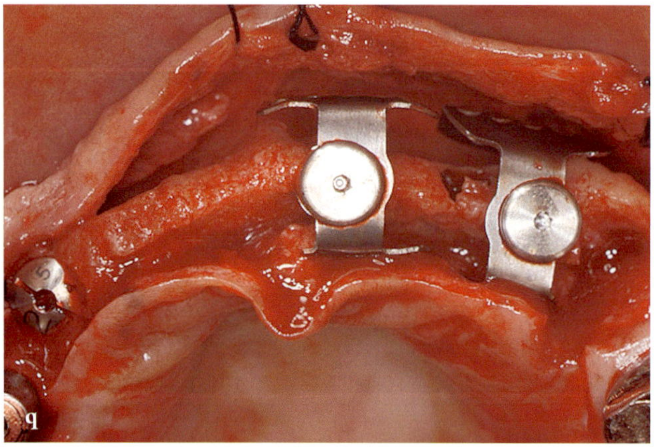

Fig 7-6q Occlusal view of FT abutment and FT wing in place.

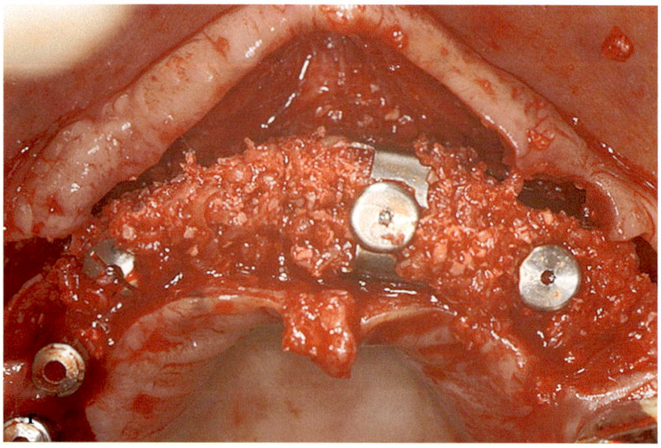

Fig 7-6r A mixture of autogenous bone and xenograft was grafted.

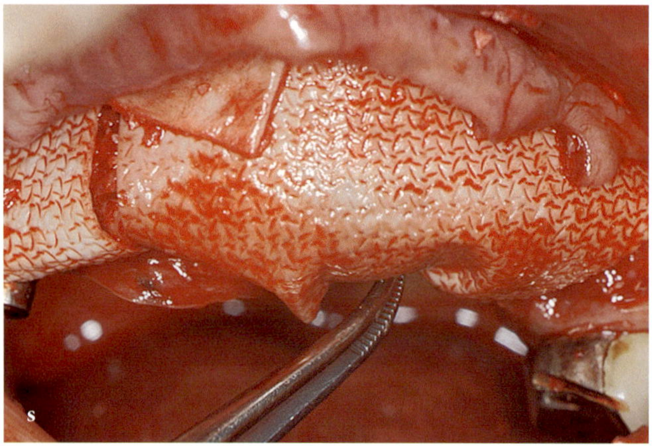

Fig 7-6s A resorbable membrane was placed and sutured.

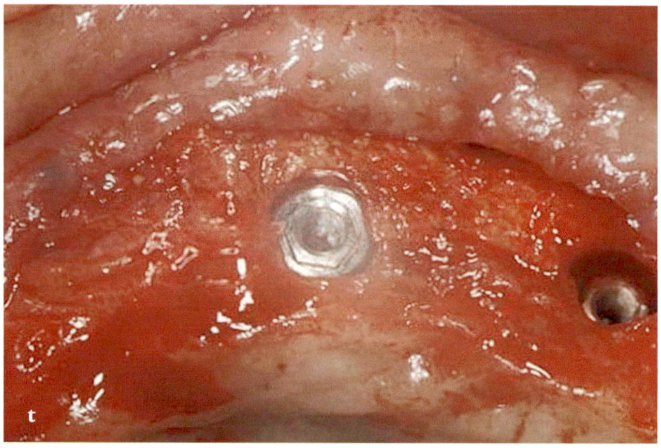

Fig 7-6t Nine months later, the FT wings and FT abutments were removed. Adequate width and height of bone was regenerated around the implants.

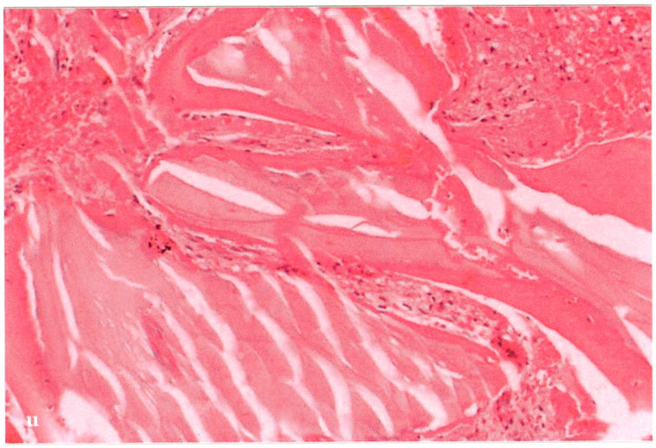

Fig 7-6u New bone formation was observed histologically. (Courtesy of Dr Takeshi Ishida.)

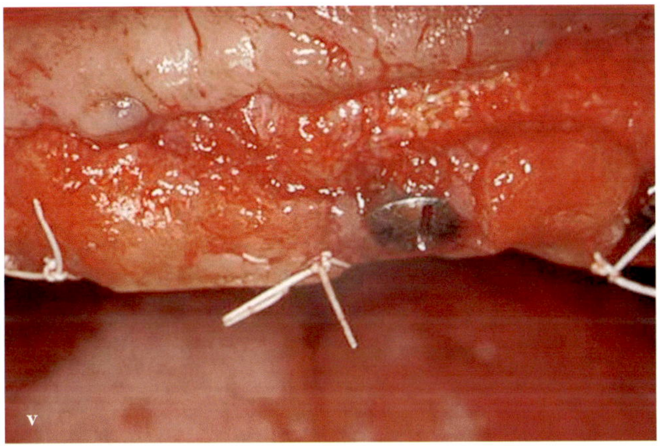

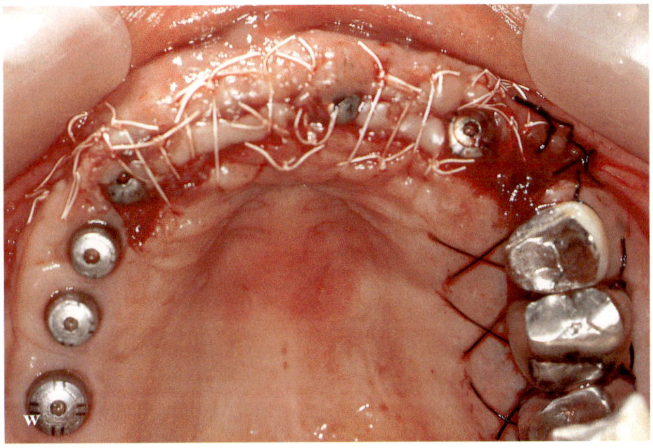

Figs 7-6v and 7-6w Stage-two surgery with interpositional graft.

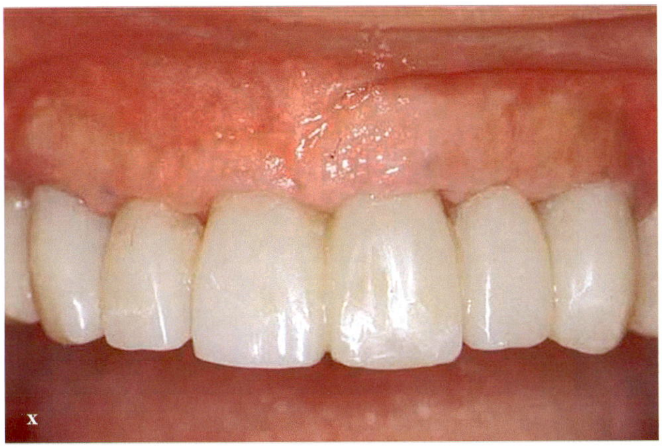

Fig 7-6x Tissue sculpting with provisional restoration.

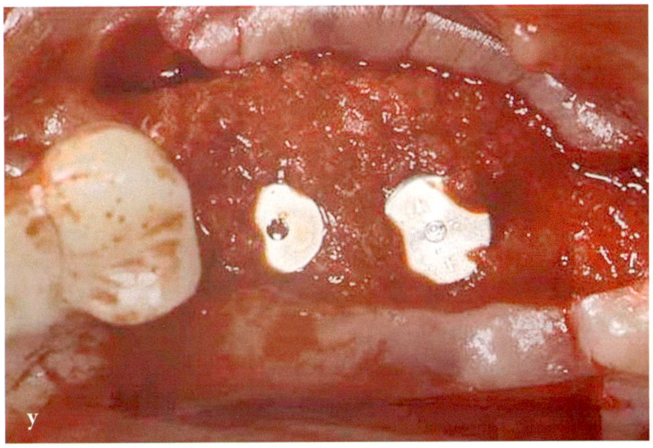

Fig 7-6y Implant placement in the left posterior maxilla, 2 months after extractions.

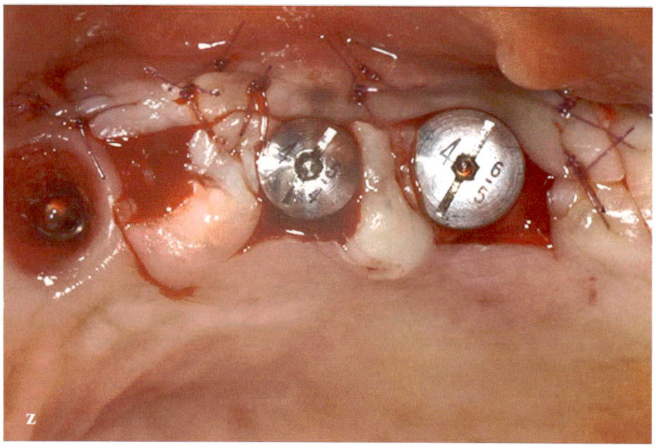

Fig 7-6z Stage-two surgery in the left posterior maxilla, 6 months after implant placement.

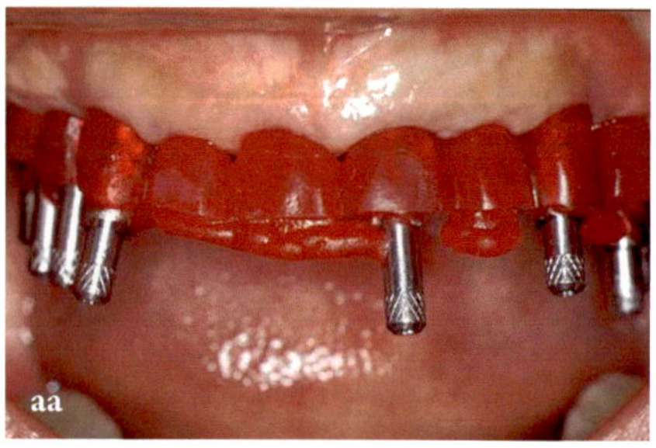

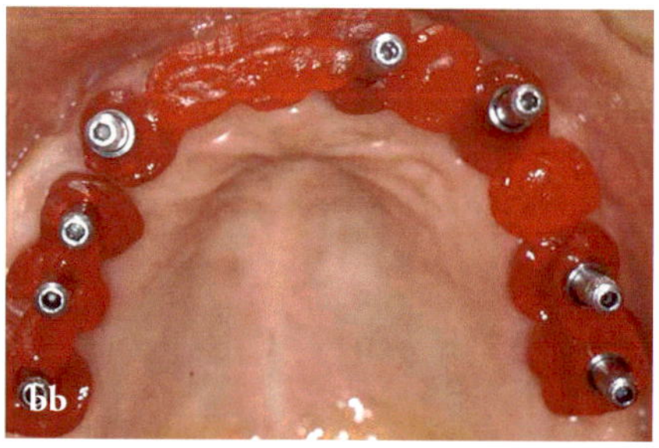

Figs 7-6aa and 7-6bb Final impression with custom impression copings after completion of tissue sculpting.

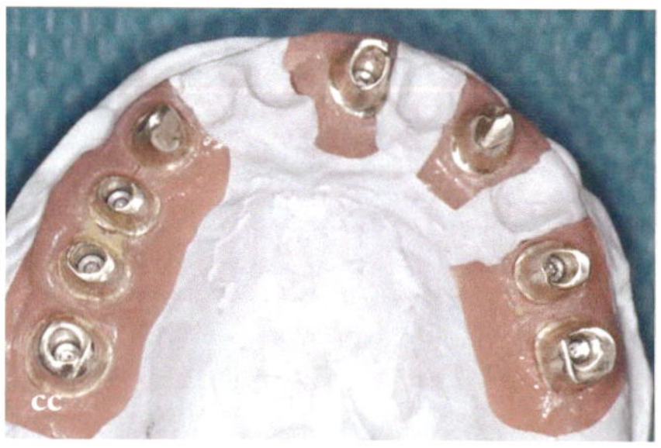

Fig 7-6cc Final gold UCLA abutments.

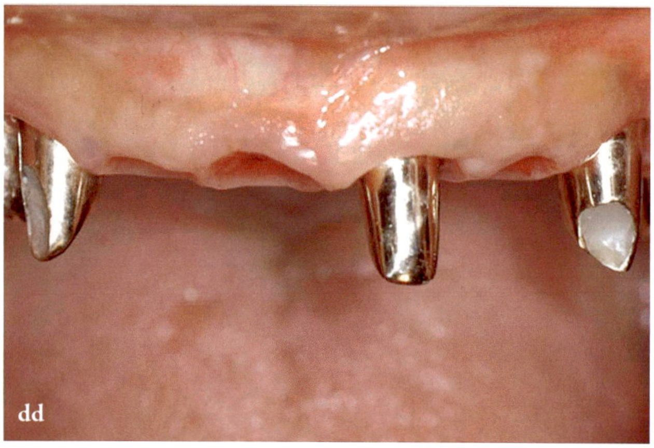

Fig 7-6dd The soft tissue profile was monitored for 6 months with final abutments and a provisional restoration in place.

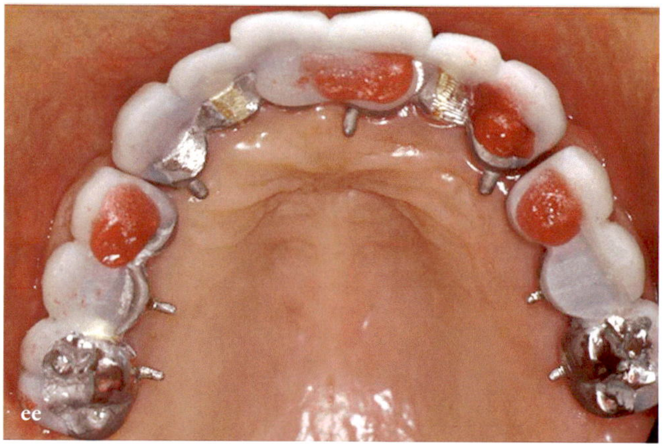

Fig 7-6ee Metal framework try-in.

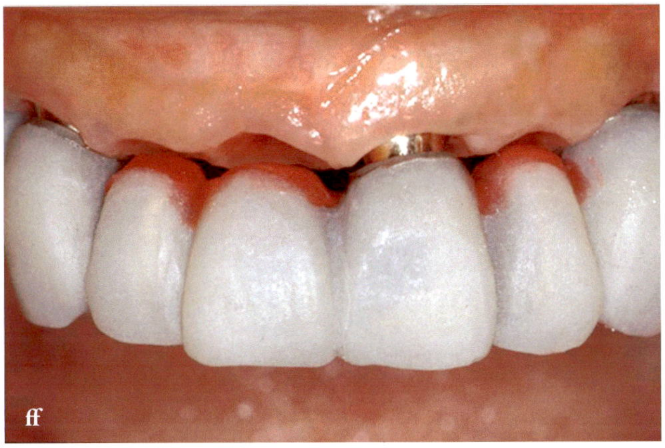

Fig 7-6ff Pressure was applied in pontic sites using resin.

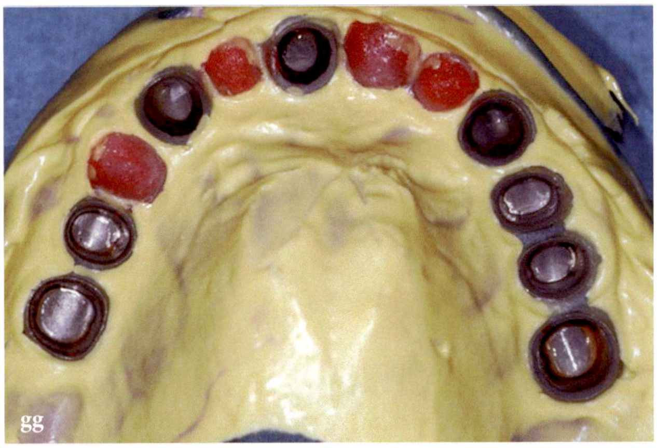

Fig 7-6gg Pick-up impression.

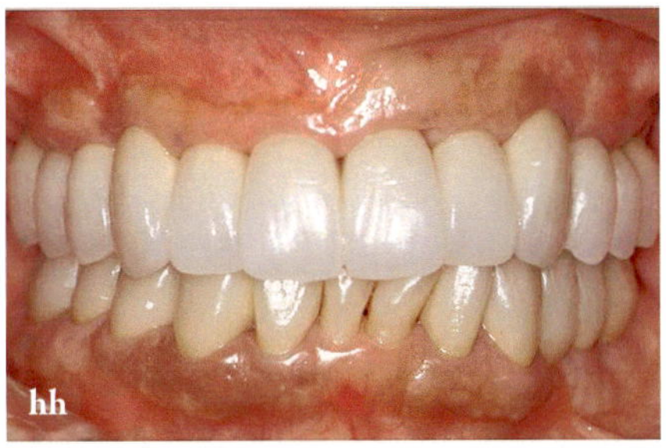

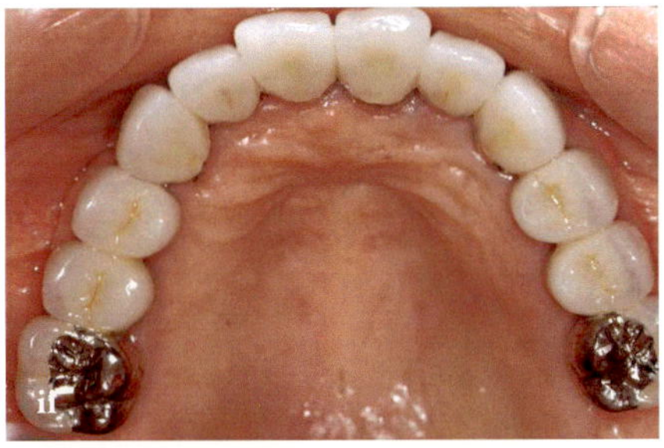

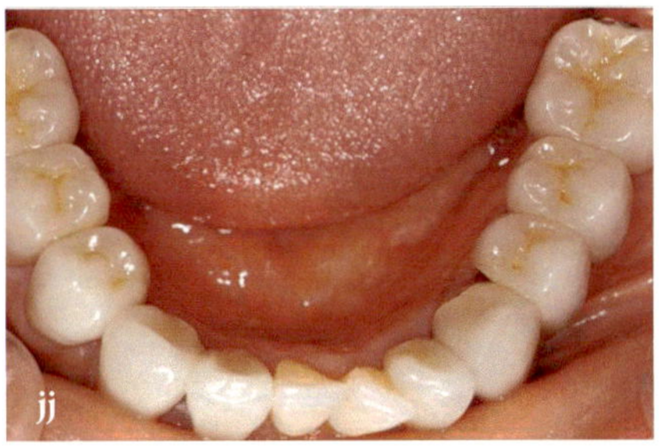

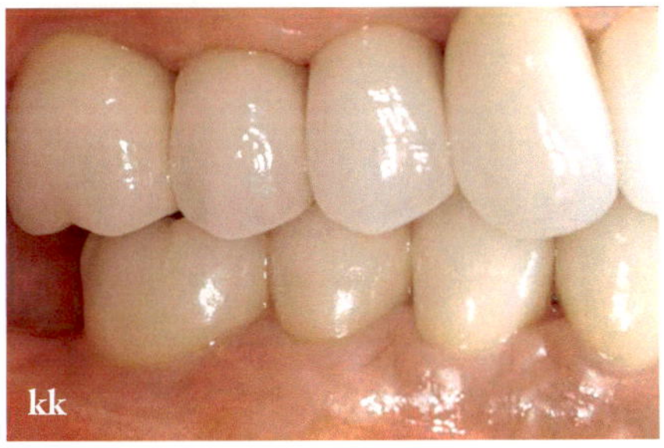

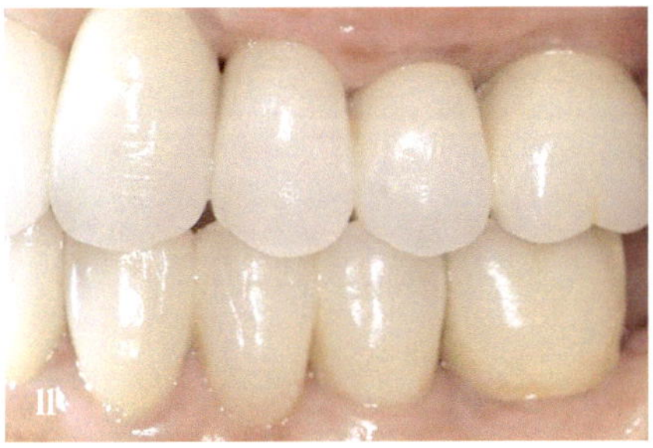

Figs 7-6hh to 7-6ll Definitive restoration.

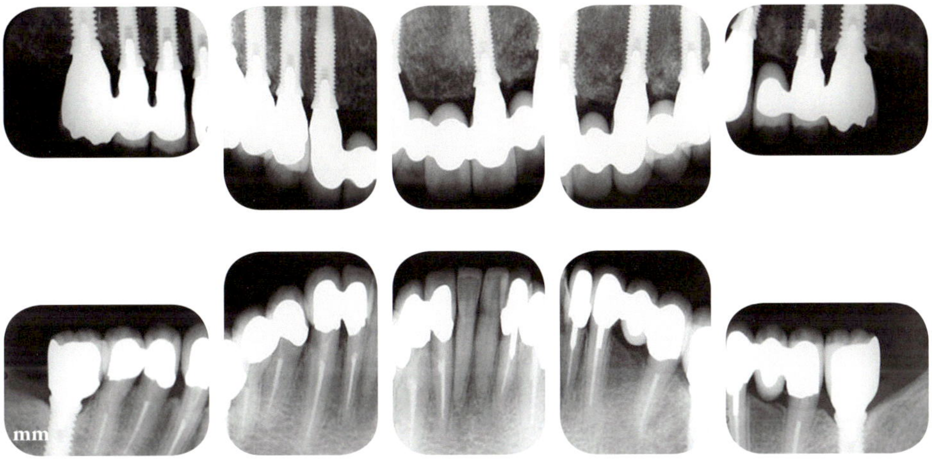

Fig 7-6mm Platform switching was selected for all the implants placed in this case.

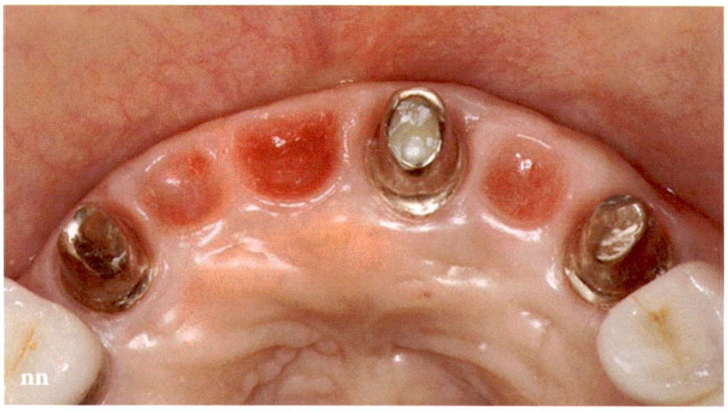

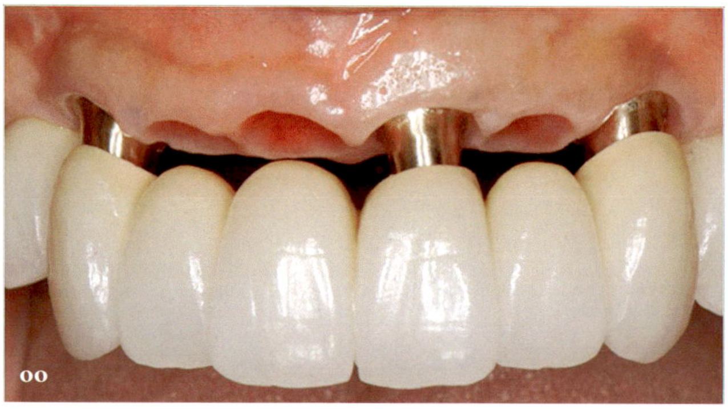

Figs 7-6nn and 7-6oo An esthetic soft tissue framework was constructed through application of the 4D concept.

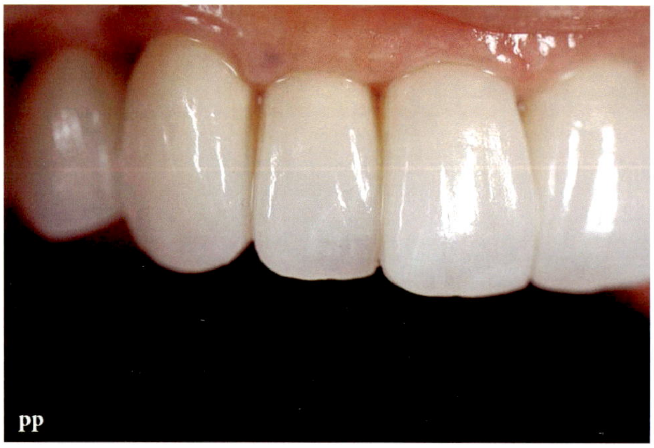

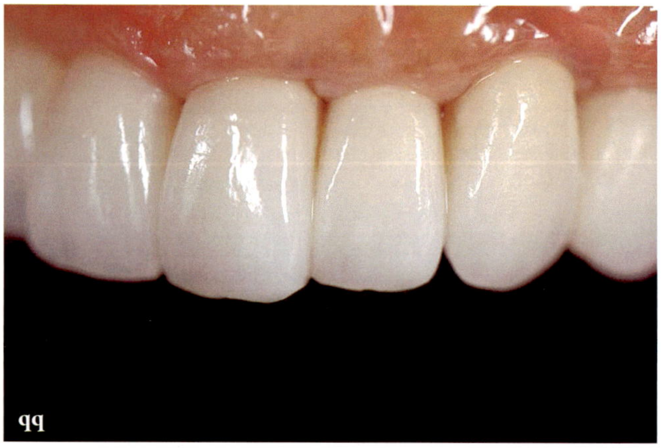

Figs 7-6pp and 7-6qq A sufficient amount of tissue and the use of pontics allowed for an esthetic definitive restoration.

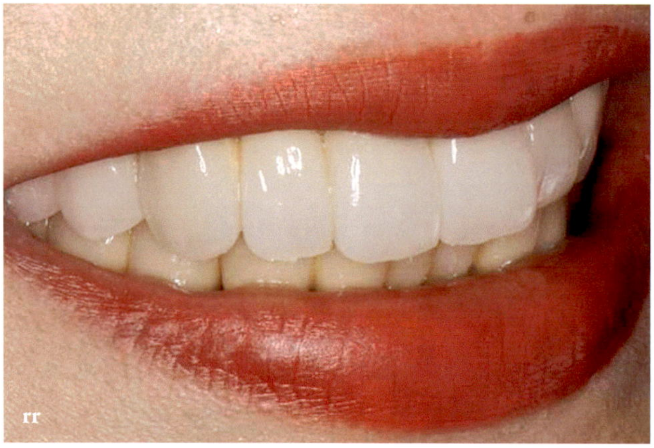

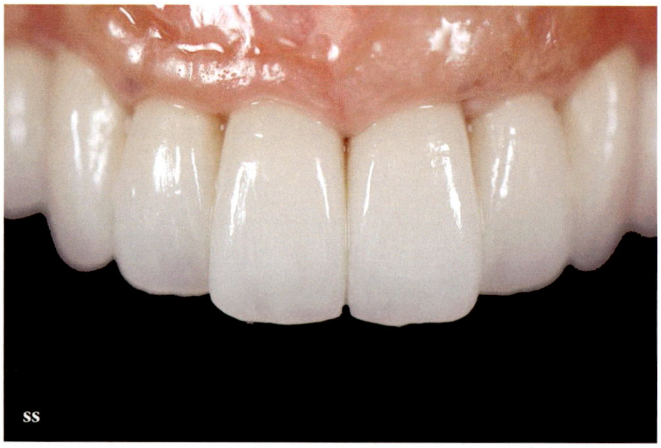

Figs 7-6rr and 7-6ss Smile *(rr)* and facial view *(ss)* with definitive restoration.

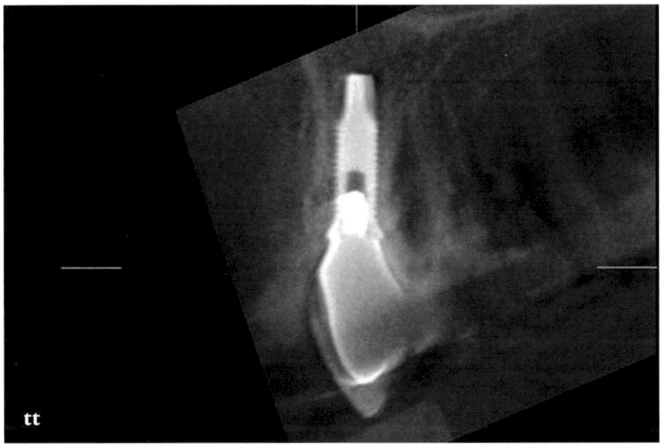

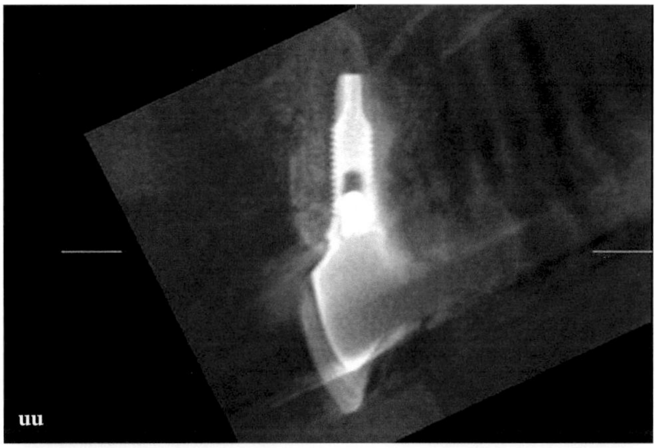

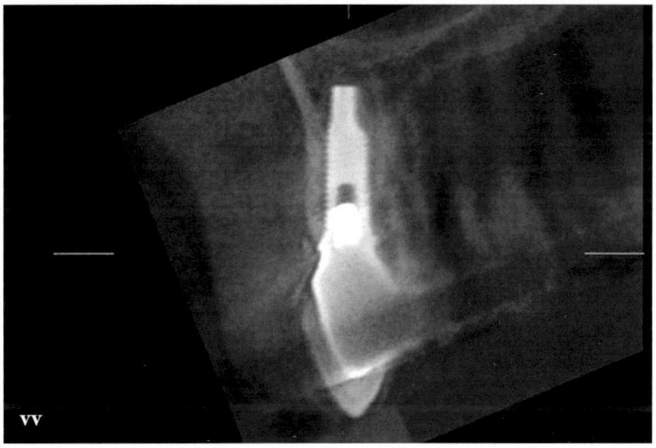

Figs 7-6tt to 7-6vv Two-year CT evaluation of implants at the maxillary right canine *(tt)*, left central incisor *(uu)*, and the left canine *(vv)* sites.

Chapter 8

4D Concept Technique Guide

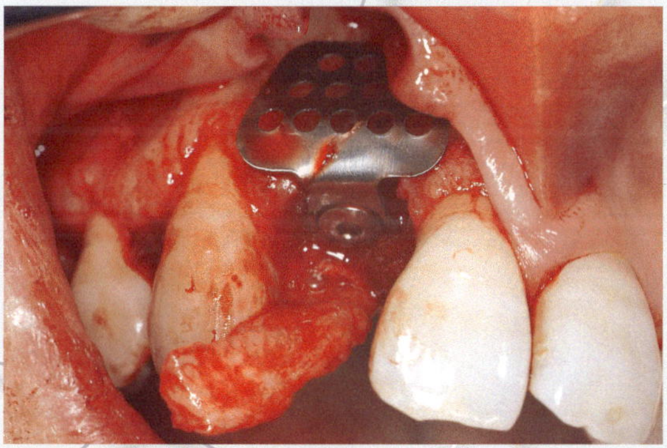

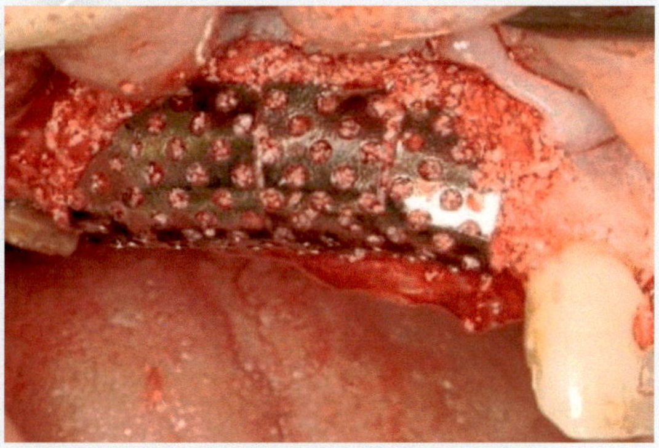

In this chapter, surgical techniques for the four-dimensional (4D) concept, including bone and soft tissue management and soft tissue sculpting with provisional restorations, are demonstrated in two clinical cases supplemented with step-by-step illustrations.

Anterior Single-Tooth Implant Case

The 4D concept applied to an anterior single-tooth implant case is demonstrated in Fig 8-1.

Initial examination

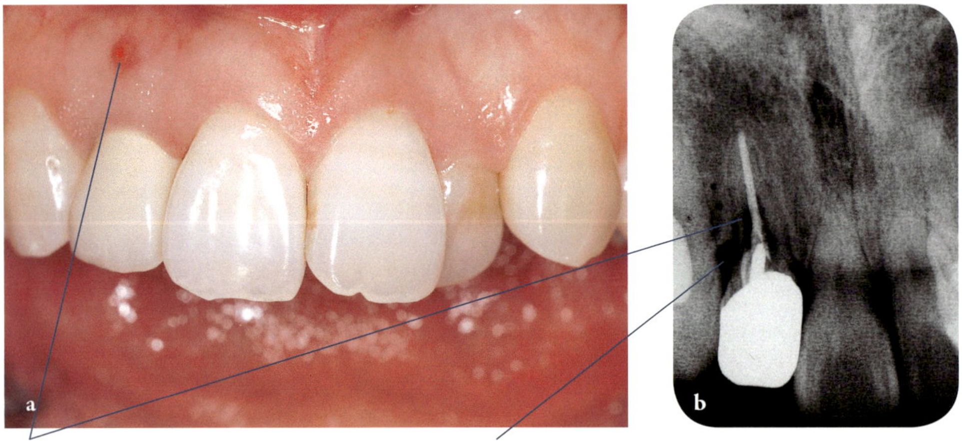

Figs 8-1a and 8-1b *(a)* Facial view and *(b)* periapical radiograph at initial examination.

! Key findings

- Because of the fistula and internal resorption, buccal bone dehiscence was anticipated; therefore, the maxillary right lateral incisor was not a good candidate for orthodontic extrusion, and early implant placement and buccal bone and soft tissue augmentation were necessary.
- The interproximal height of bone (IHB) was Class 1 on the mesial of the right canine and Class 1 or 2 on the distal of the right central incisor (see Fig 2-5).
- An esthetic final result was achievable with ideal implant positioning and buccal tissue augmentation.

Incision and flap design

Figs 8-1c and 8-1d Facial view 2 months after extraction and socket preservation with an ovate pontic *(c)* and after incision and flap elevation *(d)*.

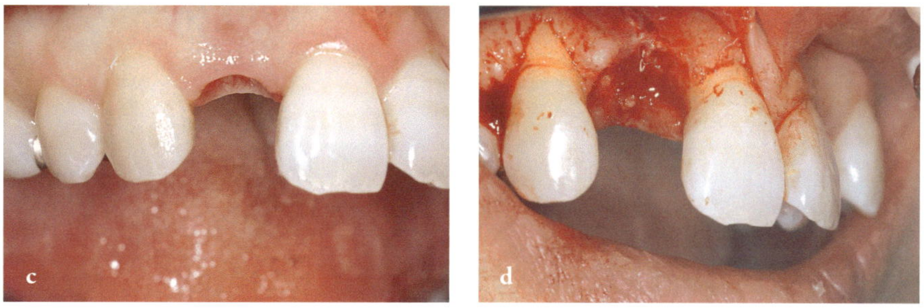

A vertical incision is made distal to the maxillary right canine at a 45-degree angle.

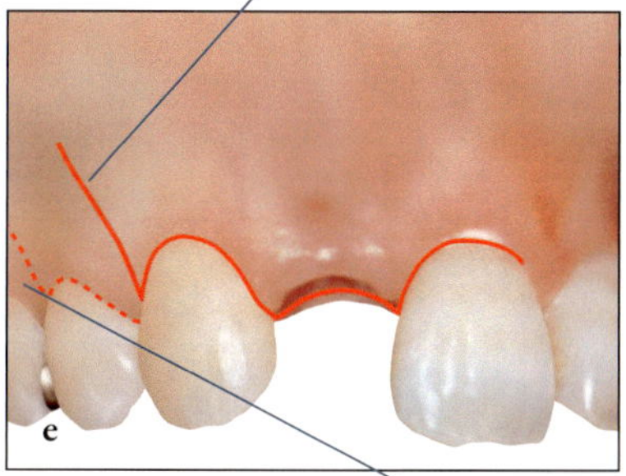

If a large amount of bone augmentation were planned, the incision would be made on the distal of the maxillary right first premolar.

When viewed occlusally, the vertical and horizontal incisions should appear to follow a single line. The horizontal incision connects at the buccal line angle of the adjacent teeth.

Avoid reflecting the papilla between the central incisors. For a large amount of bone augmentation, the flap elevation should be extended.

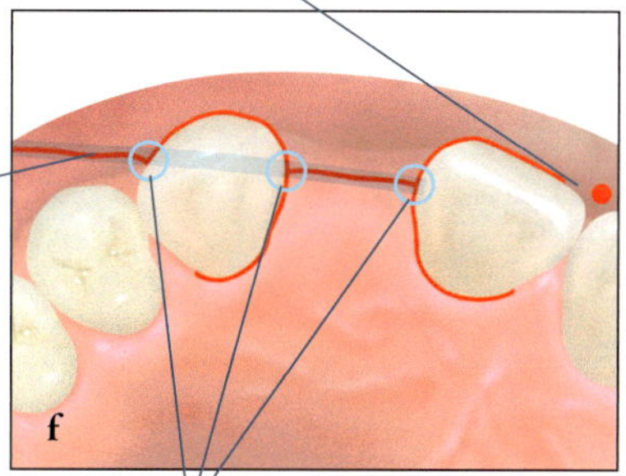

Incisions should be made perpendicular to the tooth. Intrasulcular incisions should only be made on the palatal side.

The vertical incision should extend at least 3 to 5 mm beyond the mucogingival junction (MGJ).

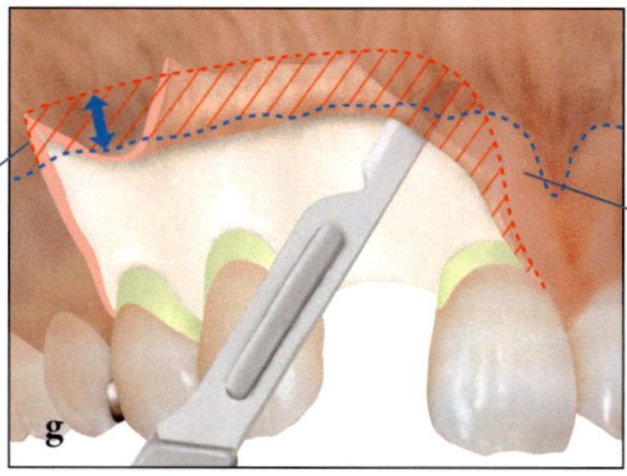

The periosteal releasing incision should be made extending distal to the left central incisor.

Figs 8-1e to 8-1g Step-by-step incision and flap design.

! Key points

- Avoid making a vertical incision in the anterior region to prevent scar formation.
- The vertical incision should be made distal of the canine or, if necessary, the first premolar.
- Make a 45-degree vertical incision to elevate a flap with a wide base.
- Take special care while performing mesial instrumentation to avoid damaging papillae and gingival tissues.

Ideal implant positioning

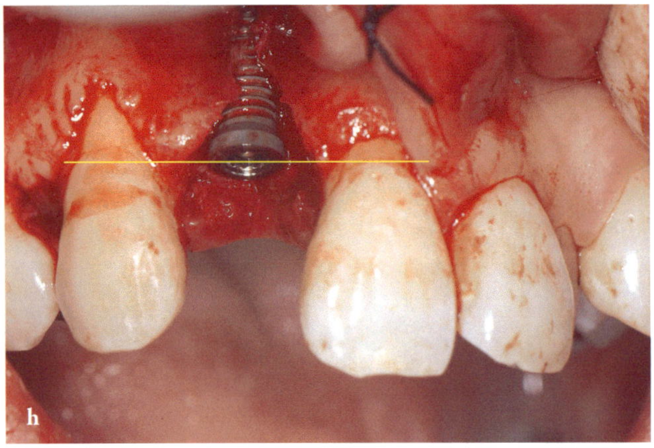

Fig 8-1h The implant platform is positioned 2 to 3 mm apical to a line across the adjacent cementoenamel junctions (yellow line).

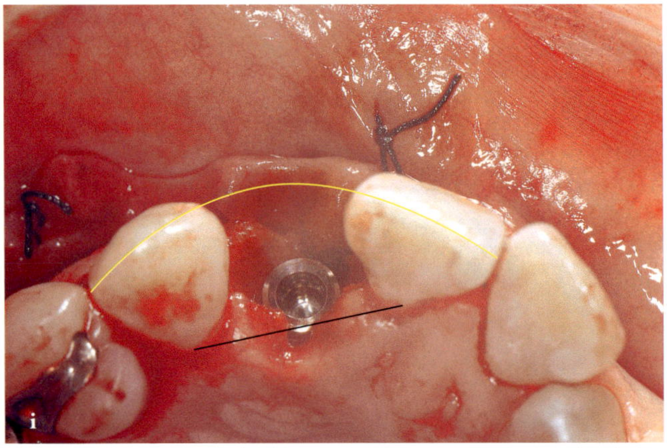

Fig 8-1i The extended long axis of the implant should be slightly lingual to a line across the adjacent incisal edges yellow line), but the implant should not be positioned palatal to a line across the adjacent palatal cervical margin (black line).

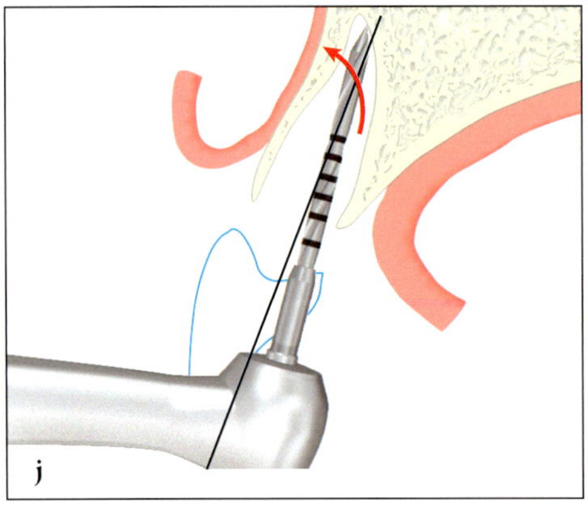

Fig 8-1j Precise drilling in the palatal wall of an extraction socket with a conventional implant twist drill is technically challenging.

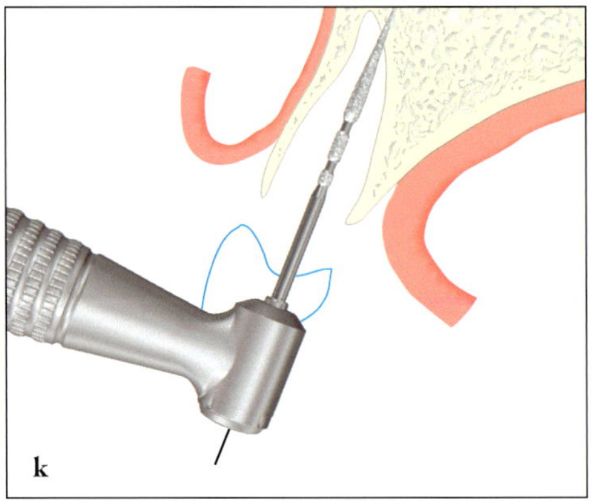

Fig 8-1k A long shank diamond bur allows precise initiation of the drilling sequence in the palatal wall of an extraction socket.

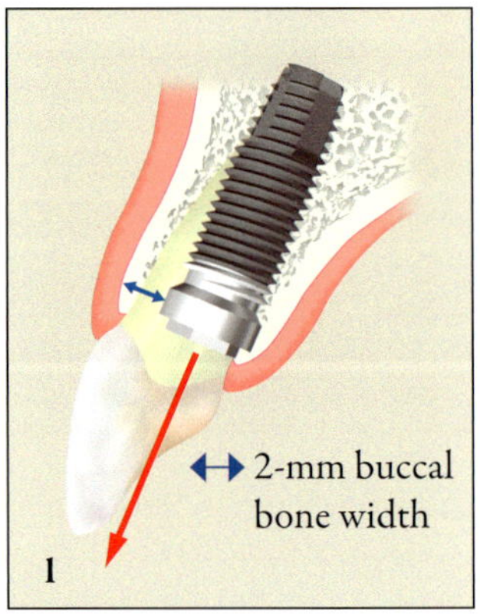

Fig 8-1l Ideal implant position.

! Technical advice

- Precise drilling in the palatal wall of an extraction socket is highly technique sensitive (see Fig 8-1j). Initiation of the drilling sequence using either a round bur to create a deep ledge or a long shank diamond bur (see Fig 8-1k) allows for a more precise implant site osteotomy.
- An ideally placed implant should be positioned 2 to 3 mm apical to the facial margin of the definitive restoration. In addition, the extended long axis of the implant should be slightly lingual to the incisal edge of the definitive restoration (see Fig 8-1l).

Buccal bone augmentation

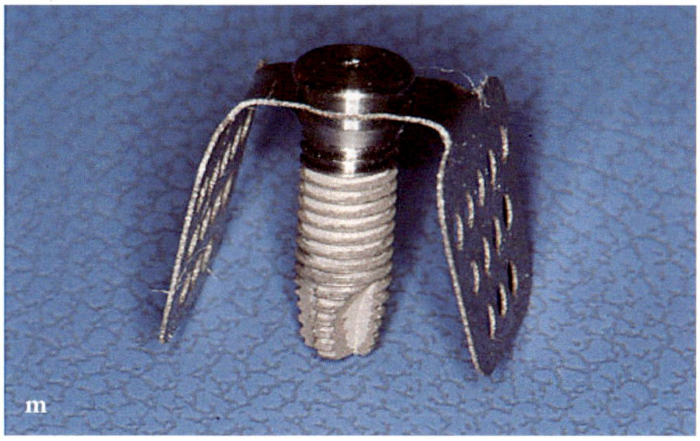

Fig 8-1m FT wing.

> **! Key point**
>
> At least 2 mm of buccal bone outside of the implant body is necessary for an esthetic definitive restoration (see Fig 8-1l). When this is not present, the clinician must select the appropriate armamentarium for predictable augmentation. In this case, an FT wing was used with the patient's consent.

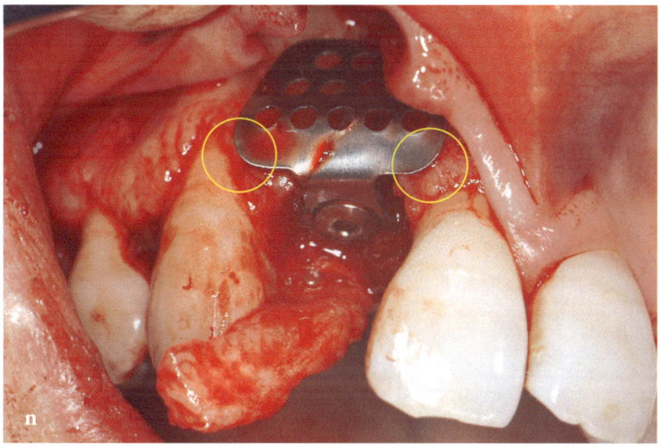

Fig 8-1n The FT wing was stabilized on the implant with a cover screw. The edges of the FT wing were well adapted to the adjacent bone *(yellow circles)*.

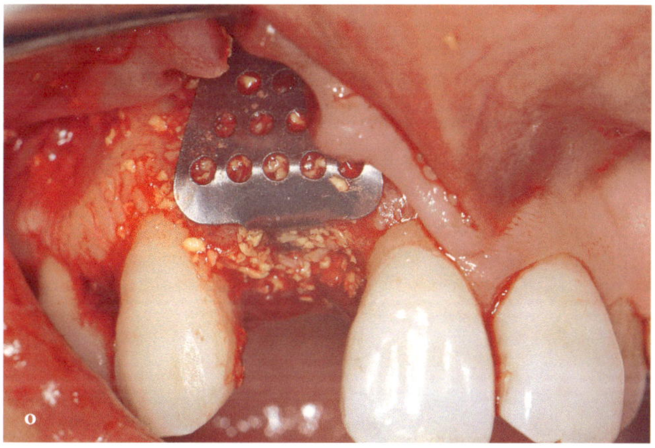

Fig 8-1o Bone graft was used to fill in the space between the FT wing and the implant.

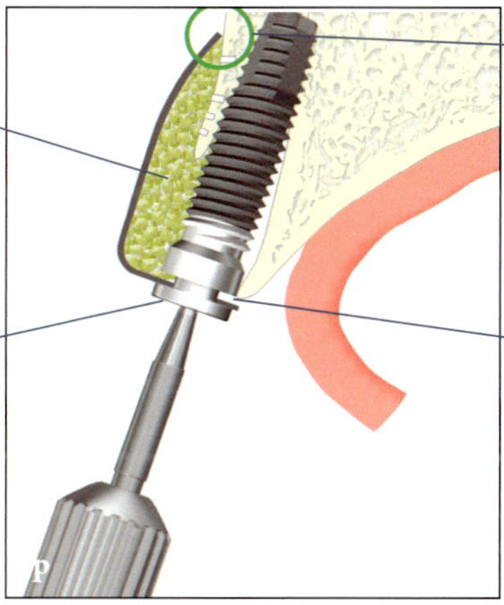

Fig 8-1p Placement of FT wing.

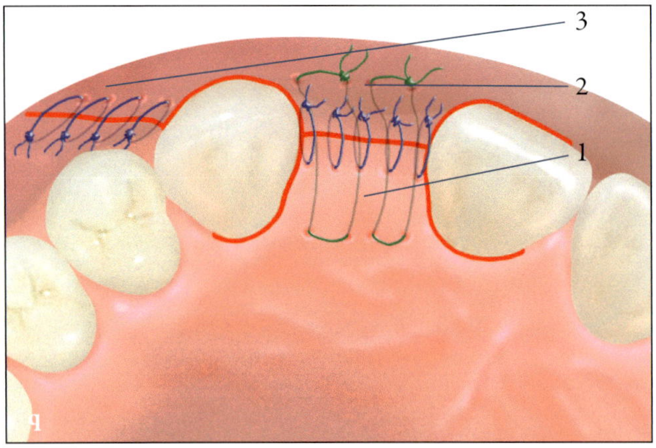

Fig 8-1q The usual sequence of suturing is *(1)* horizontal mattress suture, *(2)* simple interrupted suture, and *(3)* simple interrupted suture for a vertical incision.

! Technical advice

- The FT wing can be cut, bent, and stabilized on the implant with a cover screw (see Fig 8-1m).
- The edges of the FT wing should be well adapted to the adjacent bone (see Fig 8-1n).
- The area between the FT wing and the implant must be completely filled with bone graft.
- In this case, a cross-linked collagen membrane was placed over the FT wing, and only xenograft was placed.

Buccal soft tissue augmentation: Pedicle connective tissue graft

A pedicle connective tissue graft can be performed in a single-tooth implant case in conjunction with immediate implant placement or implant placement with guided bone regeneration (GBR).

! Key point

A coronally shifted MGJ and decreased soft tissue thickness can occur as complications of GBR. As a corrective measure, connective tissue grafting is often performed with stage-two surgery in the esthetic zone. A pedicle connective tissue graft technique can be performed with immediate implant placement to close the extraction socket and to augment thin buccal soft tissue at the same time.

! Technical advice

- Make an initial incision about 2 mm from the free gingival margin, extending from mesial of the first molar to mesial of the recipient site.
- Use sharp dissection 5 to 7 mm internally to create a partial thickness palatal flap toward the mesial of the recipient site.
- Pass the pedicle from the palatal to the buccal under the palatal tissue of the recipient site.

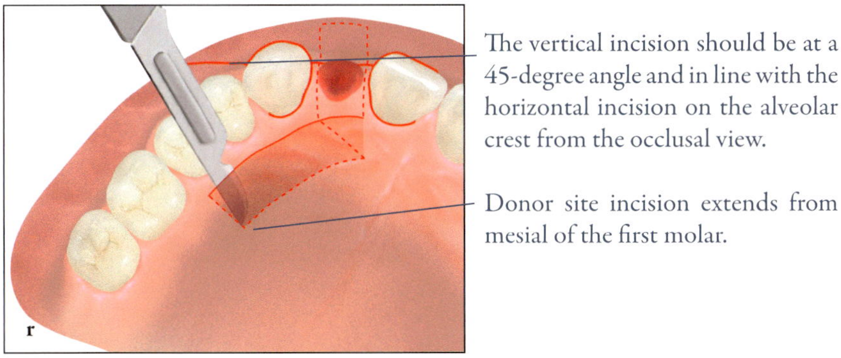

Fig 8-1r Occlusal view of incisions for a pedicle connective tissue graft.

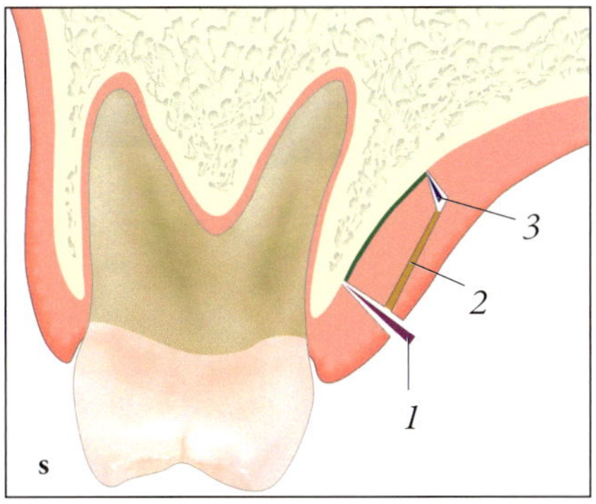

Fig 8-1s Incision sequence. *(1)* 2 to 3 mm from the free gingival margin, a perpendicular incision extending from mesial of the first molar to distal of the recipient site. *(2)* 5- to 7-mm sharp dissection toward the mesial of the recipient site. *(3)* Internal incision through connective tissue and periosteum.

! Technical advice

- The authors use JO1, JO3, and CTG-O instruments for pedicle connective tissue harvesting.
- The most distal portion of the graft should be positioned in the buccal area of the recipient site.
- The pedicle graft should extend at least 5 mm beyond the inside of the buccal flap margin for graft survival.
- The palatal aspect of the recipient site tends to become thick. This area serves as a donor site for a connective tissue graft if additional soft tissue augmentation is necessary.

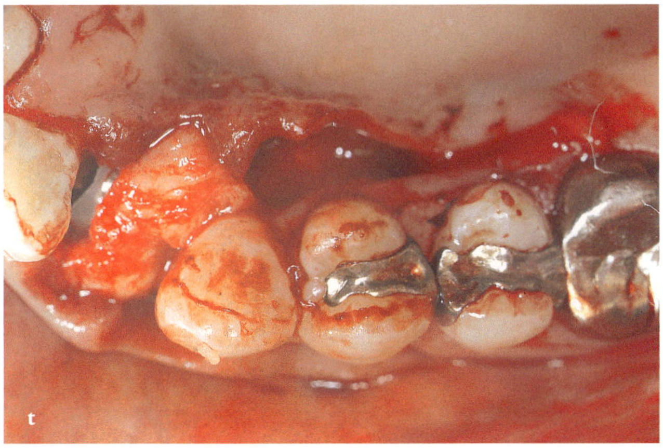

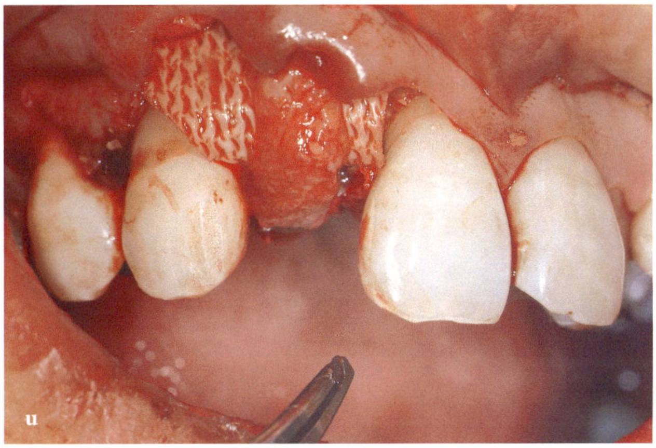

Figs 8-1t and 8-1u Pedicle connective tissue graft was harvested for buccal augmentation. Care was taken to make sure it extended at least 5 mm beyond the inside of the buccal flap.

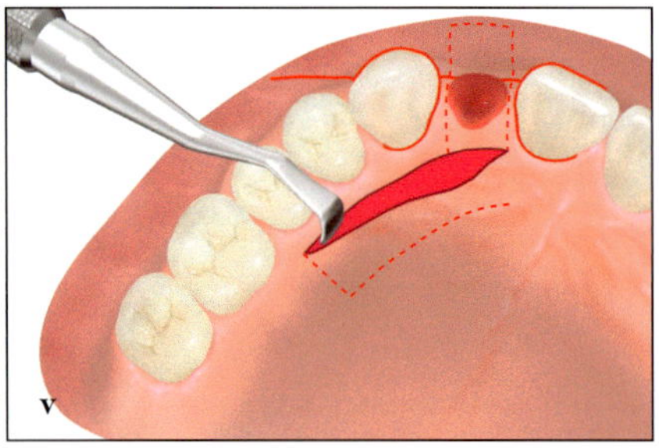

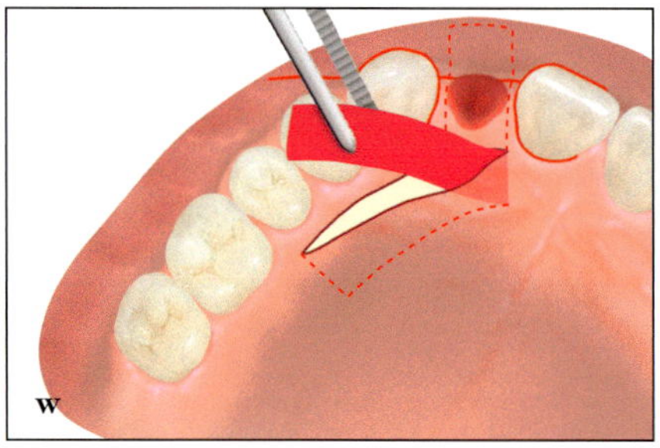

Figs 8-1v and 8-1w Pedicle connective tissue graft is reflected with periosteum using JO1 and JO3 instruments.

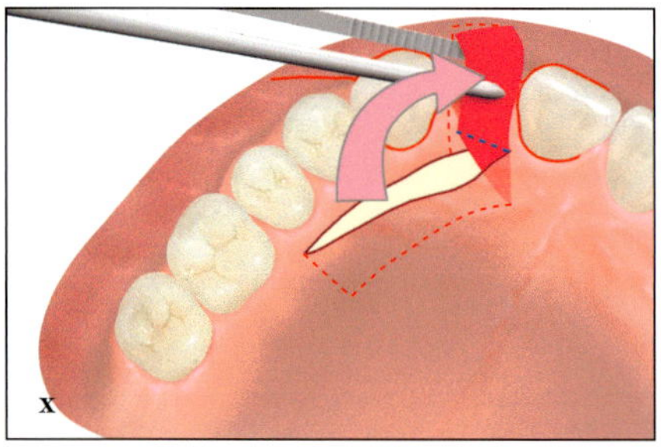

Fig 8-1x The pedicle connective tissue graft is folded and moved to the buccal donor site.

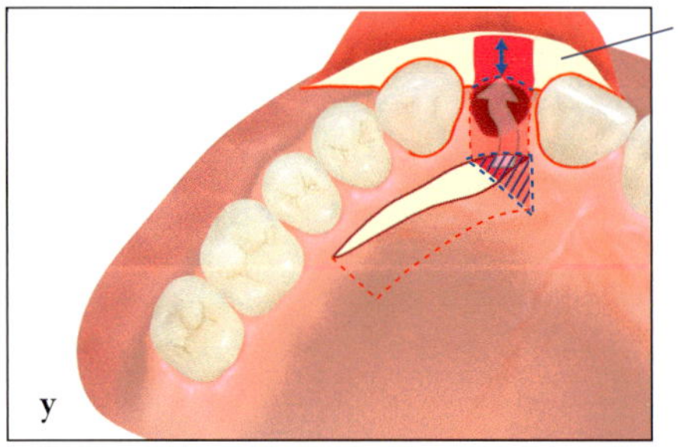

Fig 8-1y The pedicle connective tissue graft passes under the palatal tissue of the recipient site to the buccal aspect.

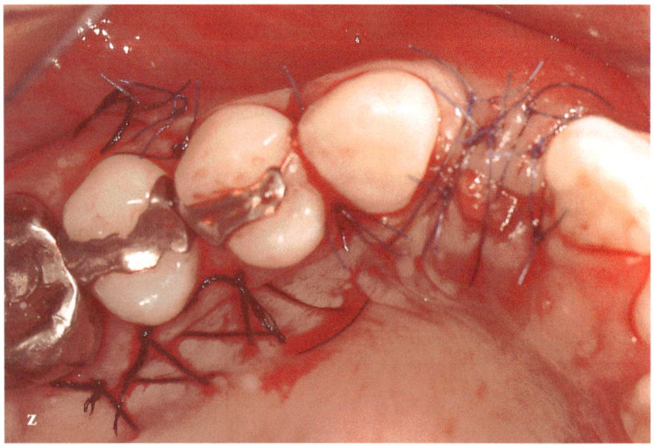

Fig 8-1z Modified mattress suture at the palatal donor site and simple interrupted suture at the recipient site.

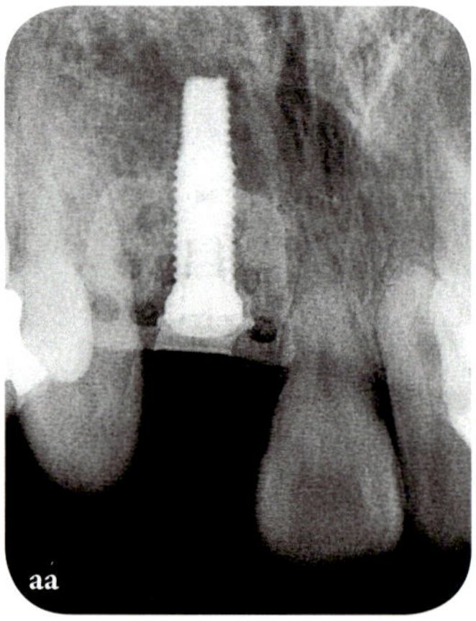

Fig 8-1aa Periapical radiograph immediately after implant placement.

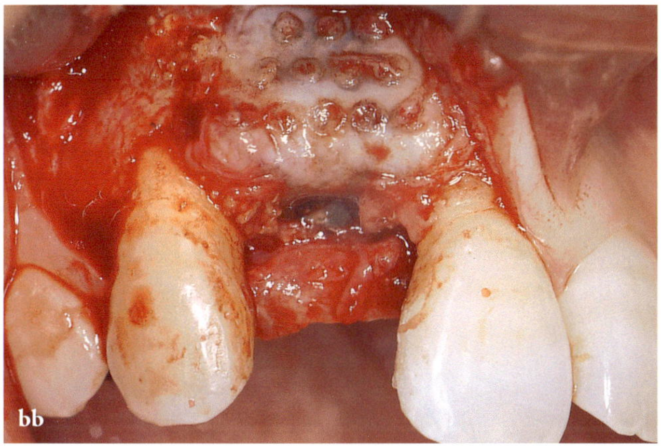

Fig 8-1bb Six months after implant placement with GBR and connective tissue grafting, the FT wing was removed. Sufficient bone regeneration was confirmed.

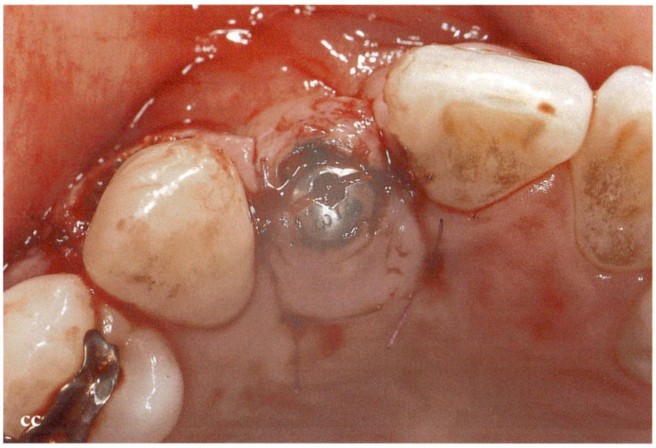

Fig 8-1cc After stage-two surgery.

Tissue sculpting

After sufficient soft tissue preservation and augmentation are performed, the esthetic soft tissue profile for the definitive restoration can be carefully sculpted using the transgingival morphology of the provisional restoration.

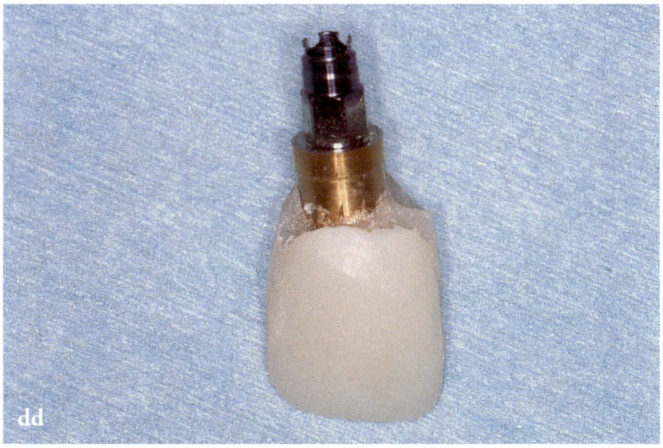

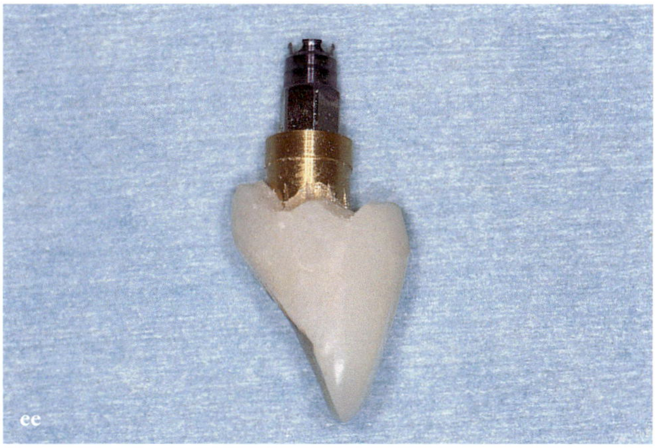

Figs 8-1dd and 8-1ee A prefabricated resin shell and temporary cylinder were cold cured in the patient's mouth. The implant was placed in a Class 1 position (see Figs 8-1l and 2-9).

! Key point

Tissue sculpting should begin 2 months after stage-two surgery or after a tissue punch technique following connective tissue grafting. This will create a smooth transition from the round implant platform to the natural root as well as a scalloped cervical anatomy. This process usually can be completed in three to four steps over the course of 2 months.

! Technical advice

After the steps described in Figs 8-1dd and 8-1ee, resin material is added to the provisional restoration to create a straight subgingival anatomy. If excessive pressure on the gingiva is observed at try-in, the subgingival anatomy of the provisional restoration should be adjusted to relieve the pressure.

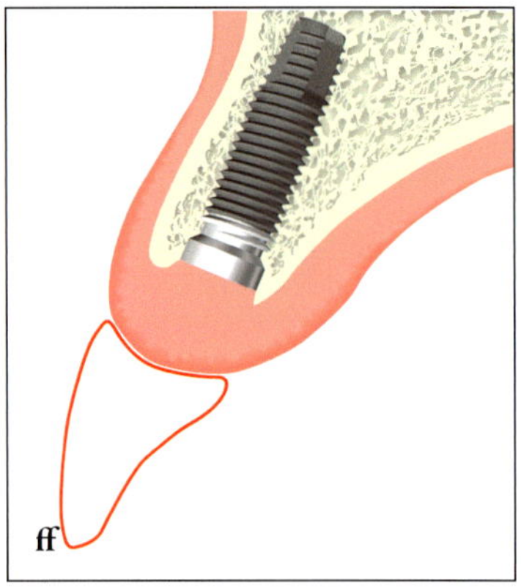

Fig 8-1ff Prefabricated resin shell of provisional restoration.

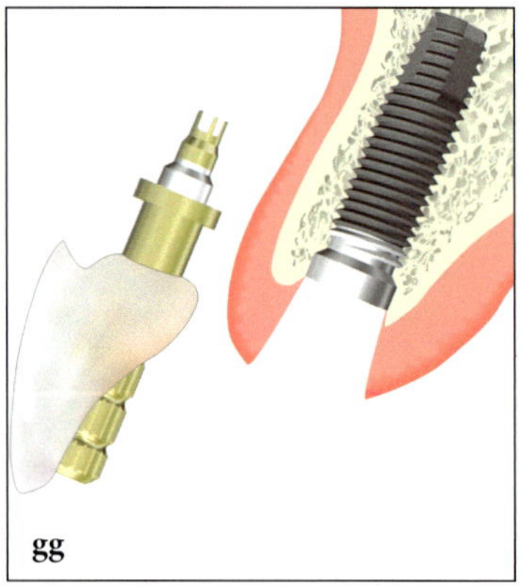

Fig 8-1gg Resin is added to create a straight profile.

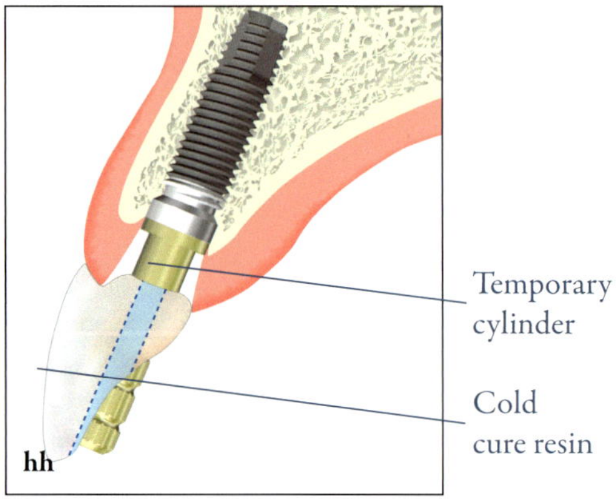

Fig 8-1hh At stage-two surgery or tissue punch, place a temporary cylinder on the implant, and then cold cure the prefabricated resin shell to the temporary cylinder.

! Technical advice

- During the first round of tissue sculpting, blanching of the peri-implant tissue due to pressure from the provisional restoration should disappear within 5 minutes.
- The access hole is located in the palatal aspect of the provisional restoration when the implant is placed in an ideal position (Class 1; see Figs 8-1l and 2-9).
- Continuing the tissue sculpting process by adding resin to increase the subgingival contour of the provisional restoration will modify the peri-implant soft tissue profile.
- The buccal subgingival contour of the provisional restoration should be reduced when buccal peri-implant bone and soft tissue volume is insufficient.

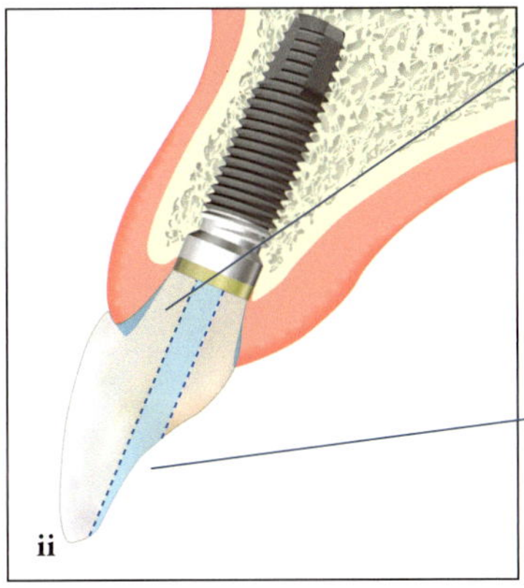

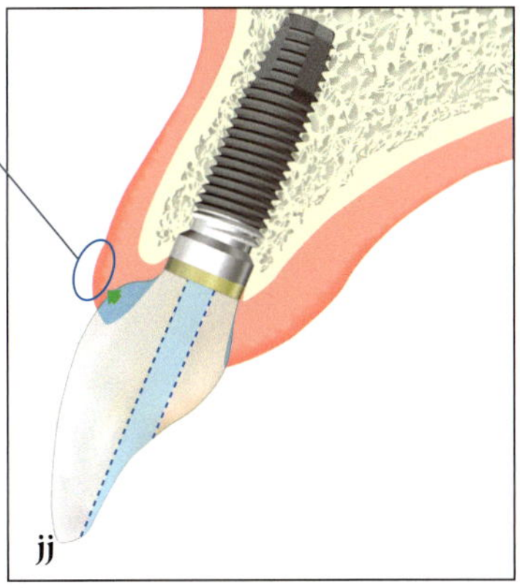

Figs 8-1ii and 8-1jj Contour and position of the provisional restoration.

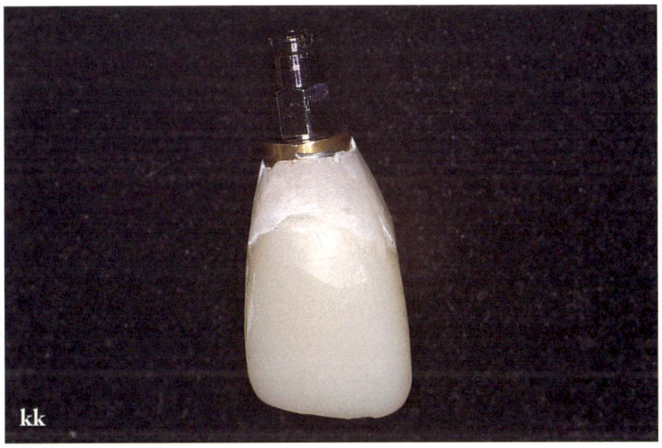

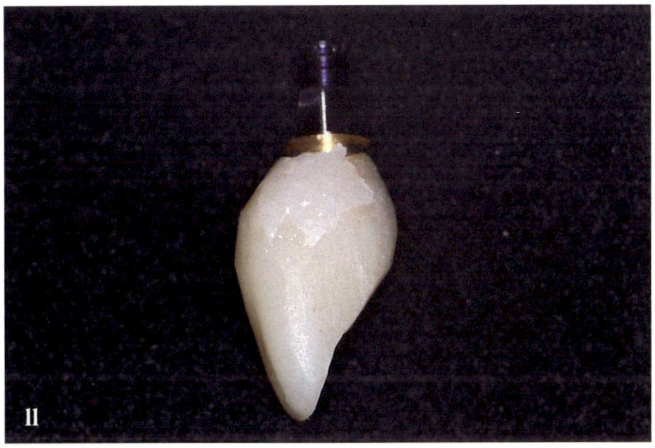

Figs 8-1kk and 8-1ll Modified provisional restoration for tissue sculpting.

! Technical advice

When buccal bone and soft tissue volume is sufficient, additional incremental tissue sculpting can be performed to establish an esthetic peri-implant tissue profile.

Custom impression coping

! Technical advice

Duplicate the transgingival morphology of the provisional restoration in a custom impression coping.

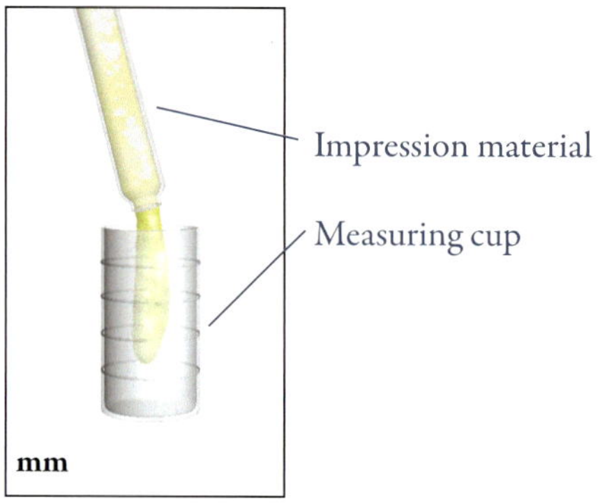

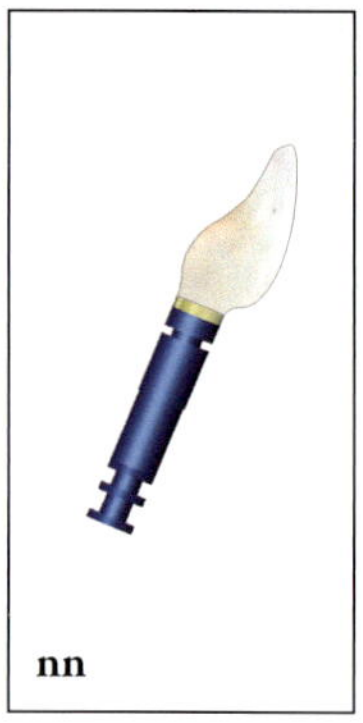

Fig 8-1mm Place impression material in a measuring cup.
Fig 8-1nn Connect the appropriately modified provisional restoration to an implant lab analog.

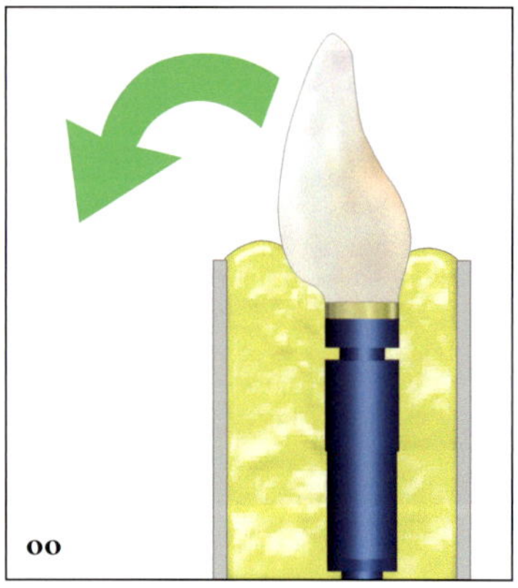

Fig 8-1oo Place the provisional restoration–analog assembly in the impression material to register the transgingival morphology of provisional restoration. When the impression material is set, reconnect the provisional restoration to the implant in the patient's mouth.

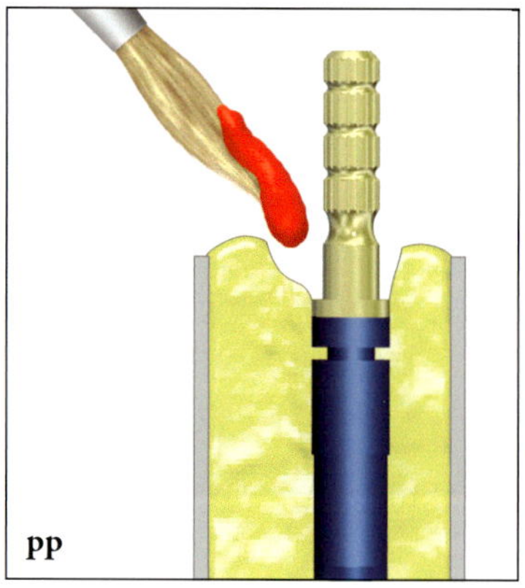

Fig 8-1pp Connect a temporary cylinder to the implant lab analog, then add resin to fill in the area sculpted by the provisional restoration.

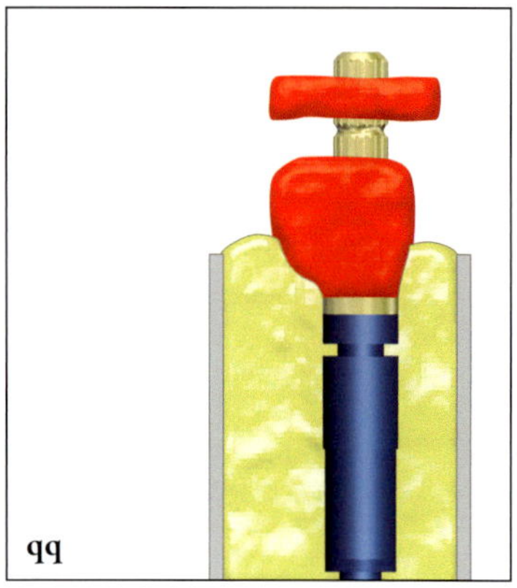

Fig 8-1qq Completed custom impression coping.

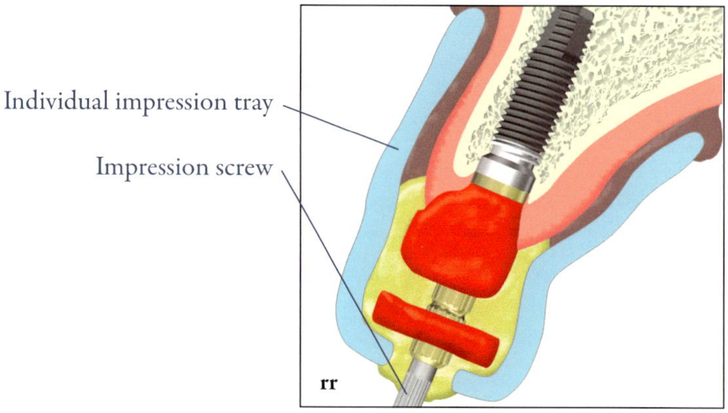

Fig 8-1rr Final impression with custom impression coping.

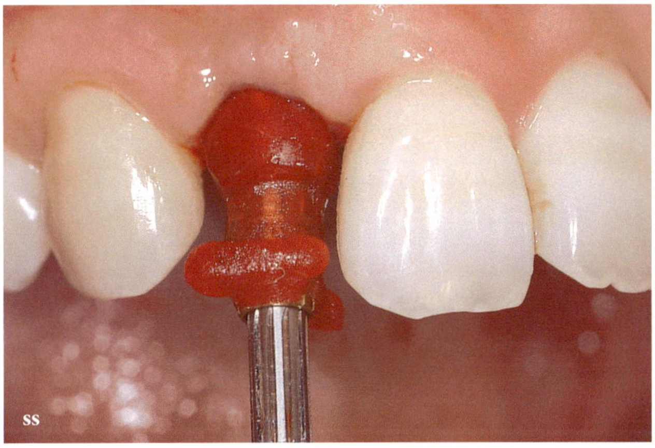

Fig 8-1ss Final impression with custom impression coping.

Final custom abutment

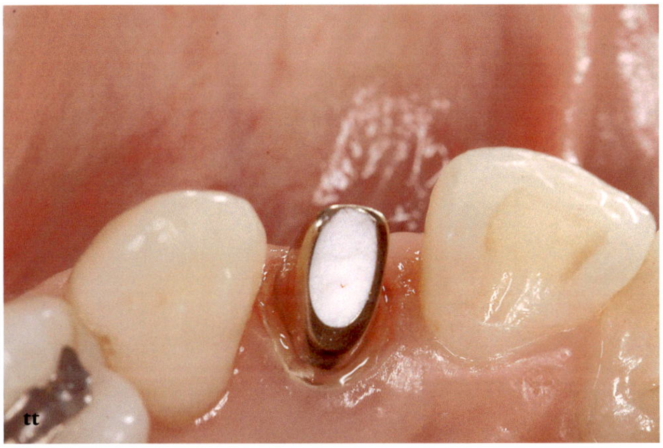

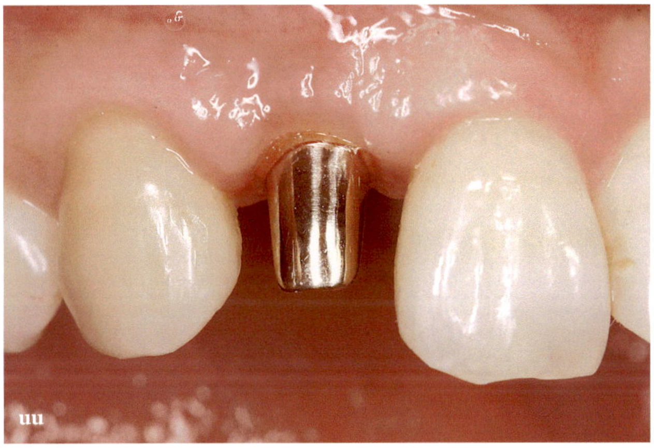

Figs 8-1tt and 8-1uu Final custom abutment in place.

Definitive restoration

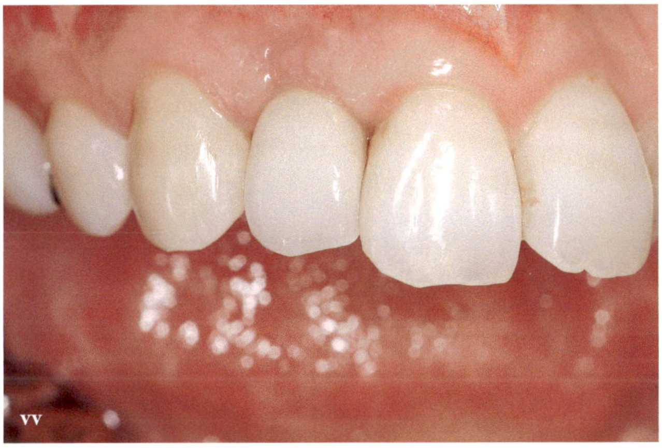

Fig 8-1vv Facial view of definitive restoration.

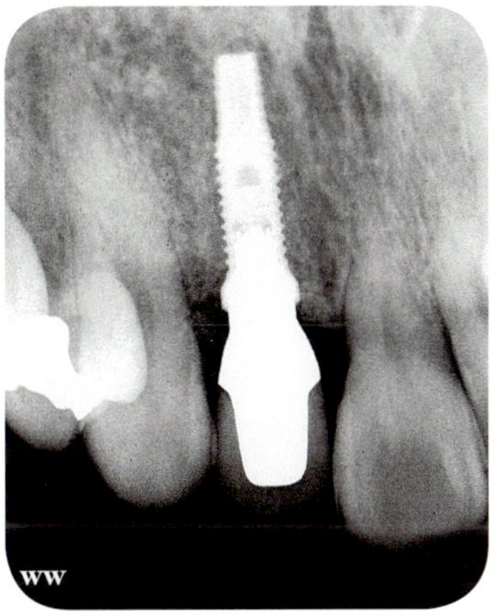

Fig 8-1ww Periapical radiograph of definitive restoration. Platform switching was used.

Multiple-Tooth Implant Case

The 4D concept applied to a multiple-tooth implant case is demonstrated in Fig 8-2.

> **! Key point**
>
> It is critical to visualize the augmentation goal using a surgical stent before and during augmentation surgery.

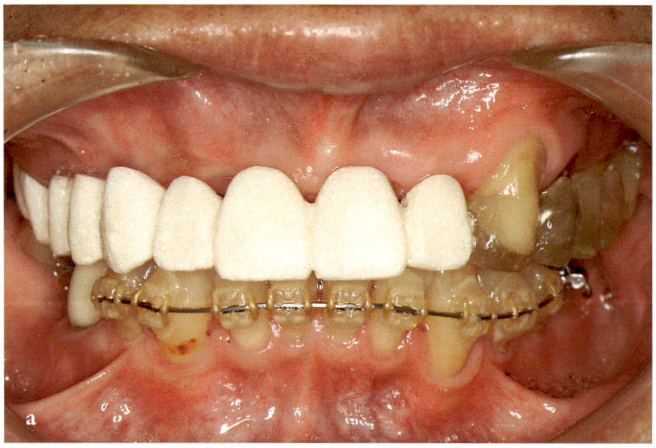

Fig 8-2a Treatment of this multiple-tooth implant case requires three-dimensional (3D) GBR.

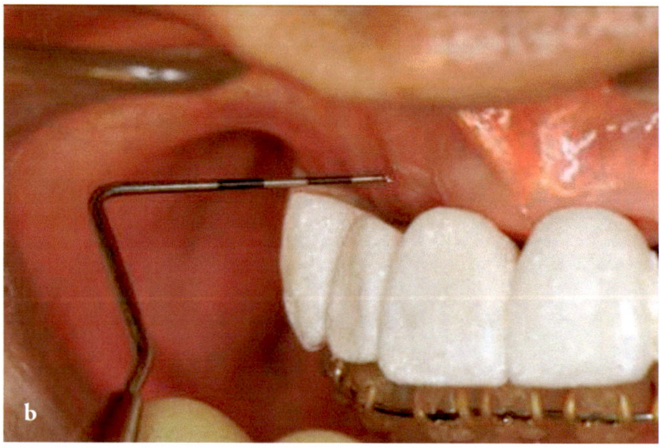

Fig 8-2b Horizontal ridge augmentation of 6 mm or more is anticipated.

Incision and flap elevation

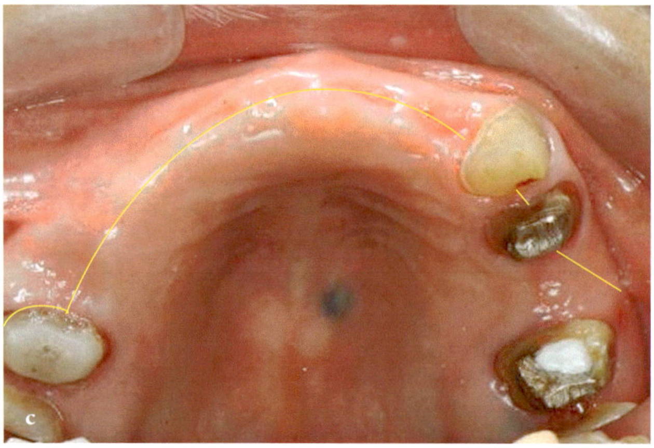

Fig 8-2c A horizontal incision should be made within the keratinized tissue over the alveolar crest. This incision should be made more facial when a large amount of vertical augmentation is anticipated. The vertical incision should be made at least one tooth distal to the targeted augmentation site and 3 mm or more beyond the MGJ. Incisions must cut through the periosteum to avoid damaging the periosteum while elevating the flap. Flap elevation should be carefully initiated with a chisel near the adjacent teeth.

Periosteal releasing incision

! Key points

- Use a new blade.
- Deepen the releasing incision to increase flap mobility.
- Maintain at least 5 mm or more distance from vital landmarks, such as the mental and infraorbital foramina.
- Take care not to damage the blood vessels while deepening the incision.

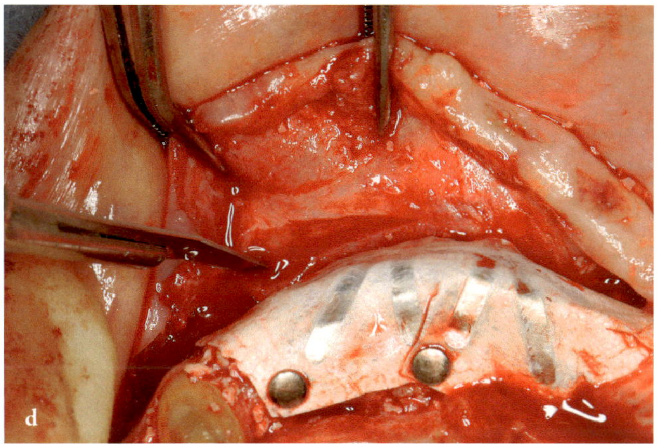

Fig 8-2d Make a periosteal releasing incision at the base of the flap (at least 5 mm from the MGJ) when flap elevation is completed. Aspirate blood from the incision area to mix with bone graft materials. Augmentation volume can be estimated at this point. Bleeding will lessen by the time of suturing.

Evaluation of augmentation volume

! Technical advice

The augmentation site should be thoroughly debrided with a chisel and a rotary instrument. Irrigation will increase visibility of the surgical area.

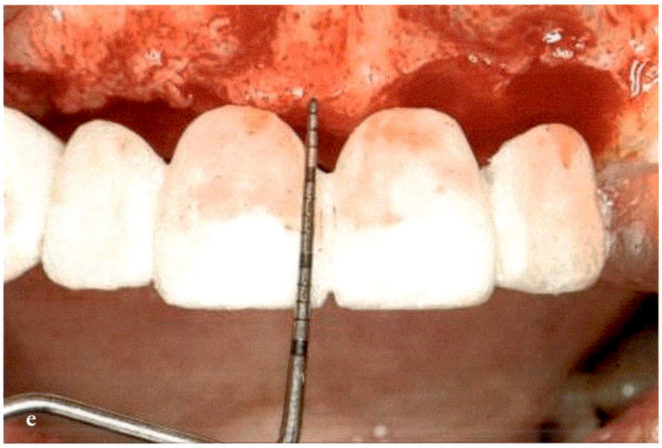

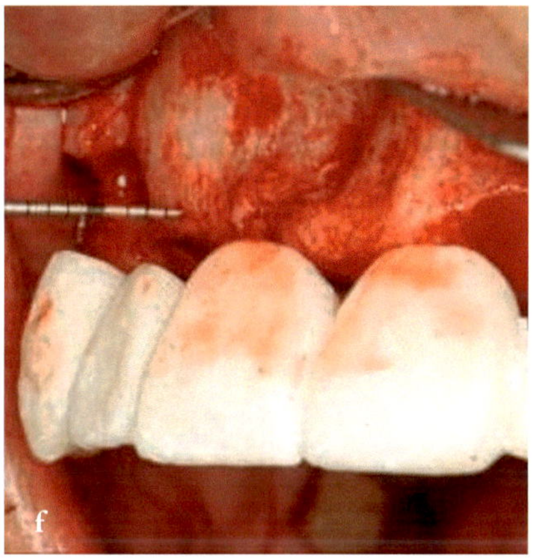

Figs 8-2e and 8-2f Use a surgical stent to determine the necessary amount of augmentation to create an esthetic definitive restoration. The ridge will need to be augmented vertically to 2 to 3 mm from the definitive restoration's contact point and horizontally to the buccal margin of the definitive restoration.

Temporary healing abutment and tenting screws

Vertical space can be maintained with a temporary healing abutment 2 to 3 mm in height (see Figs 8-2g and 8-2h) or with an FT abutment on the implant with simultaneous implant placement and GBR.

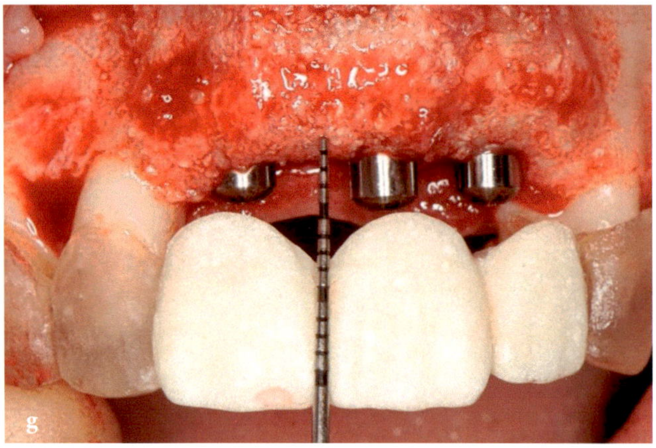

Fig 8-2g A temporary healing abutment, 2 to 3 mm in height, was placed on the implants to support vertical augmentation space.

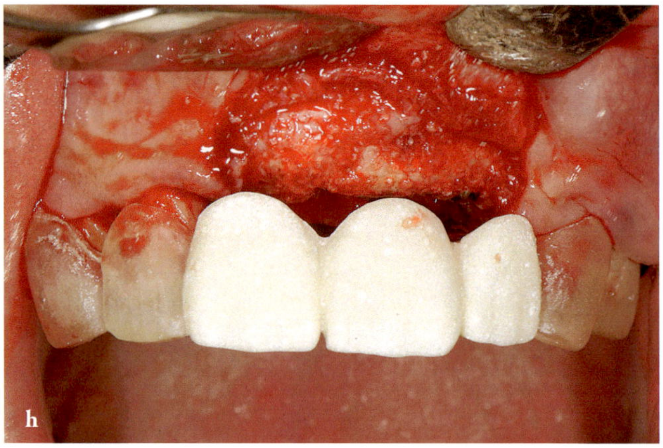

Fig 8-2h Bone was regenerated around the temporary healing abutment.

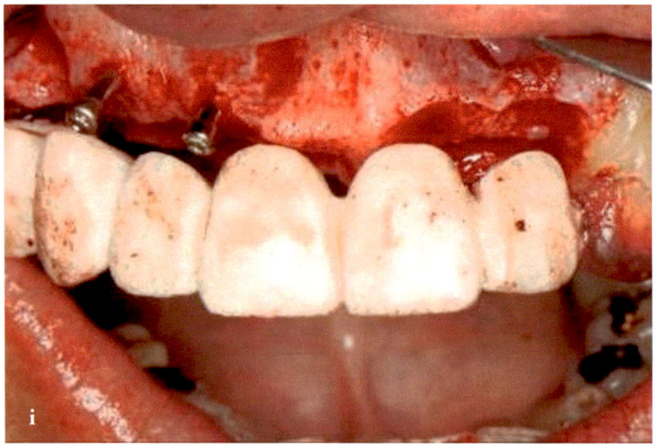

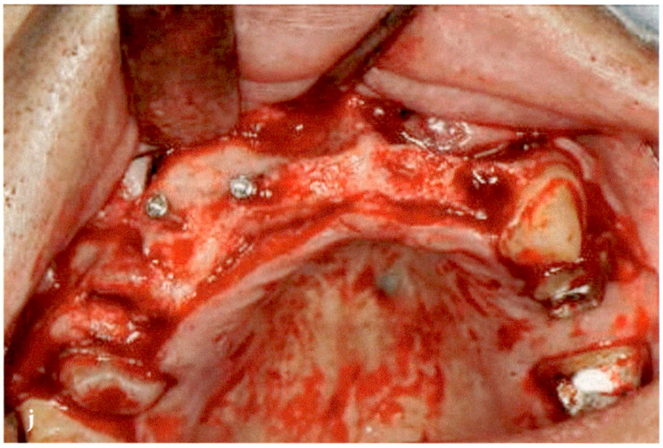

Figs 8-2i and 8-2j Tenting screws were placed to support the augmentation space with a staged approach.

Titanium-reinforced membrane

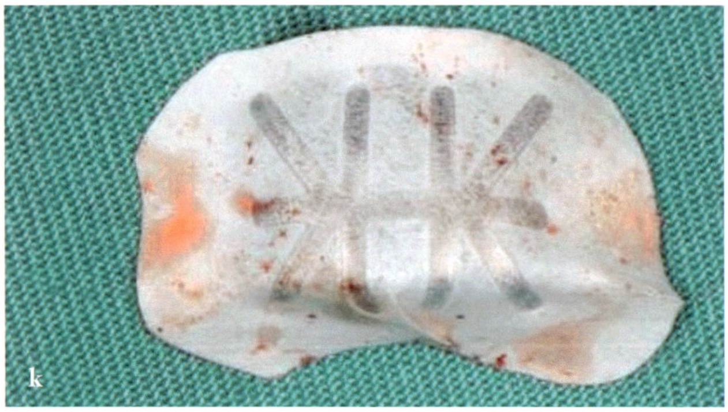

Fig 8-2k The titanium-reinforced membrane can be given a 3D form by bending the titanium frame. Keep in mind that the membrane should be at least 2 mm away from adjacent teeth, and its margin must be well adapted to the alveolar ridge.

! Key points

- Creating a slit in the titanium-reinforced membrane helps to give it a 3D form.
- Creating a slit also can remove a crease in the membrane.

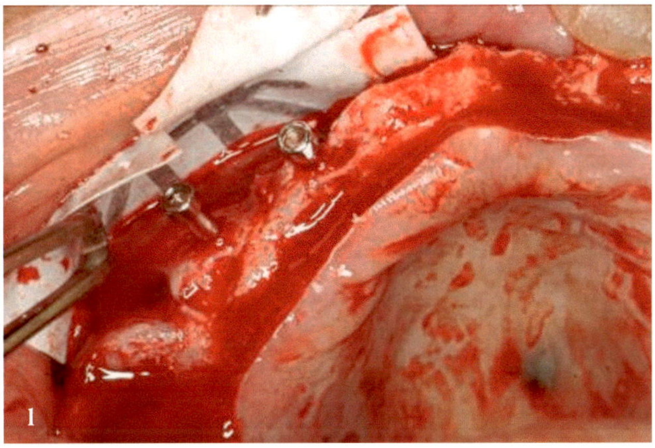

Fig 8-2l Decortication with a no. 2 round bur stimulates bleeding in the marrow space. This blood should be mixed with the grafted material to improve handling of the material.

Membrane stabilization

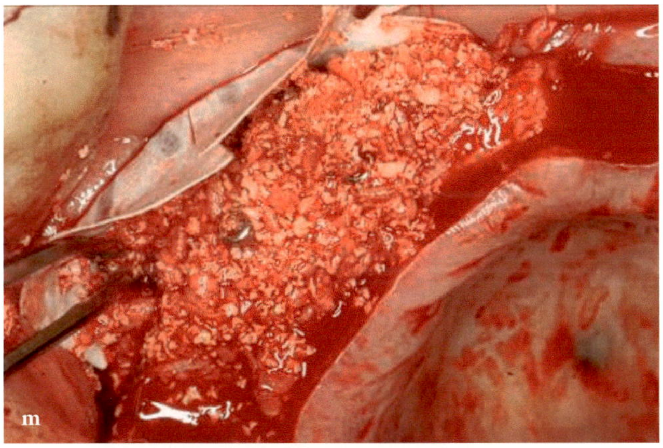

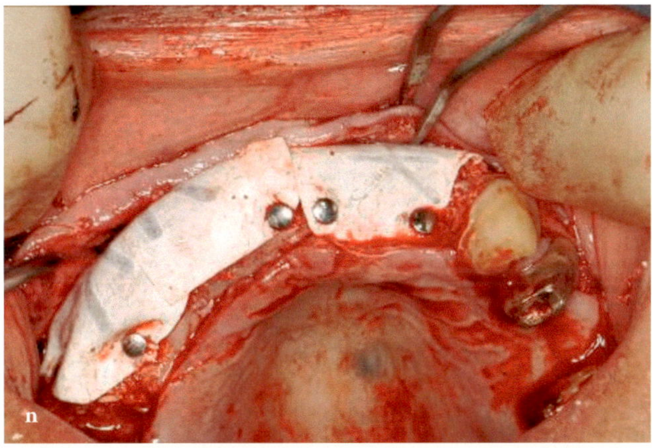

! Key points

- The bone graft should be placed soon after decortication.
- Decortication after stabilizing the membrane on one side aids the collection of blood from the marrow space.
- Use of self-tapping micro screws facilitates membrane fixation.
- Do not stabilize the membrane too apically in the palatal or lingual aspect. Micro screws seem to have better access.
- Trim the membrane with a blade after it is stabilized if necessary.

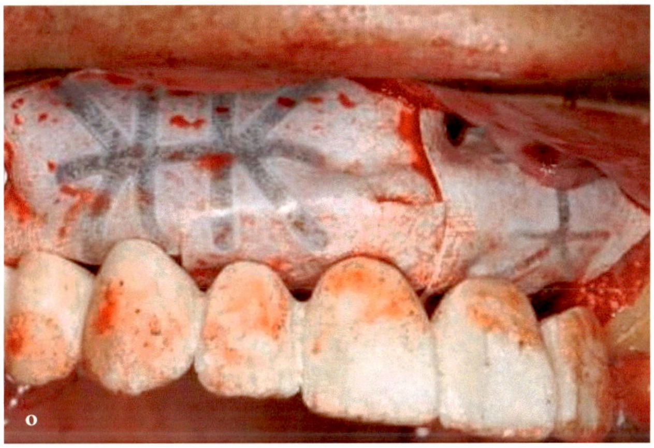

Figs 8-2m to 8-2o Use bone tacks or micro screws to stabilize the membrane at three or more locations. Care must be taken not to damage the adjacent teeth. Use a surgical stent to confirm the 3D form of augmentation.

Titanium mesh adjustment

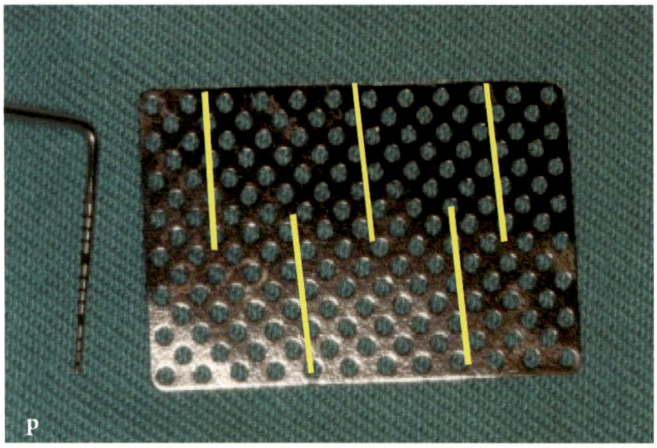

Fig 8-2p A piece of 0.1-mm titanium mesh. Long slits improve handling and allow 3D forms to be created with the mesh.

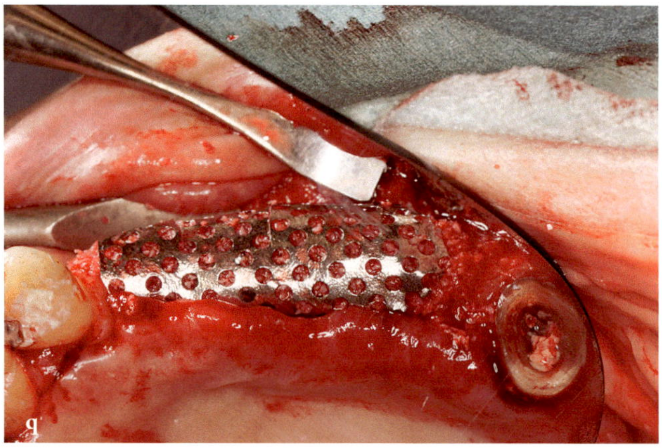

Fig 8-2q Occlusal view of adjusted titanium mesh. The buccal outline of the mesh follows the curve of the alveolar ridge.

! Key points

- Use multiple independent frames.
- Use long slits to facilitate 3D shaping.
- Adapt and adjust the mesh on a cast before surgery.
- Use thin titanium mesh.
- Stabilize the mesh (optional).

Bone graft placement

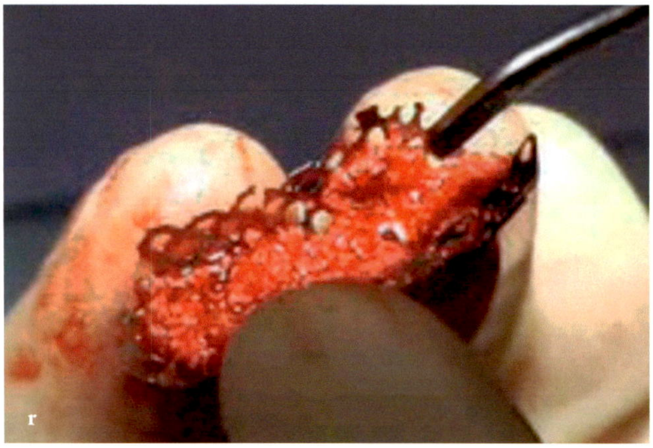

Fig 8-2r Care must be taken to place enough bone graft material in and beyond the mesh to cover the edges of the mesh and avoid open space under the mesh.

Mesh placement

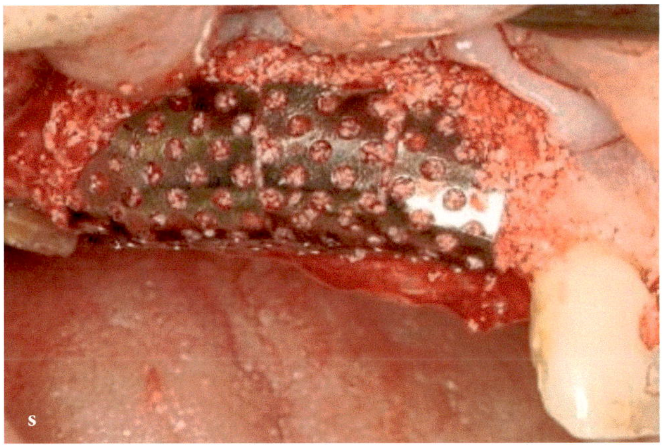

Fig 8-2s Mesh often does not require fixation, but tenting screws are necessary to aid space maintenance. A 3-mm distance is maintained between the mesh and the adjacent teeth. Enough bone graft is placed around the mesh, and there is no open space under the mesh.

Resorbable membrane placement

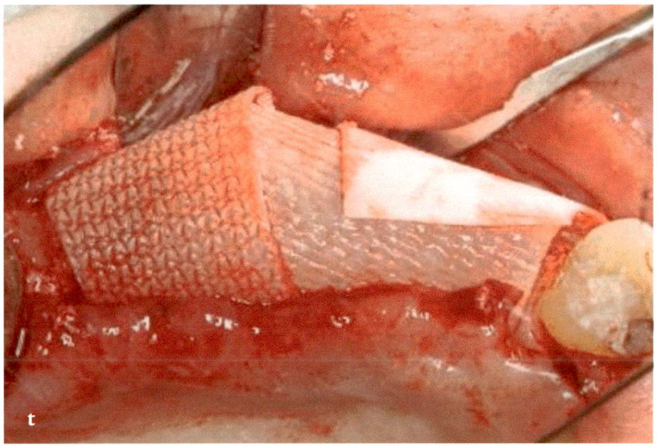

Fig 8-2t A resorbable membrane is placed to cover the entire augmentation site. The membrane must not come in contact with adjacent teeth. Placing two layers of membrane or collagen prevents mesh exposure when the flap is thin.

Releasing incision

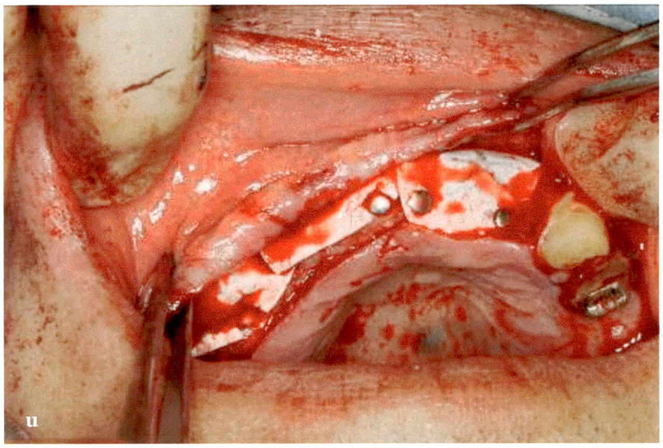

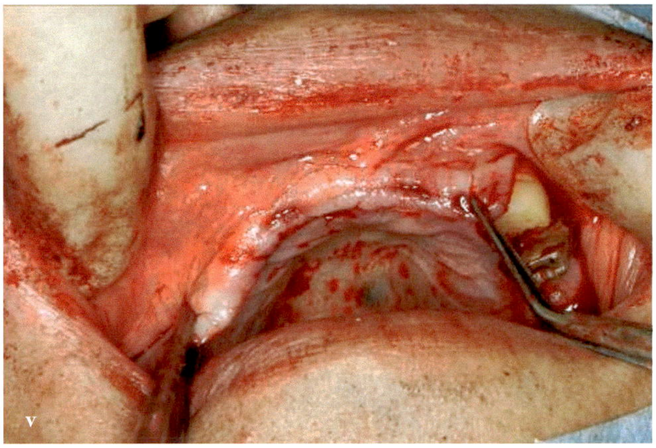

Figs 8-2u and 8-2v The buccal and palatal flaps must overlap at least 3 mm without tension prior to suturing. The buccal flap must be released if necessary at this point.

Suturing

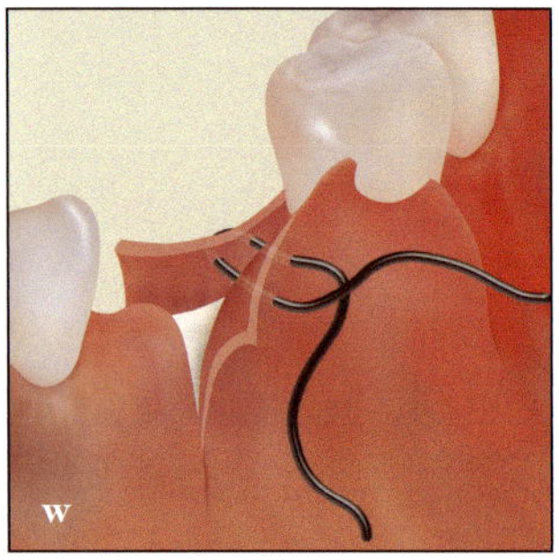

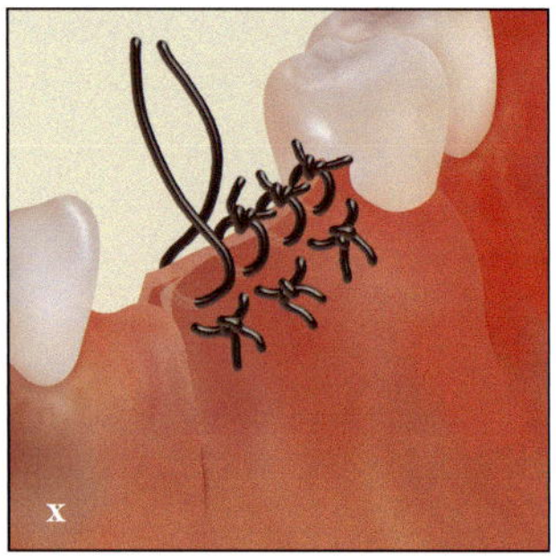

Figs 8-2w and 8-2x Use a horizontal mattress suture to approximate the buccal and palatal flap edges and to relieve tension between them. Use a simple interrupted suture to close the horizontal incision. The entrance points for the horizontal mattress suture should be 3 to 5 mm from the flap margins and from each other. The horizontal mattress sutures should be 2 mm apart.

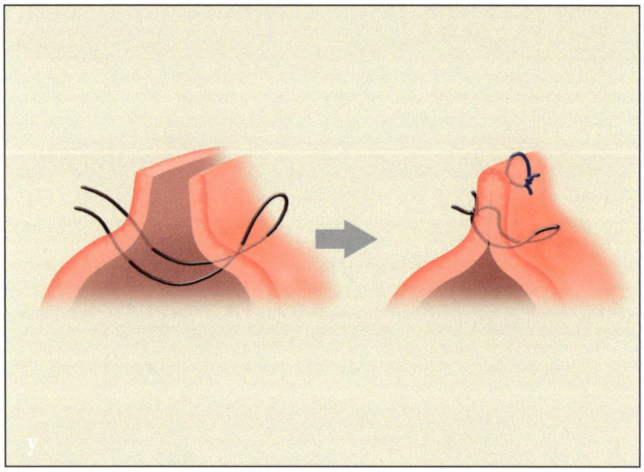

Fig 8-2y The inner aspect of the flaps should come in contact when suturing thin flaps. Horizontal mattress suture *(black)*; simple interrupted suture *(blue)*.

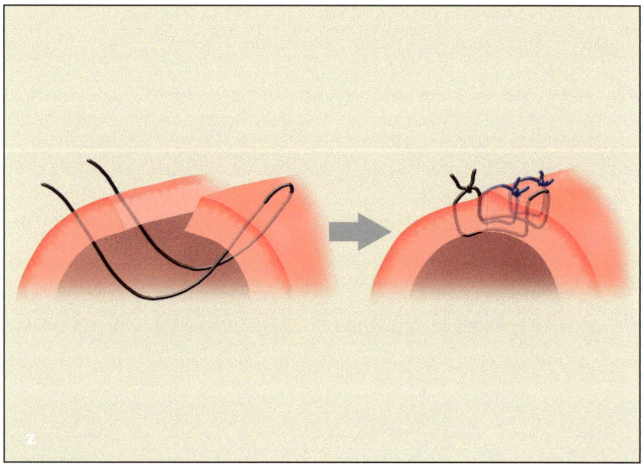

Fig 8-2z Only the flap edges should come in contact when suturing thick flaps. Horizontal mattress suture *(black)*; simple interrupted suture *(blue)*.

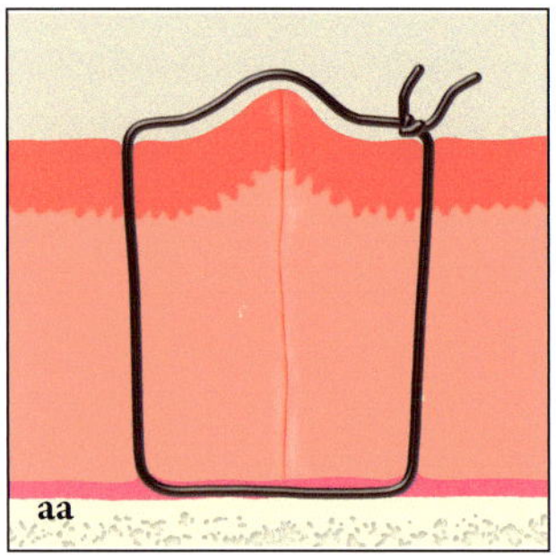

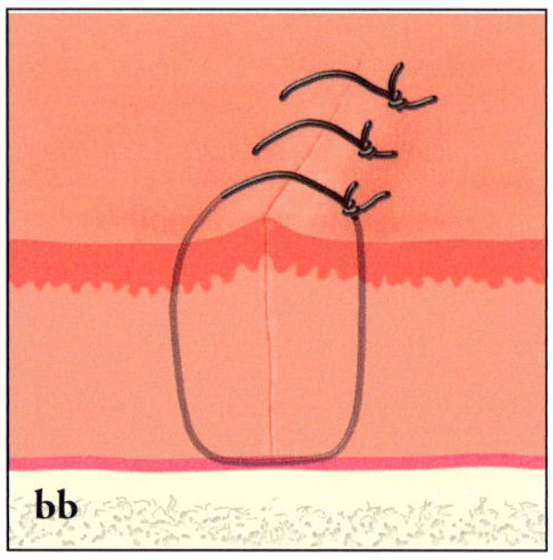

Figs 8-2aa and 8-2bb The entrance points for the simple interrupted suture should be 2 to 5 mm from the flap margin. The suture should penetrate through the full thickness of the flap.

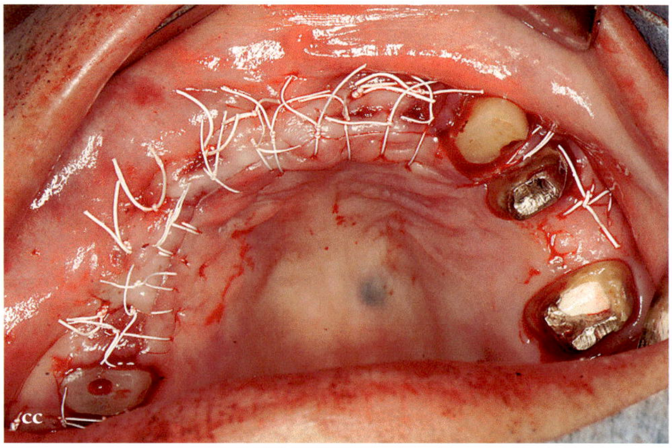

Fig 8-2cc After suturing.

Results of GBR

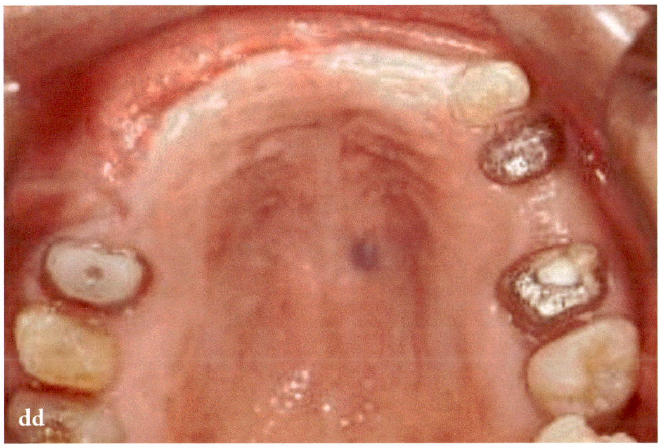

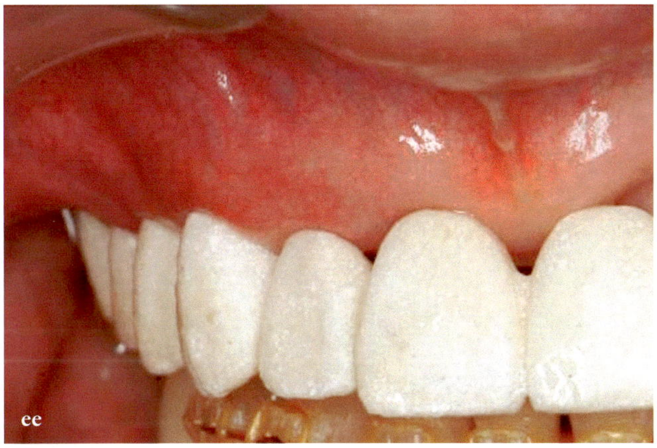

Figs 8-2dd and 8-2ee The 3D form of the alveolar ridge 7 months after GBR.

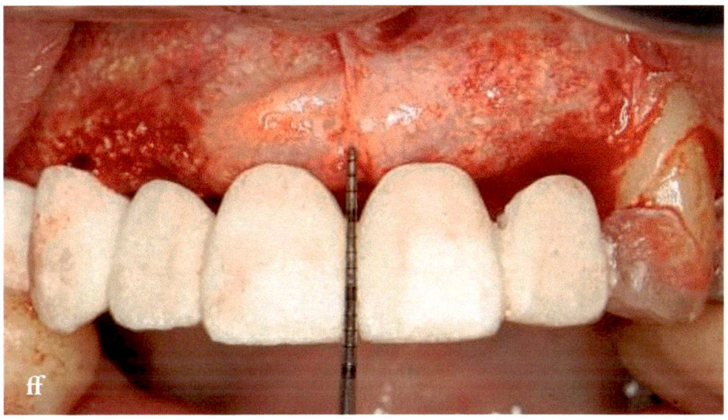

Fig 8-2ff Facial view after membrane removal. The height of the alveolar ridge is 2 to 3 mm from the contact point.

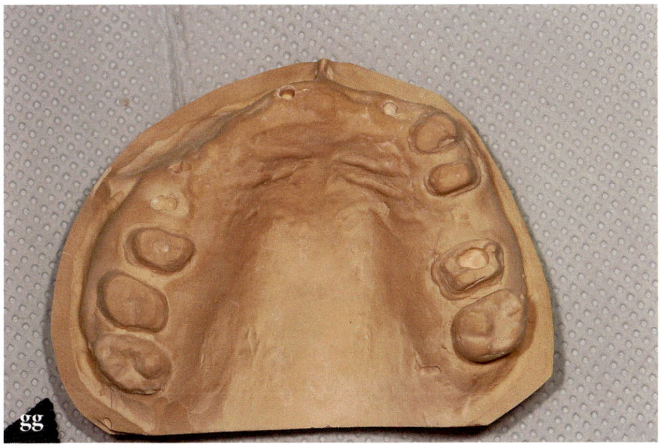

Fig 8-2gg Diagnostic cast before GBR.

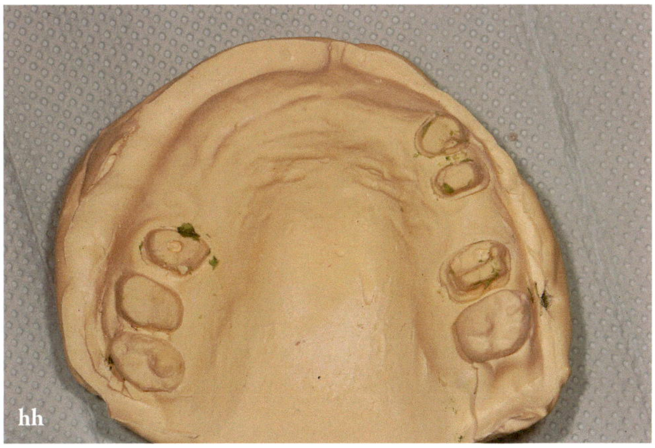

Fig 8-2hh Diagnostic cast after GBR.

A significant coronal shift of the mucogingival junction (MGJ) will often occur after a large amount of GBR, resulting in a lack of keratinized tissue at the crestal area of the alveolar ridge. In addition, the GBR barrier membrane suppresses the blood supply to the soft tissue above the membrane, which tends to decrease the thickness of this tissue. It is important to establish adequately wide and thick soft tissue around the implant to maintain underlying osseous support; greater soft tissue dimension around the implant has been noted in patients with a thick biotype. Soft tissue augmentation with connective tissue graft is often necessary after GBR, not only to augment the amount of keratinized tissue and the thickness of soft tissue, but also to create an ideal soft tissue profile for an esthetic definitive restoration. The authors often use an interpositional graft for these purposes.

Coronally shifted MGJ and lack of keratinized tissue

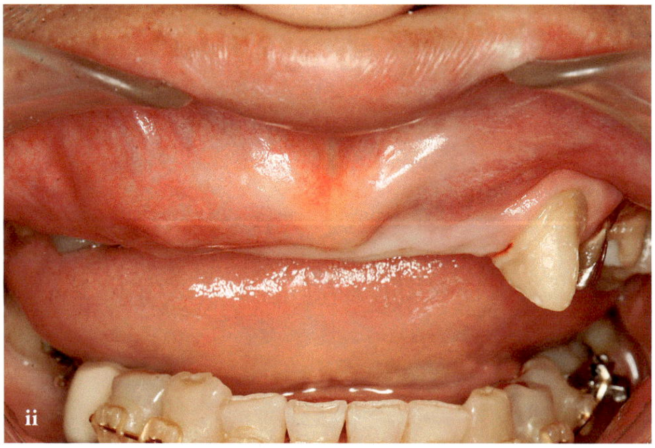

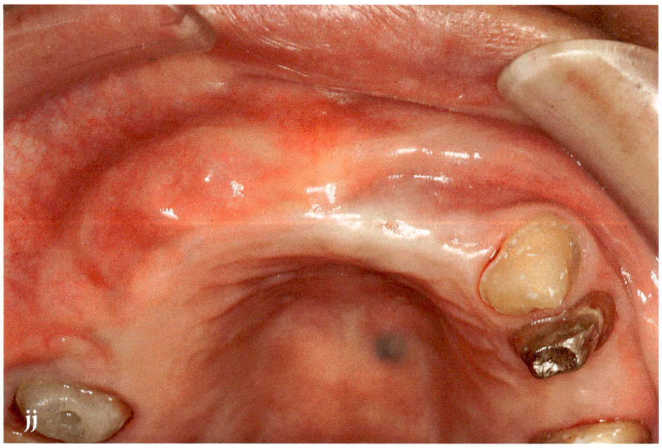

Figs 8-2ii and 8-2jj Facial and occlusal views. Coronally shifted MGJ and lack of keratinized tissue were observed after GBR.

Horizontal incision

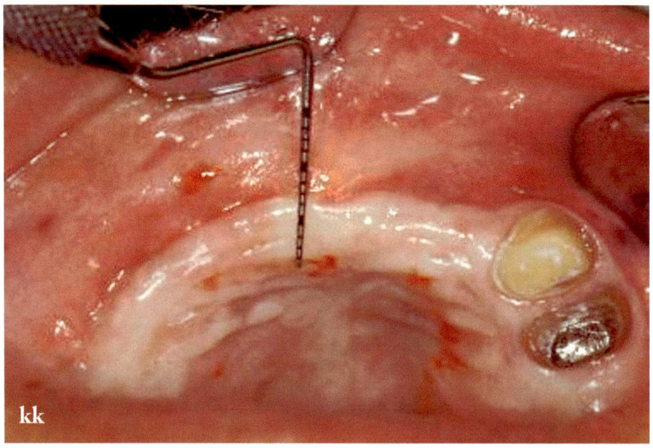

Fig 8-2kk The horizontal incision was made 5 mm from the MGJ, perpendicular to the alveolar ridge.

Vertical incision

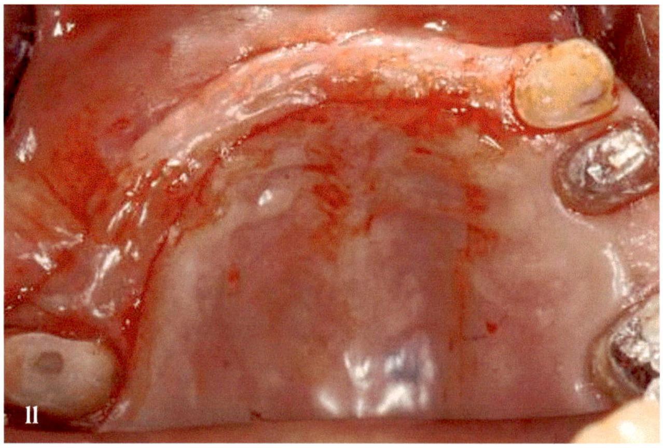

Fig 8-2ll The internal arch of the alveolar ridge is shorter than the external arch; therefore, the mesiodistal dimension of a flap created on the internal aspect of the alveolar ridge is not sufficient to cover the external aspect. Care must be taken when making the vertical incision to maximize the mesiodistal dimension of the flap by creating an inverted trapezoid shape. The full-thickness flap is first elevated from the horizontal incision, and then the partial-thickness flap is elevated beyond the MGJ.

Connective tissue graft harvesting

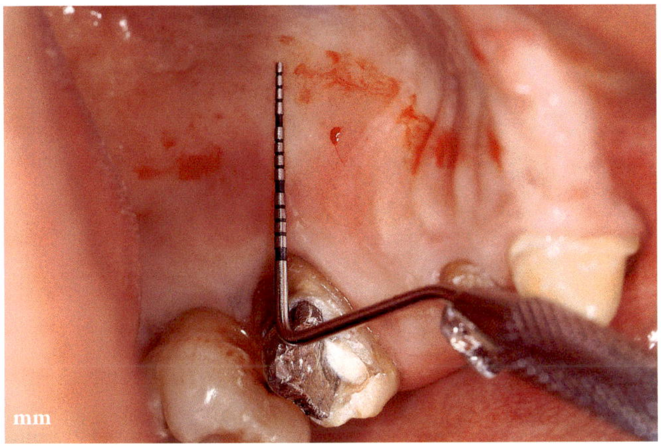

Fig 8-2mm The thickness and anatomy of the harvest site is evaluated.

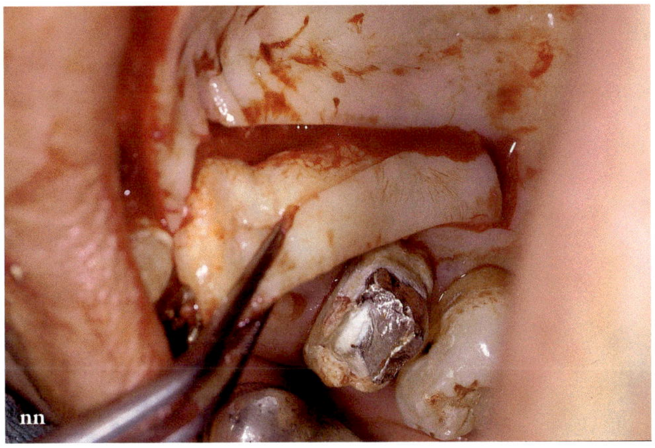

Fig 8-2nn A connective tissue graft with a 5-mm epithelial collar is harvested.

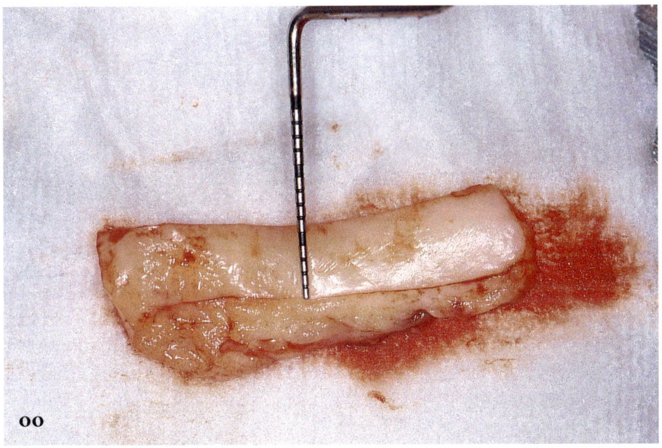

Fig 8-2oo Harvested connective tissue.

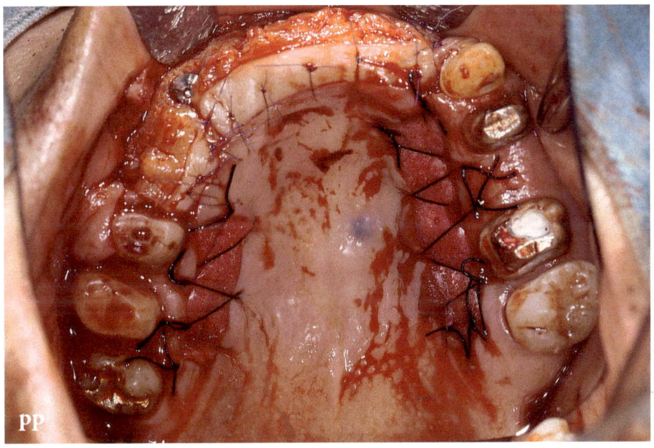

Fig 8-2pp The harvest sites have been covered with a collagen sponge, and the connective tissue graft has been positioned at the recipient site. The connection between the graft and the palatal incision line is a butt joint.

Soft tissue augmentation

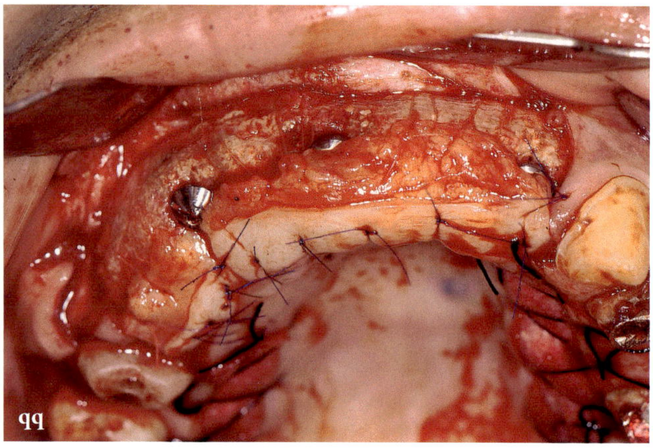

Fig 8-2qq The connective tissue graft is stabilized apically with 6-0 resorbable suture.

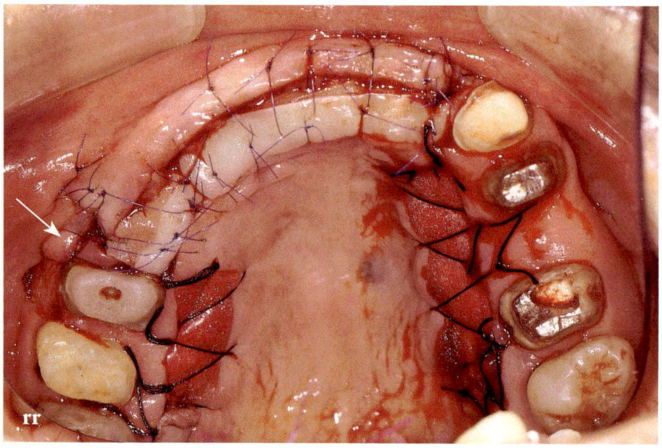

Fig 8-2rr The flap is sutured to cover the connective tissue portion of the graft. The mesiodistal dimension of the flap, which was created from the internal aspect of the alveolar ridge, is not sufficient to cover the entire recipient site. A laterally positioned flap from the adjacent area may be needed to cover the exposed area *(arrow)*.

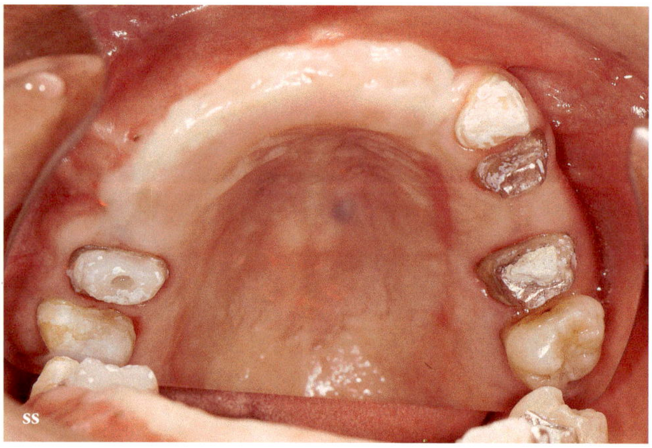

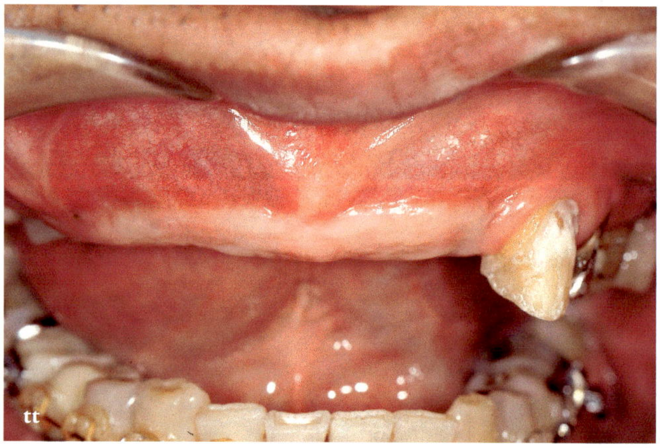

Figs 8-2ss and 8-2tt Two months after soft tissue augmentation. The palatal tissue has been moved to the facial aspect with the grafted epithelial collar positioned palatally. A sufficient amount of keratinized tissue and soft tissue thickness has been obtained.

Summary

In this chapter, protocols and clinical tips for implant placement and positioning, GBR, connective tissue grafting, and tissue sculpting were demonstrated in detail. Anterior esthetic implant treatment is challenging because every step in the process must be carefully executed.

The techniques and protocols presented in this book are the culmination of the authors' trial and error. The incision and flap design described in the text will result in fewer complications. Especially critical to successful GBR results is ensuring that the vertical and horizontal incisions form a single line from the occlusal view. In addition, the use of a combination of titanium mesh and resorbable membrane for GBR has many advantages over conventional techniques, although there is still room for improvement. The authors' experience also led them to invent a long shank diamond bur kit (2710) to facilitate ideal implant positioning.

Although achieving an esthetic result in multiple-tooth implant cases is challenging, the authors believe predictable esthetic final results can be expected through detailed examination, diagnosis, treatment planning, and sequencing of bone and soft tissue management.

Index

Page references followed by "f" denote figures; those followed by "t" denote tables; those followed by "b" denote boxes

Index

C

D

E

F

G

L

M

N

O

P

R

S

T

U

X